STEALTH Health

STEALTH Health

DEBRA L. GORDON AND DAVID L. KATZ, M.D.

How to sneak age-defying, disease-fighting habits into your life without really trying

Reader's Digest

The Reader's Digest Association, Inc.
Pleasantville, New York | Montreal

PROJECT STAFF

Editor
Neil Wertheimer

Designers
Rich Kershner
Elizabeth Tunnicliffe

Copy Editor
Jeanette Gingold

Indexer
Nanette Bendyna

Illustrators
Shawn Banner (how-to)
Scott Matthews (humor)

READER'S DIGEST HEALTH PUBLISHING

**Editor in Chief
and Publishing Director**
Neil Wertheimer

Managing Editor
Suzanne G. Beason

Art Director
Michele Laseau

**Production Technology
Manager**
Douglas A. Croll

Manufacturing Manager
John L. Cassidy

Marketing Director
Dawn Nelson

**Vice President
and General Manager**
Keira Krausz

READER'S DIGEST ASSOCIATION, INC.

**President, North America
Global Editor-in-Chief**
Eric W. Schrier

Library of Congress Cataloging-in-Publication Data
Gordon, Debra L., 1962-
  Stealth health : how to sneak age-defying, disease-fighting habits into
your life without really trying / Debra L. Gordon and David L. Katz.
      p. cm.
  Includes index.
  ISBN 0-7621-0520-8 (hardcover)
  ISBN 0-7621-0648-4 (paperback)
  1. Health. 2. Physical fitness. 3. Mind and body. I. Katz, David L.,
M.D. II. Title.
  RA776.G655 2005
  613.7--dc22
                                    2004027492

Address any comments about *Stealth Health* to:
The Reader's Digest Association, Inc.
Editor-in-Chief, Home & Health Books
Reader's Digest Road
Pleasantville, NY 10570-7000

To order copies of *Stealth Health*, call 1-800-846-2100.

Visit our Web site at **rd.com**

Printed in the United States of America
  3 5 7 9 10 8 6 4 2
US4653/IC

Note to Readers
The information in this book should not be substituted for, or used to
alter, medical therapy without your doctor's advice. For a specific
health problem, consult your physician for guidance. The mention of
any products, retail businesses, or Web sites in this book does not
imply or constitute an endorsement by the authors or by the Reader's
Digest Association.

Introduction

BETTER LIVING, WITHOUT HEAVY LIFTING

We have long heard about ounces of prevention and pounds of cure. But there is a problem with the proverb. Namely, the ounces of prevention—eating well, getting enough sleep, being physically active, avoiding stress—can require some very heavy lifting. And once you struggle to get them lifted, it can be hard to tell exactly what you've cured.

But what if those ounces of prevention could be put on a diet themselves, so they became as light as a feather? What if you could pile up tiny prevention practices, with almost no effort at all, and let them accumulate on your scale?

And while you're at it, what if you could learn more about the value of these acts of prevention and become more thoroughly convinced of all the ways they really do translate into pounds of cure? Why then, that old proverb might just be true!

It is true, and in *Stealth Health*, we've done the heavy lifting so you don't have to.

We lined up countless (well, I lost count, anyway!) valuable acts of disease prevention and health promotion, marched them into the sauna, and slimmed them down. We looked over health-promoting acts from the subtle to the stupendous to the sublime and said: No poundage! We want nothing but ounces!

And here you have the result. Prevention, on your terms; no heavy lifting. Instead, we distilled health promotion into tiny acts you can fit into your life, every day. Each one, however, is worth more than its weight in something even better than gold—health. For every tiny, stealthy act highlighted in this book is about one thing: making the quality of your life, and the quality of your health, better.

As a preventive medicine specialist, I truly believe that ounces of prevention are worth pounds of cure. But I also know that prevention isn't worth anything if it isn't practiced.

Stealth Health is about prevention you can practice on a daily basis. It's not about making room for health by building on an addition to your life; it's about finding room for prevention in the nooks and crannies of your life as it is.

Healthy living is not just something you *should* do. It is something you *can* do. With every bit of advice you act on in this book, the scales of health and happiness tip ever further in your favor. *Stealth Health* provides the elusive bridge from merely accepting the life you are living to living a life you can love and cherish, in good health, for many years to come.

I am pleased and proud to extend my personal welcome to you as you embark on this stealthy route to a healthier life.

Sincerely,
David L. Katz, M.D., M.P.H.,
F.A.C.P.M., F.A.C.P.
Yale University School of Medicine

contents

PART ONE

Stealth Health Through the Day

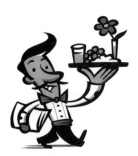

PART TWO

Stealth Healthy Cooking

PART THREE

Stealth Healthy Dining Out

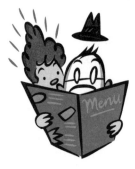

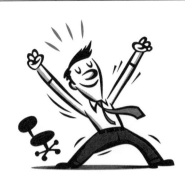
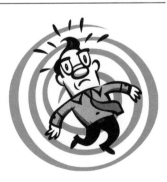

PART SEVEN

Stealth Habit Control

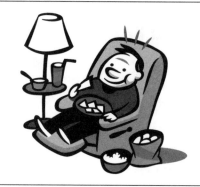

PART EIGHT

Stealth Healthy Looks

PART NINE

People and Places

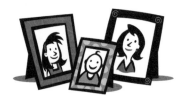

What Is Stealth Health?

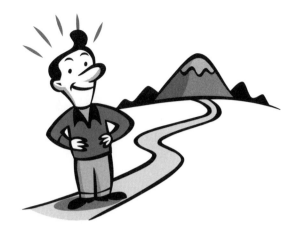

SMALL CHANGES THAT QUICKLY ADD UP

Pick up any health or diet book on the shelves these days and you come away with two impressions. First, most of us don't lead very healthy lives; there's a lot that needs fixing. And second, there's only one way to fix things—the hard way. A complete lifestyle overhaul. For example, today's most popular weight-loss programs start with truly frightening "induction phases" that involve a complete change in how you eat, including the banning of whole categories of popular foods. The discomfort and discipline involved are on a par with military boot camp—which is exactly how many popular fitness programs bill themselves today. Fitness trainers want your total submission, your total surrender.

Desire something a little more gentle? Pilates and yoga are terrific, but they require lessons, teachers, and practice, practice, practice. And woe to us if a doctor discovers something wrong with our bodies—the regimen of pills, tests, dietary makeovers, and scary talk about healthy living can often seem worse than the problem itself.

But what if there were another way—a way to get the benefits of a lifestyle overhaul without the top-to-bottom revamping? A stealthier way. A way of piling up tiny change after tiny change (so tiny you barely notice you're making them) yet emerging in the end with the kind of major change that dramatically improves your health? That wouldn't be so bad, would it? That would really deserve some serious consideration!

Welcome to Stealth Health.

Stealth Health redefines health as you know it. Living life the Stealth Health way means choosing the raisin bran, not the bagel. It's taking a five-minute walk when you get bored with your computer, rather than eating a chocolate bar. It's laughing when someone does something stupid, instead of shouting. It's going to sleep instead of watching the late movie. It's snacking on a peach, not a pie. It's kissing your partner instead of walking out the door with only a good-bye.

After all, what *is* health, anyway? As we've defined it here, health includes feeling relaxed rather than stressed; loving rather than irritated. It's finding time for yourself and your priorities that you didn't think you had. And, of course, it's also glowing, healthier skin and steady, sustainable weight control. It's more energy come afternoon and evening, less likelihood of developing diabetes and heart disease, measurably lower cholesterol and blood pressure levels, higher self-esteem, a greater sense of personal safety, and an enhanced ability to handle whatever life throws your way without falling apart.

Health is about feeling good today, and the probability of being well tomorrow. Not either/or—but both.

If all you do is think about health, you quickly get sick of it. But if you just become a little more mindful while making small decisions during your day, chances are you'll do all you'll need—and more—to take good care of your body, mind, and soul.

Here's another way to think about it: the forest and the trees. We've all been taught not to lose the forest for the trees, right? But sometimes, when it comes to health, dealing with the whole forest of choices is overwhelming. *Stealth Health*, however, offers a simple yet powerful reorientation to it all: The forest *is* the trees. Take care of the trees, and the forest will flourish.

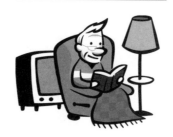

Health isn't merely the absence of disease. You are not healthy if you are perpetually stressed, frustrated or dissatisfied.

Stealth Health is the ultimate guide to the little decisions we make that add up to an enormous influence on our health. It contains more than 2,400 choices and tweaks you can make to your day, some so small as to seem almost inconsequential, yet guaranteed to make you healthier. The ideas are fresh, unusual, simple, and fast. Best of all, they work.

And they're designed for the way you live your life. For instance, we're not telling you to give up salt. Instead, we give you two dozen ways to incrementally reduce the amount of salt in your diet, until, ever so slowly, ever so *stealthily*, you find that your salt intake has hit healthy levels—and your blood pressure has dropped as a result. Instead of worrying about getting more magnesium in your diet to lower your high blood pressure, just munch on a few dried apricots every day (they're little magnesium powerhouses). No time to exercise because you spend too much time driving? We'll show you how to combine the two. Too stressed to sleep, and too sleep-deprived to handle stress? We've got dozens of simple, stealthy ways to fix both! Are you unhappy about overeating, and overeating because you're unhappy? Learn what you can sneak into even the most frenetic days to improve your mood even as you control your appetite.

Now, there will be times in this book when you will ask yourself, "How can this advice possibly help my health?" It's a

Stealthy Changes

Look up "stealth" or "stealthy" in a dictionary and the definitions contain words like "imperceptible," "unobtrusive," "deliberate," and "slow." We hope those words describe how you want to make lifestyle changes.

legitimate question. When you encounter tips that seem pretty far afield from the topic of health, like how to better organize the start of your workday or make your errand runs more efficient, chances are they will be about achieving calm or a positive attitude. There are two reasons why they are here. First, health, as we previously suggested, isn't merely the absence of disease. It involves mental and spiritual aspects as well. You are not healthy if you are perpetually stressed, frustrated, or dissatisfied. Second, your mental and spiritual health have a direct link to your physical health. Research confirms it over and over. Stress, anger and other hostile emotions and attitudes are significant risk factors for everything from heart disease to obesity.

So even if some of our advice doesn't seem to have a direct health benefit, trust us that it does help. And know that every tip in this book has come from a doctor or is doctor-approved.

Finally, you may find the occasional advice that seemingly contradicts what we've said in a different place. We are aware of these inconsistencies. In each case, it all comes down to context. For example, coffee is great for you if your goal is mental sharpness and alertness. But for a good night's sleep, coffee is nothing but trouble. We trust that you will not be confused by these occasional conflicts, and will make choices that are most sensible for your particular goals.

A Lifetime Journey

The biggest problem with intense, highly defined health programs is that they end—perhaps as fast as two weeks, maybe as long as six months. But when they end, you're back to your old ways. Which is why our obesity rates continue to rise, despite billions of dollars spent on weight-loss books and programs. And why heart disease, diabetes, and stroke—all lifestyle-influenced diseases—are rampant.

We believe that when done the right way, the pursuit of better health has a momentum all its own. One health-promoting habit will reinforce others. Chances are, after you hit some threshold of subtle, stealthy adjustments to your lifestyle, you will, in fact, have made the sweeping improvements in your health that once seemed so elusive and intimidating. In other words, take enough small steps, one at a time, and you've accomplished the equivalent of reaching Everest's peak or of circling the globe—without even getting out of breath.

Stealth Health is the roadmap to your journey. It's the directions that enable you to take one small step, followed by more small steps. Small steps that sneak health promotion into the nooks and crannies of your life, between and among the hasty moments of your days.

Bottom line: Improving your health doesn't have to be hard. In fact, it's mostly about common sense. Pick three Stealth Health tips to do a day, every day, and we promise that you will be well on your way to a lighter you, a more attractive you, a more disease-resistant you, and a more contented you. In other words, start tending a few trees, then get out of the woods and enjoy the forest!

The Everyday Health Plan

JUST SAY "THREE A DAY"!

Just as any program designed to overhaul your health would automatically be overwhelming, so, too, could Stealth Health be overwhelming. After all, we've come up with more than 2,000 tips to improve everything from the way you look to how much you weigh to your heart-health measurements to your relationships with loved ones.

Don't worry. The last thing we want to do is overwhelm you (that would be stressful, which goes against the Stealth Health philosophy).

So here's what we propose: Every day, make three pro-health choices that are outside your regular routine. That's all. Just three.

For instance, have a cup of tea instead of coffee in the morning. Substitute a bottle of water for your afternoon soda. Spend five minutes stretching in the morning while you watch the news. That's three. Call it a day. You'll do three more tomorrow.

Go ahead and make the same choices for tomorrow if you wish. But here's the one and only rule in this program: Once you've followed a choice for four days in a row, it no longer counts as one of your three choices. Instead, you should consider it a habit. It's time to add to it with a new and different pro-health choice.

Now, we know that habits are formed over months, not days. But you also know that limiting yourself to three simple changes for weeks on end won't add up to much in the long run. Your goal is to slowly, steadily, sample new health tips, and if they feel right, integrate them into your

daily routine—again, slowly, steadily, over the days, weeks, and months. Given time, you'll find that nearly every aspect of your life has changed in healthier ways—without your even noticing it!

That's it: the entirety of the Everyday Health Plan. Make three healthy choices every day. With more than 2,400 to choose from in these pages, that should be *easy*.

The Best Tips for You

Just as there is only one rule to the program, we offer you only one bit of expert advice to get you going: Focus your efforts on those areas of your health or life that need the most help. For instance, if your major health concern right now is weight, choose your three picks from the chapters that focus on healthy eating and weight loss. Having trouble sleeping? Three tips from the sleep chapter on page 79 should guarantee you a peaceful night's slumber. Which three? You pick. In *all* cases, you pick. For in writing *Stealth Health*, we began with the idea that getting and staying healthy is an option and an opportunity, not an obligation. So *you* choose—as long as you do *something,* you've taken a small step toward better health. And through an accumulation of these small steps, you will reach your goal.

As you add three more healthy choices each day, the cumulative effect will be substantial. The outcome: a sustainable, healthy lifestyle marked by fewer colds; greater energy; a leaner, more attractive body; a happier outlook; and greater resistance to chronic disease.

Focusing Your Efforts

The Everyday Health Plan is arguably the world's simplest program for weight loss, energy, immunity, and daily health. Just make three healthy choices a day! Each of us has unique health issues and goals, however. So to get you to the right changes for your situa-tion, here are our recommendations. There are nine tip-filled parts in this book, and 81 chapters with advice. In the list below, part names are in **boldface;** individual chapters are in regular type. If we recommend a part, that means any chapter within it would apply.

Health Issue/Goal	Recommended Parts/Chapters
Weight Loss	**Stealth Healthy Cooking; Stealth Healthy Dining Out; Stealth Healthy Exercise;** Burning More Calories; Losing Weight; Overeating
Managing Diabetes	**Stealth Healthy Cooking; Stealth Healthy Dining Out; Stealth Healthy Exercise;** Stabilizing Your Blood Sugar; Reduce Your Risk of Heart Disease and Stroke
Managing Stress	**Stealth Healthy Mental Relief; People and Places;** The Commute; Workplace Madness; Running Errands; The After-Dinner Routine
Improving Sleep	**Stealth Healthy Mental Relief;** The Sleep Routine
Managing Heart Disease	**Stealth Healthy Cooking; Stealth Healthy Dining Out; Stealth Healthy Exercise;** Losing Weight; Lower Your Cholesterol; Lowering Blood Pressure; Reduce Your Risk of Heart Disease and Stroke; Defusing Stress; Defusing Anger; Dealing with Anxiety; Dealing With the Uncontrollable
Managing Cholesterol	**Stealth Healthy Cooking; Stealth Healthy Dining Out; Stealth Healthy Exercise;** Losing Weight; Lower Your Cholesterol
Managing Blood Pressure	**Stealth Healthy Cooking; Stealth Healthy Dining Out; Stealth Healthy Exercise;** Losing Weight; Lowering Blood Pressure; Reduce Your Risk of Heart Disease and Stroke; Defusing Stress; Defusing Anger; Dealing With Anxiety; Dealing With the Uncontrollable
Managing Aging	**Stealth Healthy Cooking; Stealth Healthy Exercise; Stealth Healthy Looks;** Monitor Your Health; Improving Your Hearing; Sharpen Your Sense of Smell and Taste; Improving Your Vision; Improving Memory
Resisting Major Disease	**Targeted Health Goals**
Improving Appearance	**Stealth Healthy Looks**

The Stealth Health Promise

BENEFITS THAT ARE PROVEN AND SUBSTANTIAL

So just what *is* the Stealth Health promise? Well, maybe we should start with what it's not. It's *not* a promise to cut your weight by 10 pounds in two weeks. Nor is it a guarantee that living the Stealth Health way will provide you with boundless energy until a painless passing during sleep at age 107. But here's what medical studies find living the Stealth Health way *can* provide:

▸ **A leaner, healthier body for the rest of your life.** Sure, those fad diets may jump-start your weight loss, but they're nearly impossible to sustain over a lifetime. Instead, *Stealth Health*'s weight-loss tips are based on studies that show over and over again that the best way to lose weight and maintain the weight loss is through moderate daily exercise and healthy eating. Plus, we've thrown in some lesser-known research-based tips. Like eating in front of a mirror. Cutting out soft drinks. Wearing blue while you're eating. All help you eat less and/or lose weight, and all fit our definition of Stealth Health.

▸ **Better control of your blood sugar levels.** Just a brisk half-hour walk every day, or skipping sugary soft drinks and juices, or switching to whole grains, can decrease your risk of developing diabetes regardless of your weight.

▸ **A healthier heart.** It doesn't take much. One study found that just

Special Advice

There are more than 2,400 bits of health advice in this book, all of them proven, valid, quick, and effective. We stand behind them all! But we also know that it is asking too much of you to consider each and every one. So to help, we've gone through and selected tips that you might wish to consider first, and marked them for quick spotting. We marked them three ways:

 Fast Results
These are bits of advice that deliver benefits particularly quickly—in some cases, immediately!

 Easy Gains
These are tips that give the biggest value for the least amount of effort.

 Super Effective
And these are tips proven to be particularly effective through scientific research or widespread usage by experts.

The Everyday Health Plan's Top 10 Tips

If you read this book from front to back, you'll likely see some tips repeated again and again. No, we didn't forget that we used them before; it's just that certain lifestyle changes have numerous health benefits. In fact, some have so many, that we've come up with our top 10 list. Do these 10 things, and we guarantee you'll see the health benefits.

1. Drink a cup of tea in the morning.

2. Walk for 30 minutes a day.

3. Quit smoking.

4. Have a glass of wine every evening.

5. Take five minutes a day, close your eyes in a quiet room, and practice deep breathing.

6. Talk to a friend—whether in person, on the phone, or via e-mail—every day.

7. Eat fish twice a week.

8. Take a multivitamin with minerals every morning.

9. Eat whole, natural foods rather than boxed or processed foods.

10. Get a good night's sleep.

---

30 minutes of walking three or more days a week could slash your risk of heart disease more than a third.

▸ **Better control of your cholesterol levels.** Simply changing your dining habits from two large meals a day to six small meals a day, switching over to olive oil in your salad dressings, sipping a cup of tea every few hours throughout the day, and sprinkling cinnamon on your cereal can significantly improve your blood sugar levels and reduce your risk of diabetes. Simple, huh?

▸ **Stronger bones.** Here's one easy way: Tend your garden for a few hours a week. One major study found gardening to be one of the best activities you can do for maintaining healthy bones. When you're done, sip a glass of icy mineral water instead of a soda—more bone protection in yet another research-proven, Stealth Healthy manner.

▸ **More intense workouts.** No, you don't have to give up walking for running; but little things, like working out to an up-tempo musical beat, or working out in a room without mirrors, can result in a more intense workout and leave you feeling better at the end.

▸ **Improved control over stress.** Sure, a trip to the Caribbean would help, but that's hardly stealthy. How about hugging your partner, calling a friend, buying yourself flowers, and decorating the walls of your home with art? All simple changes, yet all found to reduce stress hormones in various studies.

▸ **Enhanced energy.** Studies find that just taking a 20-minute nap, a sprig of rosemary to sniff, or a brisk walk up and down the stairs can leave you feeling refreshed and energized.

▸ **Improved memory.** Studies also find that switching to whole grains, mixing blueberries into your morning cereal, and attempting the Sunday crossword puzzle can all help maintain and even improve your memory.

See how easy—and yet how beneficial—Stealth Healthy living can be?

Now, if you're ready, turn the page and embark on the easiest, stealthiest, healthiest changes you'll ever make in your life.

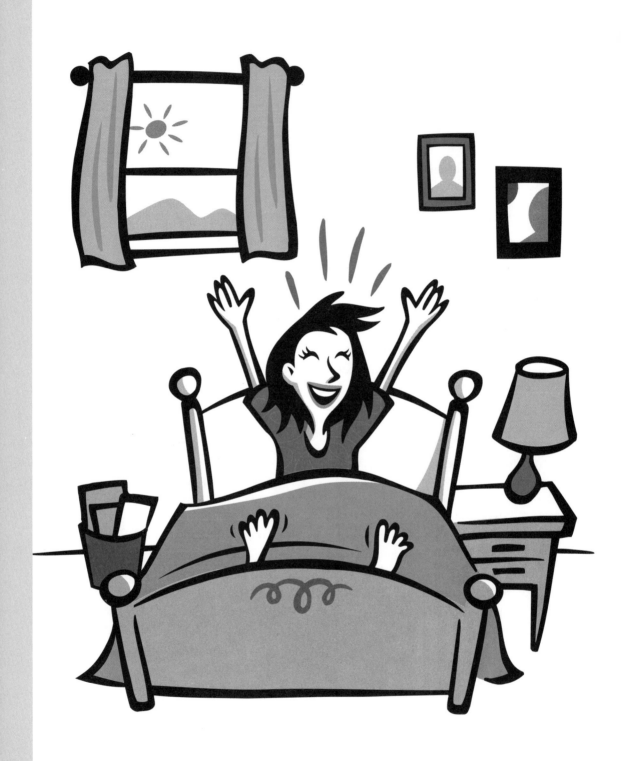

PART ONE

Stealth Health

THROUGH THE DAY

From the morning shower to the evening news, your days are full of regular tasks and routines. Here's how to make each a little calmer, a little healthier.

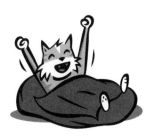

The Wake-Up Routine

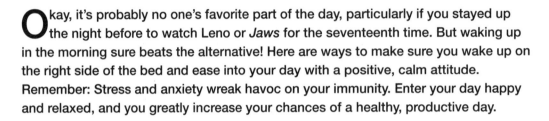

24 WAYS TO BRIGHTEN YOUR MORNING

Okay, it's probably no one's favorite part of the day, particularly if you stayed up the night before to watch Leno or *Jaws* for the seventeenth time. But waking up in the morning sure beats the alternative! Here are ways to make sure you wake up on the right side of the bed and ease into your day with a positive, calm attitude. Remember: Stress and anxiety wreak havoc on your immunity. Enter your day happy and relaxed, and you greatly increase your chances of a healthy, productive day.

1 **Go to sleep with your blinds or curtains halfway open.** That way, the natural light of the rising sun will send a signal to your brain to slow its production of melatonin and bump up its production of adrenaline, a signal that it's time to wake up. When the alarm goes off, you'll already be half awake. Even better: Go to bed early enough so that waking up when the sun shines through your window still gives you the recommended seven hours of shut-eye. If you maintain this routine, it's likely that you can start relying on your biological clock rather than an alarm clock.

2 **Set your alarm 15 minutes earlier.** This way, you don't have to jump out of bed and rush through your morning. You can begin your morning by lying in bed, slowly waking up. Stretching. Listening to the news headlines. Mentally clicking off what you're going to wear, what you're going to do, what you're going

to have for breakfast. It's just as important to prepare yourself mentally as physically for your day. These few minutes in bed, before anyone else is up, are all yours.

3 **Stretch every extremity for 15 seconds.** Try this even before you open your eyes. Lift your arm and begin by stretching each finger, then your hand, then your wrist, then your arm. Then move on to the other arm. Then your toes, feet, ankles, and legs. Finally, end with a neck and back stretch that propels you out of the bed. You've just limbered up your muscles and joints and enhanced the flow of blood through your body, providing an extra shot of oxygen to all your tissues.

4 **Stick a chair in the shower and sit in it.** Use one of those plastic chairs you can buy at any hardware store. Let it warm up under the spray for a minute, then sit in it and let the spray beat on your back. It's simultaneously relaxing and

energizing, like getting a water massage. After a couple of minutes, you can swing the chair out of the way and commence with washing.

5 **Read a motivational quote every morning.** This can provide a frame for the day, a sort of self-talk that keeps you motivated in the right direction as opposed to the negative thinking of the morning news. Another option: Use a motivational mantra that provides a meditation-like burst, or read or recite a poem that helps you focus. A good one to use: Rudyard Kipling's "If."

6 **Take a vitamin.** Keep a multivitamin out on the kitchen counter right by the coffeepot so you remember to take one every morning. More than 20 years of research led to a major recommendation in one of the country's premier medical journals suggesting that every American take a multivitamin as part of a healthy lifestyle.

7 **Eschew any decisions.** For truly relaxing mornings, reduce the number of choices and decisions you make to zero. Go about this two ways: First, make your morning decisions the night before: what clothes to wear, what breakfast to eat, what route to take to work, and so on. Second, routinize as much of your morning as possible. Really, there's no need to vary your breakfast, timetable, or bathroom ritual from one morning to the next.

8 **Cuddle with your kids.** Few things are more stressful in the morning than waking up an overtired fifth grader or a snoring high schooler. Yet this is one of the few times you can catch your child still vulnerable. Sit on his bed and gently smooth his hair as you softly waken him. Or, if you're dealing with a very young child, lie beside him and gently hug him awake. Such a moment will send a quiet surge of joy through your entire day and will become all too rare in all too short a time.

9 **Spend 5 to 10 minutes each morning listening to music** or sitting on the deck or porch just thinking. This allows the creative thinking that takes place during the night to gel and form into a plan of action, grounding you for the day.

10 **Wake to the smell of coffee.** Really great coffee. Buy the absolute best coffee you can afford—fresh beans are preferred—and put twice the amount you've been using into your coffee maker, the one you bought specifically because it has an alarm that can be set to start brewing times. The strong scent of strong coffee will pull you out of bed like a fishhook in the back of your pajamas. Plus, if you're going the caffeine route, morning is the best time for it. Caffeine is a central nervous system stimulant that acts in many ways like other stimulant drugs such as amphetamines, waking you up and

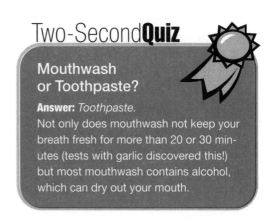

Two-Second**Quiz**

Mouthwash or Toothpaste?

Answer: *Toothpaste.*
Not only does mouthwash not keep your breath fresh for more than 20 or 30 minutes (tests with garlic discovered this!) but most mouthwash contains alcohol, which can dry out your mouth.

increasing your muscular activity. Even better: A study of 18 men found that caffeine improved clear-headedness, happiness, and calmness, as well as the men's ability to perform on attention tests and to process information and solve problems.

11 Brush your tongue for one minute.
There's no better way to rid yourself of morning breath and begin your day minty fresh and clean. After all, more than 300 types of bacteria take up residence in your mouth every night. You think a quick brush over the teeth is going to vanquish them all?

12 Take a baby aspirin.
There. You've just significantly reduced your risk of a heart attack. In one study of 220,000 doctors, those who took an aspirin every day for five years slashed their heart attack risk nearly in half. Of course, check with your doctor first to make sure this is okay for you.

13 Use real sugar in your coffee, or drink a cup of orange juice.
When researchers at the University of Virginia tested the memories of healthy 60- to 80-year-olds, they found those who had a small amount of sugar in the morning (the experimenters compared sweetened to unsweetened lemonade) even before breakfast had better memory recall that day on into the following day. We're talking small amounts, however, about a teaspoon or less; so put down that doughnut.

14 Check your morning calendar.
This is the large calendar or white board you've hung in a prominent position in your kitchen. On it, you write everything you need to know for that particular day, from kids' activities to whether the guy is coming to service the furnace to whether it's time to pay bills. Check it out carefully while you sip that first cup of coffee or morning tea; it will help you structure your day in your mind and avoid the stressful effects of forgetting something important.

15 Swallow 500 mg of calcium citrate.
Your body is better at absorbing this form of calcium than the other commonly used form, calcium carbonate, found in antacids like Tums and Rolaids. You'll need at least another 500 mg before you go to bed, but that's a tip for another chapter.

16 Drink eight ounces of water.
You've been fasting all night and you wake each morning dehydrated.

17 Create a checklist for your kids.
If you don't have kids, skip this one. But if you do, this is a biggie. To cut down on morning chaos, hang a white board in the hallway or kitchen and list all the things that must be done before the kids can leave:

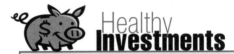

Healthy Investments

A Sun Alarm Clock Radio

Sharper Image has one, but you can find these unique alarm clocks at many electronics stores. In addition to the typical radio/alarm, the clock can be set to gradually become brighter as it gets closer to your wake-up time. The increasing light signals your brain to begin making the stress hormone adrenaline, which helps you wake up. You can also buy alarms that wake you to prerecorded messages, slowly building music coupled with aromatherapy, or alarms that gradually increase in volume.

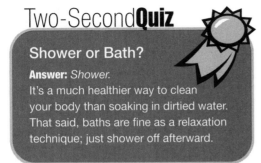

Shower or Bath?

Answer: *Shower.*
It's a much healthier way to clean your body than soaking in dirtied water. That said, baths are fine as a relaxation technique; just shower off afterward.

brush teeth, eat breakfast, get backpack together, make bed, and so on. Have them check off or erase each item once it's completed. You can do the same thing with lists printed out from your computer. Set a consequence: If all items aren't checked off 5 minutes before you need to leave, there's no TV/PlayStation/dessert/computer time that night.

18 Keep a wicker basket for yourself and each child by the front or back door. Into it go your keys, wallet, purse, and the child's backpack, papers, gloves, hats, etc. This will prevent that frantic last-minute scouring of the house as you look for lost items.

19 Split up in the morning. That means you use one bathroom and your partner uses another. Even if you are still madly in love, bathroom time should be private time. It makes for a calmer, less stressful start to your day.

20 Wash more efficiently. We spend an average of about 12 minutes in the shower. That's fine when you're preparing for date night. But in the morning, you need to get in and out quickly. If you're not into showering the night before (we do understand about bed head) try using two-in-one products like a cleanser that both cleans and moisturizes or a combination shampoo and conditioner. When you wash your body, just hit the hot spots, i.e., your groin and underarms. Everything else can just be rinsed off. The health benefit: reducing stress by saving time.

21 Prepare an emergency outfit in your closet. Include socks, jewelry, hose, etc., so on those mornings when you sleep through the alarm or simply need an extra 10 minutes, you can just pluck it off the hanger and go.

22 Dry more efficiently. Start with an oversized, 100 percent cotton bath sheet for maximum blotting. Towel-dry your hair and let it air-dry while you do your makeup or put on your underwear. Then, if you use a blow-dryer, make it a high-energy one, at least 1,600 watts. Anything else is just wasting precious time.

23 Hop on the treadmill for 30 minutes. Studies find that people who work out in the morning are more likely to stick with their exercise regimen because they get it out of the way and don't have all day to come up with diversions and excuses. Plus, you will produce endorphins that will last most of the day.

24 Kiss all the people you love in your house (including the dog and cat) before you leave. Connecting with the ones you love soothes stress and provides you with a positive start to your day, as well as keeping you focused on what's really important says therapist Barbara Bartlein, L.C.S.W., author of *Why Did I Marry You Anyway? 125 Strategies for a Happy Marriage.*

The Breakfast Routine

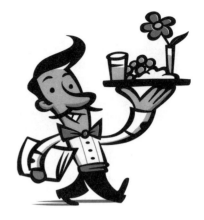

27 IDEAS FOR A HEALTHIER MEAL

There's a reason they call it the most important meal of the day. Not only is breakfast the first food and drink your body has had in more than 8 hours, but studies find that what you eat for breakfast influences what you eat the rest of the day. Additionally, people who eat breakfast are significantly less likely to be obese and have diabetes than those who don't.

The most important tip we can give you is to eat breakfast every day. Without exception. This one action alone can make a huge, positive difference in your health. But a doughnut or oversized muffin won't do it. The key is to choose energy-enhancing, health-invigorating foods. That's what we'll focus on in the tips ahead.

1 Be consistent with your portions. For most people, a perfect breakfast has three components: one serving of a whole grain carbohydrate, one serving of a dairy or high-calcium food, and one serving of fruit. Together, that would add up to roughly 300 calories. A high-protein serving (i.e., a meat or an egg) is unnecessary but certainly acceptable, as long as it doesn't add too much fat or calories to the mix. Here are a few winning combinations, based on this formula:

- A bowl of high-fiber, multigrain cereal, lots of strawberries, and low-fat milk on top.
- A granola bar, an apple, and a cold glass of milk.
- A cup of nonfat yogurt, fresh blueberries mixed in, and a slice of whole wheat toast with a fruit spread on top.

- A mini whole wheat bagel, spread lightly with cream cheese and jam; a peach; and a cup of yogurt.
- A scrambled egg, a whole wheat roll, fresh fruit salad, and a cup of low-fat milk.
- A low-fat muffin, a wedge of cantaloupe, and a cup of latte made with skim milk.

2 Have a bowl of sweetened brown rice. Consider it a takeoff on prepared cereal. Brown rice is full of energy-providing B vitamins, as well as a great source of filling fiber. Cook the rice the night before, then in the morning, put it in a bowl with a spoonful of honey, a handful of raisins, a cut-up apple, and a sprinkle of cinnamon for a unique yet delicious treat. Don't like rice? Try any of the cooking grains: barley, rye, red wheat, oats, buckwheat, quinoa, or millet.

3 Pour a cup of fruit smoothie. Simply whir a cup of strawberries and a banana in the blender, add a scoop of protein powder and a cup of crushed ice, and you've got a healthy, on-the-go breakfast filled with antioxidants. Toss in a cup of plain yogurt, and you've just added a bone-strengthening dose of calcium. An added bonus: You've just crossed three of your daily fruit servings off the list.

4 Use organic eggs. They're not much more expensive than regular eggs but are much higher in all-important omega-3 fatty acids, shown to benefit everything from your mental health (reducing risk of depression) to your heart health (reducing risk of atherosclerosis and atrial fibrillation), says Fred Pescatore, M.D., author of *The Hamptons Diet* and a physician at Partners in Integrative Medicine in New York City.

5 Sprinkle on a teaspoon of ground flaxseeds. It could be over your cereal, over your yogurt, over your smoothie, or over your eggs. Next to fish and organic eggs, flaxseeds are one of the best sources of omega-3 fatty acids.

6 Use Benecol, Take Control, or Smart Balance instead of butter. These newly developed soft food spreads contain heart-healthy plant stanols. Just 2 tablespoons daily can significantly lower your total cholesterol level.

7 Have lunch for breakfast. Instead of butter or cream cheese, top your morning (whole wheat) toast with 2 tablespoons tuna prepared with low-fat mayonnaise. The tuna is a great source of omega-3 fatty acids and an excellent source of energy-boosting protein. For the same healthy boost with a bit of variety, try lox or canned or smoked salmon (they also seem to go better at breakfast).

8 Sprinkle a whole wheat burrito with 2 ounces grated, low-fat cheddar cheese and broil for 3 minutes. While it's cooking, peel and eat an orange for valuable vitamin C. In this one small, quick meal, you're getting vitamin C and other antioxidants, calcium, fiber, and enough appetite-satisfying protein to sustain you for hours.

9 Make your own granola. Most store-bought brands are filled with sugar and fat. To make your own, mix 2 cups rolled oats with 1 cup dried fruits and seeds and a little brown sugar. Toast 3-5 minutes in a warm oven and store in an airtight container. Not interested in do-it-yourself? There are a few store-bought brands with reasonable sugar and fat levels, including Nature's Path and Familia.

10 Pour a bowlful of Kashi GOLEAN Crunch! With 10 grams of fiber, it will put you well on your way to the 25-30 grams of fiber you should be eating every day. Plus, studies find that people who regularly start their day with a bowl of cold cereal get more fiber and

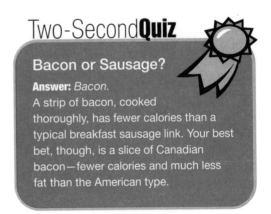

Two-Second Quiz

Bacon or Sausage?

Answer: *Bacon.*
A strip of bacon, cooked thoroughly, has fewer calories than a typical breakfast sausage link. Your best bet, though, is a slice of Canadian bacon—fewer calories and much less fat than the American type.

Chocolate "Power" Pops for Breakfast

Make up a batch of these "chocolate pops" for a yummy, yet healthy, on-the-go breakfast treat. The chocolate is really only a diversion—the inside is where the power resides. Raisins, hempseeds, nuts, and whole grains provide a rich combination of fiber, healthy oils, and protein with a great blend of flavors.

Chocolate Pops

Makes 48 pops

Pops
- 1 cup raisins (or dried apricots, dates, or figs)
- ½ cup raw shelled hempseeds (available at health food and specialty stores)
- 1½ cups low-fat nutty granola (no added oils)
- 3 cups crispy organic brown rice cereal
- ⅓ cup honey
- ⅓ cup natural peanut butter

Coating
- 2 ounces bittersweet chocolate
- 3 tablespoons skim milk
- ¾ cup rolled oats
- ⅓ cup chopped almonds

1. Place dried fruit, hempseeds, granola, and 2 cups of the rice cereal in a food processor. Grind until all is broken down into tiny pieces.

2. Place honey and peanut butter in a small pan and heat for 3-5 minutes. Take off the stove and stir until smooth. Add honey/peanut butter to the raisin-cereal mixture and grind again until a sticky dough forms.

3. Transfer the "dough" into a larger bowl and stir in the remaining cup of crispy brown rice cereal, digging in with your (clean!) hands, until well mixed. Scoop out small amounts (about 1 tablespoon) of the paste with a melon ball scooper or just with your fingers, roll it in the palm of your hand into little balls, and place on a baking sheet or large platter.

4. Meanwhile, heat milk in a pan until it boils. Take off flame. Break up bittersweet chocolate into pieces and stir into hot milk until smooth. Let cool for a few minutes.

5. Mix oats and chopped almonds in a bowl and sprinkle over an 8 x 12-inch pan lined with wax paper. Dip and roll each ball in the melted chocolate so it is evenly coated and place on top of the oats/almond mixture. Repeat until all the balls are done.

6. Stick a wood craft stick in each ball and place the pan in the freezer for at least 15 minutes so the chocolate can harden. Wrap the pops individually in cellophane, or store together in a large plastic bag and freeze.

---

calcium, but less fat, than those who breakfast on other foods. Another study found that people who ate two bowlfuls of high-fiber cereal every day spontaneously cut the amount of fat they ate by 10 percent. Don't like Kashi? Other high-fiber cereals include Raisin Bran, Multi-Bran Chex and Wheat 'N Bran Spoon Size (8 grams), Kellogg's All-Bran Original (10 grams), and General Mills Fiber One (14 grams).

11 **Eat half a grapefruit twice a week.** Grapefruits are loaded with folate, found to significantly reduce the risk of stroke. However, be cautious if you're taking regular medications. Grapefruit and its juice can interact with medications that have to be processed through the liver. Check with your doctor about any possible interactions between grapefruit and any medications you're taking.

12 Sip a cup of green tea with your breakfast. In addition to its heart-protective benefits, green tea may also have some weight-loss benefits, with one study finding it appears to raise the rate at which you burn calories and speed the rate at which your body uses fat.

13 Top your cereal with soy milk. Packed with potent phytoestrogens, soy has been credited with everything from protecting your heart to promoting stronger bones. But make sure that it's fortified with calcium; otherwise you're missing a great opportunity to get some bone-building calcium.

14 Host the breakfast equivalent of "build your own sundae." Who says breakfast has to be boring? Choose a selection of sliced fruit, yogurt, whole grain cereals, and/or whole grain pancakes or toast, and let everyone mix and match to create their own toppings. Lay everything out on paper plates (for easy cleanup).

15 Add a vitamin. Take any and all supplements with breakfast, suggests nutrition expert Shari Lieberman, Ph.D., author of *The Real Vitamin & Mineral Book*. Taking supplements with food reduces the chance they'll upset your stomach, and improves the absorption of minerals.

16 Spread apple slices with peanut butter. The protein and fat in the peanut butter provide a good start to the day, while the apple and the quercetin it contains provide fiber and protection against some cancers and heart disease.

17 Have a breakfast sandwich. Top a whole wheat English muffin with melted low-fat cheese (part-skim

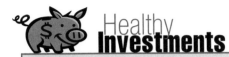

Healthy Investments

A Blender

Why? Blenders are great for making breakfast smoothies in the morning. You can toss in any kind of fruit—fresh, canned, or frozen—along with cottage cheese or yogurt for your calcium portion, a handful of nuts or seeds for heart-healthy fats, and a sprinkle of cinnamon for extra flavor. Add a cup of crushed ice in the summer for a frosty drink, or warm it in the microwave for 30 seconds on cold winter mornings.

mozzarella is a good choice), a sliced tomato, and a sliced, hard-boiled egg.

18 Crush cold cereal in a Baggie, add a peeled banana, and coat with the cereal. Voilà! Breakfast on a banana (as well as a healthy dose of potassium, beneficial in preventing strokes).

19 Hit the vegetarian section of the grocery. Soy bacon and sausage, gardenburgers, and soy crumbles make great sources of protein for breakfast without the saturated fat of their meat originals.

20 Make a blob. From nutritionist Alana Unger, R.D., of The Lifestyle Center in Visalia, California, comes this sounds-weird-but-tastes-great idea for an on-the-go breakfast. Mix ½ cup peanut butter, ¼ cup nonfat dry milk, 3 cups crushed flake cereal, and 2 tablespoons honey. Form into "blobs" (should make 10 blobs). Wrap each blob in plastic wrap and refrigerate. Grab a couple with a travel cup of skim milk and go!

21 Sprinkle ½ cup of blueberries on your cereal. Studies find the tiny purple berries are loaded with valuable antioxidants that can slow brain aging and protect your memory. Not into cereal? Try baking blueberries into oatmeal to create your own oatmeal-blueberry granola bar, or mixing them into whole wheat pancake or waffle batter.

22 Drink three cups of unsweetened orange juice every morning. The vitamin C in OJ not only boosts your immunity, but also improves your cholesterol levels. One study found that drinking three glasses of orange juice a day for four weeks raised levels of HDL, or "good" cholesterol, by 21 percent. If three cups is too much for you, substitute a couple of oranges. For the best Stealth Health effect, make it calcium-fortified juice.

23 Eat a bowl of sliced strawberries three times a week. Loaded with vitamin C, strawberries have numerous health benefits, one of them being protection for your eyes. One study of 247 women found that those taking vitamin C supplements were 75 percent less likely to get cataracts than those who didn't take it. It's better, though, to get your vitamin C from food. Other health benefits packed into berries: They're rich in a wide variety of antioxidants, low in calories, and even have a low glycemic index (shown to better maintain steady blood sugar levels).

24 Slice two kiwifruits into your morning smoothie. You may have just reduced your risk of premature death by as much as 30 percent, since a British study found that every ounce of vitamin C-laden fruits you eat a day reduces your risk of premature death 10 percent. Want an even easier way to eat a kiwi? Just slice the top off and scoop out bitefuls with a teaspoon. It's delicious, fun, and fast.

25 Get at least five grams of fiber during breakfast each morning. If you don't get off to a good start with your daily fiber intake, you'll never reach the recommended amount (15-25 grams per 1,000 calories). Plus, fiber is quite filling with no extra cost in calories. You can get those five grams in just a few bites with a large raw apple, ½ cup of the high-fiber cereals mentioned earlier, ½ cup of blackberries, or two slices of dark, whole grain rye bread.

26 Choose these toppers for your (whole wheat) bagel or toast:
- Two tablespoons nonfat cottage cheese sprinkled with flaxseed
- One slice low-fat cheese melted over a slice of mango
- Two tablespoons soy butter with a sliced banana
- One slice baked ham and one sliced tomato

27 Shave one ounce of dark chocolate over a cup of nonfat yogurt. Mix. The calcium-rich yogurt can actually help in your efforts to lose weight, while the antioxidant-loaded dark chocolate can help reduce the stickiness of "bad" LDL cholesterol and keep your arteries more pliable. Plus, who can resist starting the day with chocolate?

The Pill Routine

9 WAYS TO BETTER MANAGE YOUR MEDICINES AND SUPPLEMENTS

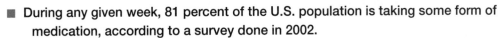

We are a nation of pill poppers. The numbers are staggering:

- During any given week, 81 percent of the U.S. population is taking some form of medication, according to a survey done in 2002.

- An estimated 4 billion prescriptions were filled or refilled in 2004. In addition, Americans currently buy 5 billion over-the-counter drug products a year, or roughly 18 per person.

- About 26 percent of adults take a multivitamin every day. While a large-scale poll hasn't been conducted on the subject, estimates of the number of people taking a vitamin, herb, or natural supplement on any given day exceed 50 percent.

- Small wonder that about 17 percent of hospitalizations among the elderly are the result of medication reactions.

As that last item suggests, too often we're taking our medicine incorrectly. We don't take it when we should, we take it with things we shouldn't, we mix it up and mix it around. The National Council on Patient Information and Education estimates that about half of prescriptions filled each year are not taken correctly. In fact, about one in five patients never even fill their original prescriptions!

By following some simple solutions outlined here, however, you can make sure you take your drugs properly, avoid interactions, and learn what to look for when buying over-the-counter drugs on your own.

1 Every time you visit a new doctor, or visit an old doctor after several months, bring every pill you're currently taking. Throw into a plastic bag every prescription medicine, vitamin, herb, supplement, and over-the-counter drug—even the aspirin—that you take in a typical day. Insist that your doctor look over it all to see if there are any problematic combinations or redundancies.

2 Ask your health-care professional if there is a way to streamline the medications you take. Some medications can be given once a day in sustained release, rather than having to take them three times a day. Others can be taken once per day or in a combination product that can decrease the numbers of drugs you're taking overall. Some can even be taken once a week!

3 Ask your doctor these questions about any new prescription:

- What is this medicine for?
- What side effects might I encounter?
- What side effects are dangerous and should impel me to stop taking this medicine and call you?
- If I have to stop this medicine because of side effects, is there another that I can take instead?
- What are the dangers for me if I don't take this medicine?
- What time of day should I take it?
- Should I take it with food or without?
- Can I take it with any kind of liquid, or only with water?
- How will I know if this medicine is working?
- How long should it take to begin working?
- How long should I continue taking this medicine?

Remember: While only a doctor can prescribe medicine, you are the one ultimately responsible for your health. Taking a prescription drug is your choice, and doing it smartly is your responsibility.

4 Consolidate all your prescriptions to one pharmacy, and then meet

with the pharmacist. Pharmacists are more than just prescription fillers. They are specially trained in understanding possible medicine interactions, including interactions with herbal supplements. When you consolidate all your prescriptions, your pharmacist can be watchful for just such things. In addition, some pharmacists receive special training in managing diseases like hypertension and diabetes and can provide counseling sessions. They are also a great resource for insider information on the best over-the-counter drugs.

Choosing the Right Vitamin

Been vitamin shopping lately? If you have, you probably needed to visit the pain-relief aisle afterward for something to deal with the headache all the choices caused. Here's what clinical nutritionist Shari Lieberman, Ph.D., author of *The Real Vitamin & Mineral Book,* recommends to make it easier to choose the right ones:

- Choose natural versions, rather than chemically synthesized versions, when buying fat-soluble vitamins like A, D, E, and beta-carotene.

- Avoid additives like coal tars, artificial coloring, preservatives, sugars, starch, and other ingredients that you simply don't need with your vitamin.

- Don't worry about chelated minerals. Chelation means the minerals have an added protein to enhance absorption. But they're often more expensive, and the studies on whether they really are absorbed faster than nonchelated minerals are sparse.

- Don't worry about time-release formulations. These supplements may actually take longer to be absorbed and provide you with lower blood levels of the vitamin or mineral.

---

5 Then consolidate all your medicines at home to one location.

It is generally wiser to have everything together rather than scattered around the house, car, purse, or briefcase. Choose a space that is dark, and that is perpetually at room temperature (unless instructions call for medications to be refrigerated). It should be accessible to adults, but not children. While you are doing this, check each container to see if any have passed their expiration dates. Throw out any prescription medication that you no longer need. Saving those last few antibiotics for the next infection is absolutely the wrong thing for you to do!

6 Create a rigid pill-taking routine. You want to take your pills at the same time and place every day, and you want a trigger to remind you to take them. Some ways to proceed:

- Buy a pill box or other medication gadget, and each Sunday evening, restock it for the coming week. Place the pill box at your preferred pill-taking site, and do not move it!
- Link your pill taking to a part of your morning ritual, such as brushing your teeth, or drinking your first glass of water or juice for the day.
- Set the alarm on your watch, computer, cell phone, or personal digital assistant to beep when it's time to take a pill. Then,

no matter where you are, or how busy you are, you'll get a reminder.

7 Watch out for shift work. Working different shifts can create timing problems when taking your medications. Try to take them when you would normally have a shift change so the timing is similar whether you're going to bed or to work.

8 Buy measuring spoons just for your medicine, and store them with your medicine. A kitchen teaspoon or tablespoon is rarely accurate.

9 Follow the golden rules of medicine. None of the following tips are particularly clever or surprising, but all bear repeating—and adhering to:

- Provide full disclosure to your doctor and pharmacist: that you have allergies, that

---

Buying Medicine Over the Internet

The Internet has been a boon for prescription medications and over-the-counter drugs and supplements. But since it's hard to know exactly whom or what you're dealing with in cyberspace, you need to take some special precautions.

- Check the validity of the pharmacy Web site. Legitimate drug-dispensing Web sites are certified through the National Association of Boards of Pharmacy's (NABP) Verified Internet Pharmacy Practice Sites (VIPPS) program. To be VIPPS certified, pharmacies must comply with the

licensing and inspection requirements of their state and each state to which they dispense pharmaceuticals. Additionally, pharmacies displaying the VIPPS seal comply with NABP criteria related to privacy, security, drug authenticity, quality assurance, and customer consultations. You can get a list of VIPPS-approved pharmacies by going to nabp.net or by calling 847-698-6227.

- Beware of purchasing drugs that aren't normally available in the U.S. You

may wind up with counterfeit medications that can make you sick, or "sugar pills" that will do nothing for your condition.

- Do not order a prescription through any site that just has you fill out a questionnaire or form, rather than seeing or talking to a doctor or pharmacist.

- Only do business with sites that provide direct access to a registered pharmacist. Use this pharmacist for the same kind of information you would get from a pharmacist in a retail store.

you are pregnant, that you have particularly high or low blood pressure, that you are prone to nausea, that you are on a diet. All can affect a drug's efficacy.

▶ When you pick up your prescription, open the bag immediately to verify that the medication you received is the correct one, at the right dosage, for the correct duration.

▶ Always ask your doctor or pharmacist if a medicine or supplement should be taken with or without meals.

▶ Take only the amount of medication prescribed or listed on the label.

▶ Get your prescriptions filled during slow times for the pharmacist, to avoid mix-ups.

▶ Whenever you purchase a supplement, ask your pharmacist if it has any potential interactions with prescription or over-the-counter drugs you're taking.

▶ Don't use or share medications prescribed for someone else.

▶ Don't take your medicine in the dark or without glasses or contacts if you need these aids to see.

Do**Three**Things

From Karen L. Kier, Ph.D., M.Sc., R.Ph., professor of clinical pharmacy and director of drug information at Ohio Northern University's College of Pharmacy comes this advice on managing medications:

1. Find out from your pharmacist if the medication can be put into different containers such as pill box reminders. Some medications are light sensitive or may not be compatible with plastic.

2. Try to fit taking your medications in with your daily routines. It is best to be able to associate your medication with a daily activity, like washing your face.

3. Make a chart or have a pharmacist make a chart of each medication and the times at which you take those medications. Hang the chart on the refrigerator door.

▶ Keep your medications in their original packaging with the full instructions, even over-the-counter and herbal products.

REMINDER

 Fast Results
These are bits of advice that deliver benefits particularly quickly—in some cases, immediately!

 Easy Gains
These are tips that give the biggest value for the least amount of effort.

 Super Effective
These are tips proven to be particularly effective through scientific research or widespread usage by experts.

The Commute

21 TIPS FOR A HAPPIER JOURNEY

If you're like most Americans, it takes you about 25 minutes to get to work, up from 22 minutes in 1990 and about 9 minutes in 1980. If you live in New York, New Jersey, or Maryland, your commute is even longer, averaging about 30 minutes. Over the course of a year, then, you're spending about five workweeks—208 hours—just getting to and from work!

It's enough to give a yoga teacher ulcers.

So it should come as no surprise that in one of the few major studies ever conducted on commuters, researcher Meni Koslowsky, Ph.D., a psychology professor from Bar-Ilan University in Israel and author of the book *Commuting Stress,* found commuters experienced significantly high levels of stress. However, Dr. Koslowsky also found that not all commuting is created equal, nor is the stress a foregone conclusion.

The tips below are designed to help make your commute less stressful, saving precious wear and tear on your heart, brain, immune system, and emotions. And, we promise, providing a calmer start or end to your day.

1 **If at all possible, take public transportation.** Here's why. Dr. Koslowsky's research found that it's not the commute per se that is so stressful, that is, the time we spend in the car. The real stress comes from the issue of control. If you drive your own car to work, part of the reason you do it is to feel that you're in control. So if you get stuck in traffic, you feel that you have *lost* control of your commuting experience, which is where the stress comes in. By taking public transportation, be it the train, streetcar, or bus, you have already given up control of your commute. If you get stuck, then, you won't be blaming yourself for the delay. Nor will you be torturing yourself to solve the situation.

2 **If at all possible, take the train.** Going back to that control issue again, Dr. Koslowsky's research found that another major cause of commuter stress is uncertainty. And there is far more uncertainty in driving a car, or even commuting via bus or carpool because of traffic accidents, traffic jams, etc., than in taking a train, when arrival times are more concrete.

3 **Consider carpooling.** Now, we're not telling you to definitely carpool, because here the research is ambiguous. On the one hand, Koslowsky's research finds that carpooling can reduce stress, both in terms of the "giving up" of control side of the issue, and in terms of the social interaction that occurs. But if you're

an introvert who prefers a quiet commute so you can read or think or listen to music, then carpooling with people who expect conversation could just stress you out all the more. Bottom line: If you're an outgoing, people kind of person, try the carpool. If you're an introvert, stick to your regular transportation system.

4 **Avoid rush hour, any way you can.** It's such an obvious way to improve your commute, and yet the fact that the streets are clogged every rush hour shows few people are bothering to find an alternative. What are viable alternatives, other than moving or getting a new job?

- Seek a one-hour shift in the time you start and end work.
- If your company has satellite offices that are closer to home, see if you can work there on occasion.
- Drive in before the crowds, and create a constructive pre-work ritual for yourself, such as exercising, taking a walk, eating a leisurely breakfast, running errands, whatever.

5 **Take the route with the least stop-and-go traffic.** Longer is better if traffic flows smoothly and you avoid lots of lights, turns, and crosswalks. For most of us, no form of driving is as stressful as trying to move quickly on crowded surface streets.

6 **Above all, lose the "race" mentality.** All that weaving, darting, and surging rarely gains you more than a few minutes, but at a huge price to your stress levels (not to mention the extra wear and tear on your car and lousier gas mileage). Drive calmly, without abundant lane changes, speed surges, or rapid

braking, and your commute will become so much more pleasant.

7 **Don't be judgmental about thy fellow driver.** Funny thing about high-stress drivers. When someone passes them, they get angry. When someone is going slower than they are, they get angry. They get angry when others forget to signal a turn, or if their car is larger, or has its brights on, or they're playing their music too loudly. Fuggedaboudit. Overreacting to other drivers is a sure road to stress, headaches, and anger. The better approach: Be a defensive driver, and never let what other drivers do bother you one bit.

8 **Learn while you drive.** You've always been meaning to learn to speak Spanish or read the latest bestsellers. Now's your chance. You can rent books on tape from the library or subscription services, or download them from the Internet and burn them onto CDs or upload them onto your MP3 player. Even bumper-to-bumper traffic is bearable when you're in

Two-Second**Quiz**

Manual or Automatic Transmission?

Answer: *Automatic.*
The two main public-service arguments for a manual transmission—you'll burn more calories and less gasoline—don't hold up. Shifting gears and pushing a clutch pedal don't add up to exercise unless you're driving an 18-wheel tractor-trailer. And on new cars, automatic transmissions have gotten increasingly fuel-efficient. From a stress standpoint, an automatic will make driving much easier.

Sniffed Your Car Lately?

If you're the type of person who uses your car as a moving trash can, you're putting more than your upholstery at risk. Dirty cars can become a rolling Typhoid Mary, filled with insects, germs, mold, pollen, and other irritants and pathogens destined to have you sneezing, itching, watering, and just plain sick. Just consider the fact that if you're like most Americans, you spend an average of 75 minutes a day in your car. That's several times more than most people spend in the bathroom!

To keep your moving living room as healthy as possible, follow these tips:

● **Sniff the air.** If your car smells like dirty socks, you've probably got mold. Check the air-conditioning coil, which may harbor mold, the carpeting in the car and trunk, and that old blanket you threw in the backseat after your son's soccer game last weekend—the game they played in the pouring rain. Then do battle: Remove the mold or moldy items, use the strongest cleanser you can without spotting the fabric to clean what remains, and do all you can to dry the car's interior thoroughly.

● **Clean your car regularly.** Remember that when it comes to health, a clean interior is more important than a clean exterior, so a run through the car wash doesn't count. Be sure to steam clean the carpeting and upholstery (unless you have leather upholstery) every couple of months, wipe down the interior with a damp cloth, throw out any trash daily, and be diligent about clutter control.

● **Roll the windows up—especially if the weatherman calls for rain.** Dampness and carpeting are a dangerous mixture. The result—mold—can cause a plethora of health problems, ranging from allergy and asthma exacerbation to wooziness and even neurologic problems.

● **Make sure the air-conditioning system is draining properly.** If the moisture builds up and doesn't drain out, it provides an ideal breeding ground for mold.

● **Keep the air circulating.** Say you're driving a friend around who has a cold. If you don't crack the window or open the outside vents, you're just recirculating germ-laden air throughout your car, possibly setting yourself up for your own infection.

---

the thick of an exciting mystery story. Dr. Koslowsky's research also found that commuting is less stressful when you're doing something else while driving the car (and no, painting your fingernails or filling out your tax forms is not appropriate).

9 **Use the cell phone for personal conversations only.** While cell phones are definitely a boon to the commuter, Dr. Koslowsky's research finds that using your cell phone for work-related tasks, such as setting up meetings, only *increases* your stress because it increases your workday. Instead, set your phone on speakerphone and voice-activated dialing and use it to keep up with relatives, check on your college-age kids, arrange a dinner party with the neighbors, or just fill in your mother about your recent successes. An added bonus: If any conversation gets too stressful, you can just say you're heading into a tunnel and ring off.

10 **Create a selection of music just for the commute;** one for going to work and one for relaxing on the way home from work. Workout experts know that music can serve many purposes and that each selection needs to be tailored to an individual's needs, says psychologist Patricia A. Farrell, Ph.D., author of *How to*

Be Your Own Therapist. Play the selection on an MP3 player if you ride the train or bus or in the stereo of your car. Conduct, if you want, or sing along, if you're in your car. No need to be shy. The music has another benefit if you're driving; one study found that people who listened to music when stuck in a traffic jam were less likely to get angry and violent than those who didn't listen to music.

11 Practice good automobile ergonomics.
That means more than just buckling up. Before you head out of the garage, make sure your headrest is set directly behind your head, aligned with the top of your ears. Adjust your seat and steering wheel for maximum comfort. Check each mirror to make sure you don't need to lean or crane your neck for best vision. Now you can strap up.

12 Leave 30 minutes earlier than normal.
Do this both coming and going. Studies find that the less sense of "time urgency," or worry about being late, you have, the less stressed out you'll feel during your commute.

13 Lift your legs up and stretch them for 30 seconds.
Now, obviously, we only want you to do this when you're stopped in traffic. But this movement is important, because it reduces the risk of blood clots from sitting too long in one position. Also put one arm behind your neck and stretch it by holding on to the elbow with the opposite arm. Switch sides. Do one of these stretches every time traffic comes to a halt.

14 Play a game.
Remember the old "I Spy" games you used to play when you were a kid on interminable road trips? Invent your own version. Maybe you track the number of women you see applying makeup while driving. Or the number of people you see picking their nose. Or the number of people you see on cell phones. Begin keeping track each day and see if you can beat your previous day's record.

15 Equip your car.
Make sure you have the following with you: A spill-proof coffee cup filled with your favorite brew. A bag of nonperishable snacks (try protein bars, dried fruit, juice boxes or bottled water, and pretzels) in case you get caught in traffic just as your blood sugar plummets. Something to read in the event traffic comes to a complete halt, and a fully charged cell phone with headset.

16 Use your dashboard as a bulletin board.
Tape up a family photo, or a favorite motivational passage, or a list of reasons you like being in your car, or something to remind you of your next vacation. Look at it frequently when traffic slows.

17 Develop five alternative routes for your commute.
Again, this gets back to the control issue. If you know you can go a different way, you have automatically given yourself more control over the situation.

18 Prepare for your commute the evening before.
Check the weather report and national, state, and local Web sites for information on highway construction. Listen to the local radio traffic report for warnings and updates. Again, this puts the control back into your hands.

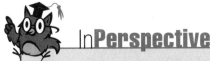

In Perspective

Why Stress Affects Your Health

You might think commuting has very little to do with health. But the stress that comes from commuting most certainly can affect your well-being. Here's why.

Every time you're confronted with a stressor—whether it is a traffic jam, a fire, or a bounced check—your body releases a cascade of stress hormones such as epinephrine, adrenaline, and cortisol. They, in turn, send a volley of signals to various parts of your body to ready them for action. For instance, your liver releases glucose to provide instant energy to muscle cells. Your lungs expand, your heart beats faster, and your blood pressure rises to send more oxygen-rich blood throughout your body. Your bowel and intestinal muscles contract. And so on. All of which can lead to common stress-related conditions ranging from chronic hypertension, angina and gastric reflux, to constipation and irritable bowel syndrome, to depression, anxiety, and fatigue.

Stress can even make you fat. Cortisol is not only a powerful appetite trigger, but chronically high levels of cortisol actually stimulate the fat cells inside the abdomen to fill with more fat, creating a life-threatening form of fat called visceral fat, which puts you at higher risk for heart disease and diabetes.

Stress also inflicts its damage in more insidious ways by affecting the very system that is supposed to guard your health: your immune system. Turns out that, like most systems in the body, the immune system has a feedback loop. After it finishes attacking foreign invaders with inflammatory chemicals, the brain sends out cortisol, the stress hormone, to shut down this inflammatory response and send the immune system back into a quiet, or homeostatic, state. But if your body is releasing cortisol all the time—as it does under chronic stress, the kind that comes from commuting—then your immune system is constantly being suppressed, increasing your risk of illness.

19 **Relax before you get into the car.** Instead of scarfing a scalding cup of coffee and choking down a bagel in the car, get up early enough so you can have a leisurely breakfast before beginning your commute. Once you arrive at work, take another few minutes to sip a cup of tea or coffee before diving into your work. On the way home, stop by the coffee room before you get into your car and just sit quietly with a drink for five minutes before heading home.

20 **Multitask via the radio.** Set your car radio to both a favorite music station and a news station. Use travel time to get caught up with the news, then switch to music before you arrive to relax or get "pumped," as circumstances warrant.

21 **Work out in your car.** Do isometrics while driving by tensing and relaxing your leg muscles, tensing your arm muscles against the resistance of the steering wheel, and/or tensing your abdominal and chest muscles. When done correctly for bouts of 10–15 seconds, these toning exercises can make an appreciable difference in your appearance, improve your fitness, and mellow you out without your ever breaking a sweat and without adding an extra minute to your packed schedule.

Starting Your Workday

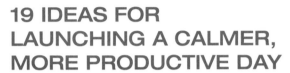

19 IDEAS FOR LAUNCHING A CALMER, MORE PRODUCTIVE DAY

Have you ever been guilty of ending a lousy workday by snapping at the kids, being rude to your spouse, gorging on junk food, vegging out in front of the TV, or turning to alcohol? A bad workday may not seem unhealthy unto itself, but it can serve as the domino that starts a whole chain of destructive actions.

The way you begin your workday sets the tone for the rest of the day, not only at work but also at home. A few simple measures taken at the start of the day can make all the difference to how it ends. We've compiled the following tips to help you get off to the right—and healthy—start.

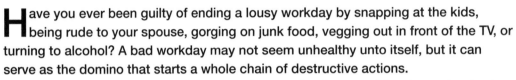

1 Limit your work-starting routine to 15 minutes. That is, don't spend more than 15 minutes getting coffee, settling in, reading e-mails, checking messages, or looking at newspapers. You are often at your freshest and most productive at the beginning of the day. A prolonged morning routine takes the positive edge off you and makes your afternoon more stressful. Better that you jump into the important work quickly, and read the nonessential e-mails after you've covered lots of ground.

2 Write *two* to-do lists. The first should contain everything that you need to get done soon. It should be a comprehensive list of short-, medium-, and long-term projects and work, and you should constantly adjust it. The second to-do list should be what you can reasonably

expect to get done today, and today only. Be fair to yourself. Factor in the disruptions, meetings, phone calls, and travel hassles that are interwoven in our days. Make the tasks as specific as possible (i.e., conduct online research for ostrich meat market) and assign a time you plan to devote to it (20 minutes). Print the list out on brightly colored paper; this keeps it from getting lost on your desk. By prioritizing your work and slicing it down to small, achievable pieces, you greatly increase the chances that you will be satisfied with your day's accomplishments.

3 Take a few moments to assess the day's emotional challenges. Almost as important as your to-do list is a "be prepared for" list. Inventory the tough phone calls, boring meetings, challenging customers, frustrating red tape, infuriating rush-hour drives, droning detail work, and other mental challenges you are likely to face. Then accept that they are inevitable, and prepare yourself to get through them without anger, frustration, or impatience. Remember: It's usually not our work that gets us down—we all should enjoy our work!—but rather the challenges that lie along the periphery of the job.

4 **Visualize your day.** Taking that last point further, you might wish to start each day by closing your eyes for 10 or 20 seconds and visualizing how you want it to go. See yourself making a stellar presentation at the board meeting. Experience the great feeling you're going to have when you finally make the sale or deliver the goods or get that report off your desk. Hear yourself providing positive feedback to your employee, or even your boss. If you are religious, make this a prayer.

5 **Schedule some social time come midmorning.** Most likely, you work with people whom you like and know rather intimately. In fact, camaraderie is what makes many jobs great. So build into each morning a ritual in which you can spend a few moments of social time with colleagues. Make it short, at an

appropriate time, and don't let a day go by without getting to it. Avoid phone calls if you can; they can unexpectedly turn into big time-eaters.

6 **Likewise, schedule some reading time.** There's not a job that doesn't require at least some reading, be it about the company, the industry, the marketplace, the economy, the price of tomatoes. Create a ritual that gives you 15 minutes or so to review newspapers, electronic newsletters, industry magazines, company memos, and other reading. Be disciplined—this is not the time to read the funnies or do online shopping! You'll find that being up-to-date on your business has many advantages, just one of them being a sense of control about your own situation.

7 **Keep essentials nearby.** If you have storage space for private stuff where you work, stock up on the following:

- A case of low-fat granola bars (the perfect snack or substitute breakfast)
- A case of bottled water (keeps you away from the soda machine)
- Bags of slow-dissolving mints or candy (helps prevent needless snacking)
- Supplements, including a multivitamin, B-complex, C and E vitamins, and echinacea (good for when cold season hits or you forget to take vitamins at home)
- A box of tissues (always handy)
- At least five family photos (which always lift the spirits)
- A snack pack (an array of nutritious snacks).

8 **Make sure you have the right equipment for a healthy day** in the office. If you're deskbound, that means:

- Headphones for the telephone so you're not leaning your neck to one side when you talk on the phone.
- An antiglare filter on your computer screen to reduce vision problems. One study on filter screens found they improved the quality of the screen image and significantly reduced the percentage of people with tired eyes, fatigue, itchy or watery eyes, dry eyes, and headaches.
- A wrist rest for your computer so that you keep your wrists elevated, thus avoiding pressure on the nerves that go through your wrist, which can cause carpal tunnel syndrome.

If you are in sales or service, you are likely to be on your feet much of the day. Comfortable, supportive shoes are just a start. Good socks and underwear, a steady supply of breath mints, and braces or other support for your back, knees, or any other problematic joints are also important. Finally, establish a safe place to keep your keys, cell phone, and other pocket stuff. Full pockets can affect your posture and movement.

9 Set your watch or computer alarm to go off every hour.
This will be your signal throughout the day to take a break, get up and stretch, walk around the building, etc.

10 Sit up straight.
One common cause of fatigue, carpal tunnel syndrome, and back pain is our tendency to slump while we're typing or sitting. Every time your alarm beeps or your phone rings, consider it a reminder to straighten that back, throw back those shoulders, and lift up that neck.

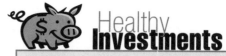

Healthy Investments

A 16-Ounce Freezer Water Bottle
Use it to keep cold water on your desk all day long. This ensures you stay hydrated with a healthy, noncalorie liquid vs. sugar-filled sodas, juices, or sports drinks.

11 Loosen your tie (if you're wearing one).
Researchers at the New York Eye and Ear Infirmary found that tighter ties increased eye pressure, a risk factor for glaucoma.

12 Spend a few moments sparking your creativity.
Here's a good way if you have a computer. Each morning, pick a random word or name. It could be "Eduardo," or "shad roe," or "aquamarine." Spend five minutes exploring the word on the Internet. (Is there an "aquamarine.com" Web site? Yes—it's all about a modern fish farm.) Don't have a computer? Then pick up a dictionary, open it to a random page, and look for interesting words. Creative exercises like these blow the night's cobwebs from your mind and set your brain up to embrace new information—even in a job you've been doing for years.

13 Record your message for the day.
Effective use of voice mail "can eliminate many inefficiencies concerning business communications," says Marilyn Chalupa, a business education and office administration professor at Ball State University in Muncie, Indiana. Her advice: Change your message each day, and make it specific and useful. For instance, you might leave a message saying that you're in the office, but in meetings most of the day, and

A Packed Lunch or A Purchased Lunch?

Answer: *Packed lunch.*
It'll be healthier, it'll have fewer calories, it'll be cheaper, and it'll save you lots of time that you can use walking, reading, or socializing.

so won't be returning calls until the next morning. Or you could leave a message saying that you're in the office, but working on a major project all day, and will only be checking messages at lunch and 4 p.m. You can even leave a voice mail for one person if you know someone is calling for specific information. Some phone mail systems enable you to leave this information in a separate place on your voice mail.

14 Plug in your cell phone as soon as you get to work. That way, it's fully charged and ready to go regardless of what happens the rest of your day.

15 Start your day with a cup of hot cocoa while you tackle your most creative work. Research finds that one cup of cocoa a day for five days can increase blood flow in the brain, hands, and legs, and helps regulate blood pressure. Choose a brand that isn't loaded with sugar or hydrogenated oil, such as Ghirardelli's.

16 Get to work an hour before everyone else. That precious hour of calm—before the e-mails start pouring in, the phone starts ringing, and the problems start piling up—is more valuable than diamonds in terms of your overall work performance and accomplishments. An added bonus: You'll get to leave early.

17 Find a compliment you've received from a coworker, boss, or client via e-mail, print it out, and tape it inside your top drawer. Whenever you're feeling overwhelmed, discouraged, or useless, open the drawer and take a peek to remind you of what others think of your abilities.

18 Keep fresh flowers or plants at work. A study from Texas A&M University found that live plants increased creative thinking.

19 Block off 30 minutes on your calendar at the end of the day. This might seem like a strange thing to do when you're starting your day, but this is your time to begin your transition from work to home. During this last half hour of your day, you'll finish answering any e-mail, update your to-do list for the next day, and clean off your desk.

Workplace Madness

36 WAYS TO CALM THE CHAOS

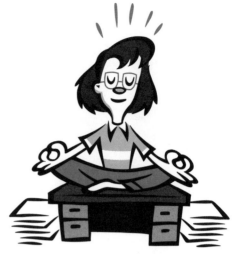

Most days of the week, you get up, get dressed, eat breakfast, and head into one of the unhealthiest places in the world. Problems at work are more strongly associated with health complaints than any other life stressor—even more than financial problems or family problems. In fact, researchers at Ohio State University have found the first-ever link between stress and back pain. Turns out that people who get upset when they're criticized in the workplace use their muscles in ways that might lead to injury over time. That helps explain why people with certain personality types—namely, introverted people and those who dislike performing repetitive tasks—are more likely to report back pain on the job.

Here is a wide spectrum of Stealth Health tips to help you better cope with workplace stress (without taking out your boss).

1 **Work on one thing at a time.**
Today's office worker changes tasks an average of *every three minutes,* a lightning-speed day of interruptions helped along by the multitasking made possible with computers. Working on eight things at once might seem impressive, but it isn't. Rather, it is exhausting, inefficient, and highly stressful. So instead of constantly checking e-mail, having two or three documents open on your screen at one time, or returning voice mail messages as they come in, structure your day to focus on one thing at a time. In particular, start your day by blocking out two uninterrupted hours for hands-on work. During this time, do not answer your phone or check e-mail. Then check e-mails and respond all at once. Go to lunch. Then structure your

afternoon the same way. Designate a time immediately after lunch and an hour before you leave for returning phone calls.

2 **Work in short bursts.** The flip side to multitasking is that it is hard to sustain creativity or intensity over one task for long stretches. Rather, our brains work in cycles of creativity, then rest. So work this way. After an hour or so of concentrated work, get up for five minutes, stretch, walk around, do some calisthenics. Not only will this help the quality of your work; by the time you finish your day, you'll have snuck in 30 minutes of stress-reducing exercise.

3 **Give your colleagues a grade.** A "D" is for people who drain your energy, and an "F" is for people who fill

you up with energy. Now make sure that you avoid the D's as much as possible throughout the day. Conversely, when you're feeling drained, take a few minutes to connect with an F, suggests James Campbell Quick, Ph.D., professor of organizational behavior at the University of Texas in Arlington.

4 **With difficult workplace relationships, deal directly, but constructively.** "Toxic people" are those whose negativity, intensity, or demeanor always seems to drain or annoy you—the D people from above. They can be your boss, your assistant, your colleagues—in other words, they are people with whom you frequently interact. After a negative encounter with a toxic person, the temptation is to be angry and accusatory. But that leads nowhere. Instead, try this direct, honest, and disarming approach: "I am finding our interactions stressful because of ____ and am feeling bad about ____. I would like our working relationship to improve. What suggestions do you have for me?" Even if you feel that the other person is the one who should change, by asking for her suggestions, you avoid putting her on the defensive. If she is even

a little reasonable, this will likely lead to, "Well, I guess there are some changes I could make too."

5 **Praise yourself at least once a day.** "We don't take enough time to praise ourselves for doing things well," says Dr. Quick. So when you've completed an interim or long-term goal, tell yourself—out loud—what a good job you've done. You'll get a psychic burst of energy and confidence that will go a long way toward helping you maintain your cool amid the workplace madness.

6 **Be creative in motivating yourself.** Here's a good one: Write a check to some organization you loathe, put it in a stamped, addressed envelope, and tell a trusted friend to mail it if you fail to meet an important deadline or complete a vital task. Or go the positive route: Give the friend something you really cherish or desire and only let your friend give it back to you if you achieve your goal.

7 **Forgo the coffee during team meetings or group work.** A study sponsored by the British Economic and Social Research Council found that when men drank coffee while working together in a group, it tended to make the group less effective. The study also found that just the perception that the drink contained caffeine—whether or not it actually did—also increased the men's feelings of stress and their heart rates.

8 **Stand against the wall and slide down it as if you were sitting** in a chair. Stay there for a few minutes without looking down, just feeling your spine against the wall. Breathe deeply (in through your nose, out through your

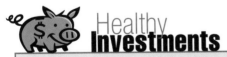

Healthy Investments

An Indoor Water Fountain

The sound of running water is calming, the view of running water oh-so-pleasant. Plus, a fountain on or near your desk acts as a humidifier amid the dry, overprocessed air of many offices. Small fountains are available for as little as $25. Usually you just add water, plug them in, and keep an eye on the water level as the days go by.

mouth) and focus on one peaceful thought (waves crashing on the shore, taking a walk through the woods, a glass of wine by a roaring fire). Press your feet into the ground as you hold this position and picture the stress oozing out of your body into the ground. When you stand up, shake out your arms and legs and return to work refreshed.

9 Keep a vacation file on your desk. Fill it with brochures of places you would like to visit. When you're feeling stressed, daydream your way through the file. It will help remind you of one reason you're working, and provide a few minutes of virtual vacation.

10 Read a poem out loud twice a day. The cadence, words, and images will soothe your soul. Not into poetry? If you're a religious person, try reading a Psalm or other sacred writings. If you love music, listen to a few of your favorite songs.

11 Make an altar or display in your office to remind you of your life outside the office. Include pictures of your spouse, children, and/or pet, a photograph of yourself doing something fun, plus a memento that reminds you of a special occasion. When you feel yourself getting overwhelmed and stressed out, take five minutes and simply stare at the display. Recall the day each picture was taken. Hold the memento and return in your mind to the place where you got it. Now you're ready to return to the workaday world.

12 Keep a work journal. This is a journal you keep in your desk drawer (preferably locked). Write in it

whenever you feel your temper rising, your frustration growing, or your despair increasing. In it, you can write all the things you'd *like* to say to the boss/client/colleague so you get it out of your system without losing your job. It will also help you understand in a more realistic manner what it is about your job and your day that really drives you crazy—and what you actually enjoy. Do not, however, keep said journal on your computer.

13 Keep a Nerf gun in your office. And try to get some of your coworkers to do the same. When the stress feels overwhelming, hit the halls shooting. It is a completely fun, cathartic, and non-destructive way to let off steam.

14 Fill your office with plants and make sure you cluster them within eyesight, near your computer. Studies find that plants significantly lower workplace stress and enhance productivity.

15 Schedule a sick day. If you're experiencing an unusual number of headaches, sore neck, sore back, or other aches and pains; find you have trouble falling or staying asleep; or are snapping at

Are You a Workaholic?

Sharon Lobel, Ph.D., professor of management at the Alber School of Business and Economics at Seattle University, has an interesting perspective on workaholism. Rather than saying that all workaholics have a problem, she divides them into two types: Happy Workaholics, who don't wish for a different lifestyle, and Unhappy Workaholics, who complain regularly that they do want a change.

"Happy Workaholics value work more than other aspects of life and arrange their lives accordingly," she says. "If someone loves to work and spends most of her waking hours at work, that's not a problem, in my opinion. On the other hand, if someone wishes that he had more time to devote to family, fitness, or hobbies but is prevented from doing so because he works too many hours, that person is an Unhappy Workaholic."

So how can you tell which category you fit?

"People who say they're working to 'advance at my job' or 'to buy a house' are probably not Unhappy Workaholics," says Dr. Lobel. "Unhappy Workaholics are likely to say their employer makes them work long hours and they're likely to express resentment toward the employer." Feeling overwhelmed, depressed, and tired are other telltale signs of the Unhappy Workaholic.

And what do you do if you find you're in this latter category?

"I think everyone needs to ask themselves what really matters in their lives," says Dr. Lobel. "Which values are most important? Achievement, wealth, social justice, health, relationships? What gives you the most rewards? Then you need to look at how you're living your life. Do you devote time and energy toward what you most value? If the answer is yes, then there isn't much of a problem. If the answer is no, then it's time to implement some change strategies."

your coworkers for no reason, it's time for a day off. Check your calendar for the upcoming week and pencil in the day you're going to call in sick. This is not lying—you *are* sick. It's just mental rather than physical. But if you don't take the day and spend it doing something you enjoy, you can bet you *will* be sick before the month's end. Don't believe us? Just consider that up to 80 percent of visits to primary care physicians are for stress-related complaints.

16 Schedule 10 minutes of "worry time." This is time to close your office door or go sit in an empty conference room and focus on what is stressing you out. You can bring your journal or just a sheet of paper. Divide the paper into three columns: My Worry; Why It Worries Me; Worst Thing That Could Happen. Once you confront the worst thing that could possibly happen—and realize that it's highly unlikely it ever *will* happen—you can get back to work with your worry load lightened.

17 When things feel like they're falling apart all around you, take five minutes and draw. Seriously. Grab a pencil and some blank paper and sketch the chaos around you, or something funny, or something peaceful, or a caricature of the bad guy of the moment. Using another part of your brain and focusing on something outside of the chaos itself will provide a much-needed break.

18 Manage your e-mail. With about 5.5 *trillion* e-mails sent each year, an amount that increases 40 percent annually, this electronic form of communication has become a major source of workplace stress. One study out of

Canada's University of Western Ontario found that managers spend more than an hour per day on e-mail, extending their workweek by an average of five hours. The study also found that only 17 percent of e-mail users can answer their e-mails in the same day. To cope:

▸ Read e-mails once, answer immediately, delete if possible, or move them to folders, suggests leadership expert Zach Kelehear, Ph.D., of the University of Alabama at Birmingham. Overflowing in-boxes are depressing, and take too long to read and sort.

▸ Insert e-mail responses in the subject line whenever possible rather than composing a new message each time, and reply to e-mail only when you have something to say, notes Dr. Kelehear.

▸ Never send an e-mail if you're angry. You can write it (preferably in your word processing program) then save it until you feel calmer.

▸ Use the automatic signature function in your e-mail so people can call you or send you information via snail mail.

▸ Don't waste time acknowledging receipt of e-mail. Also, don't e-mail and phone with the same message.

▸ Don't insert the recipient's address first before composing the e-mail message, says Christina A. Cavanagh, Ph.D., professor at the University of Western Ontario and author of *Managing Your E-mail: Thinking Outside the Inbox*. Doing so could mean you mistakenly send a message before it's finished or when it's saying something you didn't want it to say.

 In**Perspective**

Why Is Work So Stressful?

Lots of reasons. The National Institute for Occupational Safety and Health (NIOSH) has even compiled a list of them.

● **How tasks are designed.** Heavy workloads, infrequent rest breaks, long work hours and shift work, and hectic and routine tasks that have little inherent meaning, don't utilize workers' skills, and provide little sense of control are all stress provoking.

● **Management style.** If your workplace (or manager) eschews worker participation in decision making, micromanages, has poor communication, and lacks family-friendly policies, you're working in a potentially toxic environment.

● **Interpersonal relationships.** Do you get support and help from coworkers and supervisors or do you feel like you work in a pit of vipers? If it's the latter, consider your workplace stressfully sick.

● **Work roles.** If you have conflicting or uncertain job expectations, get too much responsibility heaped upon your shoulders (particularly without the authority that should go along with it) or feel you are wearing too many hats, you're working in a toxic waste dump when it comes to stress.

● **Career concerns.** Job insecurity and lack of opportunity for growth, advancement, or promotion; rapid changes for which you're unprepared; and continued rumors of layoffs and belt tightening can all send you to the doctor with a stress-related illness.

● **Environmental conditions.** Unpleasant or dangerous physical conditions such as crowding, noise, air pollution, or ergonomic problems can turn even the most laid-back work environment into a stress pit.

Complain or Be Quiet?

Answer: *Complain.*

Complain effectively, by being specific and positive, focusing on how correcting the problem will help the company, and by providing at least one viable solution to the problem. Any sensible business wants to do things better. If your boss or company is so insecure or political that you can't speak honestly about things needing to be fixed, it's time to move on.

▸ Use the rule of three: If you've gone back and forth three times on a topic and you're still confused or have questions, pick up the phone.

19 **Listen to Muzak in your office.** A study from Wilkes University in Wilkes-Barre, Pennsylvania, found that newspaper reporters who listened to Muzak (any kind of mellow tune will do) substantially reduced not only their feelings of stress but also their levels of stress hormones.

20 **Go talk to your best friend at work.** Studies find that social support at work is associated with lower blood pressure during the workday and smaller blood pressure increases even during work-related stressful moments.

21 **Rub a drop of lavender oil on your inner wrist.** The aroma of lavender (or cucumber oil) is a known relaxer. Close your eyes, hold your wrist up to your nose, and sniff deeply, picturing as you do a field of lavender in Provence, the purple stalks waving in the breeze.

22 **Put four drops of Bach Rescue Remedy, a flower essence formula, in a glass of water and drink it down.** This natural remedy is believed to soothe stress, relieve impatience, and reduce worry.

23 **Leave the office for lunch every day.** Getting out of the office, away from the stress and into a totally different environment, clears your mind and helps you put some perspective on whatever hassles are dogging your day.

24 **Eat three Brazil nuts.** They're an excellent source of selenium, a mineral that may help prevent depression. And given the state of today's workplaces, we need all the help we can get.

25 **Munch on a handful of pumpkin seeds.** Rich in iron, they can help counter the iron-depleting effects of a stressful workplace.

26 **Eat a peppermint patty.** The chocolate is stress relieving, the peppermint provides a burst of minty energy, and the tiny sugar rush might be just enough to get you over the hump. At the very least, it's better than slamming your office door, kicking your computer, or reacting in otherwise self-defeating ways to a madness-filled workplace.

27 **Pour a cup of boiling water over a handful of chamomile** leaves or a chamomile tea bag. The herbal mix, long known for its gentle, soothing properties, will help you to de-stress and center yourself.

28 Try some beverage leverage. Increase your productivity and decrease your stress by keeping an invigorating beverage handy at your workstation: hot tea or coffee in cold weather; iced tea, iced coffee, or perhaps just fruit-flavored mineral water in the heat. Choose something that feels just a bit indulgent, but doesn't contain a lot of unwanted sugar or calories. Sip frequently.

29 Hold one nostril closed with a finger and blow strongly out through the other (blow your nose first). This is a yoga movement believed to reduce stress.

30 Walk and talk slower. This tricks your body into thinking that things are calmer than they actually are, says Patricia A. Farrell, Ph.D., author of *How to Be Your Own Therapist* and moderator for WebMD's anxiety/panic board.

31 Examine your real feelings. If you love what you do, the stress related to your job will be far less damaging than if you don't (this is the "good" stress vs. "bad" stress theory). So if you hate your job, it's time to explore other options. Spending a few minutes each evening rewriting your résumé, researching other job options, or contacting potential employers can help you better handle the stress at your current job.

32 Build rewards into your work-week. Having something to look forward to makes every difficult task more bearable. It might be a special dinner, a movie, a game of racquetball, or a massage. Put it in your schedule wherever it will help the most and think of working hard in advance to get to that reward.

33 Offer feedback. As they say, it's better to give than to receive. Provide praise and recognition to others at work whenever appropriate. You will feel good by making others feel good, and the good feeling will tend to spread.

34 Have a "perspectivizer" handy. Work may seem overwhelmingly stressful at times, but your troubles are likely smaller than they seem. Keep a picture in your office—the earth taken from space, a starry night, or the ocean—and look at it whenever you feel overwhelmed. Amid countless stars and the timeless crashing of waves against the shore, how important is that deadline, really? Now take a deep breath and return to work with a refreshed sense of perspective.

35 Plan ahead. When work is challenging, devote some of your downtime—weekends, evenings, or even using a tape recorder in the car—to delineating a sequence of tasks. This is a standard technique during medical residency training, when the task list of the day can stretch for 36 hours. Make a list, place boxes next to each item, and check off the boxes as you move through the list. You will avoid forgetting anything, you'll stay on task, organization will make you efficient, and (we know from personal experience) it's very satisfying to check off those boxes.

36 Socialize your work. Consider a once-a-week lunch gathering with coworkers where you talk about a particular work issue. Use the collective brain to figure out how to do something better, improve the work facilities, enhance productivity, or improve relationships.

The Lunch Hour

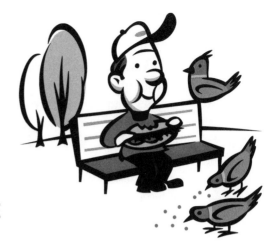

15 WAYS TO MAXIMIZE YOUR MIDDAY BREAK

For too many of us, the lunch hour has become just another extension of our already overburdened day. Although the lunch hour was originally designed for just that—lunch—today we spend our midday break running errands, pecking away at a computer keyboard, or returning personal phone calls. When we do actually sit down and eat, it's often to consume whatever comfort food we can scrape together from the company vending machine or cafeteria. Yet your lunch hour offers the perfect time to break this hectic cycle. Rather than spend the hour stressing over what you still need to accomplish or quickly inhaling fatty, salty, high-calorie foods, consider the following advice.

1 Go outside. If you work in an office or a retail establishment, you likely are stuck in the same building all day long. Now's your chance to escape. Soak in the sun, watch the rain, or feel the wind. Breathe some real air, and disconnect for a moment from the job. At least once every workday you should make the time to step outside, even if just for two minutes. It will recharge your body and your mind.

2 Daydream for 15 minutes—and then eat, run errands, or return to work. "Creative daydreaming is not only a way to get out of the daily lunch hour grind, but also a way to put your creative juices to work," explains Patricia A. Farrell, Ph.D., psychologist and author of *How to Be Your Own Therapist*. If you're feeling particularly stressed about a project, spend your 15 minutes mentally exploring

ways you can tackle it. If you feel mentally stale and burned out, spend the 15 minutes in la-la land, on a mini vacation. Imagine yourself strolling the beach, climbing a mountain, or generally spending time in a location that makes you happy. "Take yourself somewhere and have an adventure," says Dr. Farrell.

3 Nap for 10 to 15 minutes. Studies increasingly show the value of short naps during the day, and progressive employers are becoming more lenient about them. So if you can, curl up under your desk, nod off in your car (unless you're driving!), or otherwise arrange yourself in your office chair so you can snooze without anyone noticing. "Your nap will refresh your mind and put a whole new perspective on the afternoon, because it breaks the tension of the day," says Dr. Farrell.

4 **Pack a frozen dinner.** They're not just for dinner anymore. You can pop your dinner into your break room microwave for a quick-and-easy meal that allows plenty of time to run errands or power walk during the rest of your lunch hour. Today's frozen food aisles include organic, vegetarian, low-fat, low-carb, and numerous other healthy food options. Look for a frozen dinner that supplies fewer than 400 calories, 15 grams total fat, 800 milligrams sodium, and 15 grams added sugars. It should contain at least 8 grams fiber and 7 grams protein. The fiber and protein will give you staying power during the afternoon, preventing the post-lunch refrigerator raid. The protein will also keep you alert. Good options include Amy's Country Dinner, Celentano Eggplant Rollettes, Linda McCartney Southwestern Style Rice and Beans, Seeds of Change Spicy Peanut Noodles, and Taj Ethnic Gourmet Chicken Tikka Masala.

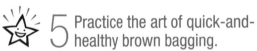

5 **Practice the art of quick-and-healthy brown bagging.**
Packing your own lunch need not take a lot of time or creative energy. Include a source of lean protein, fruit or vegetables (raw carrots, celery, broccoli or cauliflower florets with a bit of low-fat ranch dressing work great), and whole rather than processed grains. Leftovers from last night's dinner work wonders, as do the following quick-and-easy sandwich options:

▸ Peanut butter and banana sandwich: two slices whole wheat bread topped with two tablespoons peanut butter and half a sliced banana.

▸ Chicken or tuna salad sandwich: six ounces water-packed tuna or ½ cup cooked chicken breast pieces mixed with

one tablespoon light mayo and relish or shredded carrots, served between two slices of whole wheat bread.

▸ A whole wheat pita "pizza": one pita stuffed with low-fat pizza/spaghetti sauce, part-skim shredded mozzarella cheese, carrot shreds, broccoli pieces, peppers, tomatoes, spinach, mushrooms, or other veggies of choice, Canadian bacon, and fat-free veggie sausage. Melt in the microwave before eating if desired.

▸ Tortilla roll-up: one whole wheat tortilla spread with one tablespoon fat-free cream cheese, topped with two slices fat-free lunch meat and various veggies such as chilies, lettuce or spinach, tomatoes, onion, cucumber, sprouts, or shredded carrots.

▸ Veggie sandwich: two slices whole wheat bread spread with one tablespoon fat-free mayo or mustard and stuffed with one slice low-fat or fat-free cheese, along with lettuce, sprouts, and sliced avocado, tomatoes, and peppers.

Two-Second**Quiz**

Lunch or Graze?

Answer: *Graze.*
Nibble food throughout the day, rather than having a large, formal lunch. Spreading out your calories stabilizes blood sugar and insulin levels, provides more frequent relief from stress, tension, and boredom, and avoids the post-meal fatigue, because there is no big meal. Plus, you never get *really* hungry, and so are less likely to make regrettable food choices that result when you're starving. Best reason: All-day grazing frees up lunchtime for other things, such as a walk, or catching up on work so you can get home a bit earlier and go for a walk then.

6 **Pack ready-to-eat soup.** Your grocery store stocks numerous healthful soups sold in microwavable cartons. According to research conducted at Pennsylvania State University, broth-based soups weigh down your stomach, enabling you to feel full on fewer calories. Toss a bean and vegetable soup along with a cheese stick and a carton of skim milk into your lunch bag. In just a few seconds, you'll have packed all the protein and fiber you need to power your body and brain through the afternoon.

7 **Get away from your desk—even if it's just for 15 minutes.** No matter how pressing that big project is, physically remove yourself from your office for at least 15 minutes. Walk the hallways, chat with a friend, or as mentioned, go outside. The time away from the desk will refresh your mind, allowing you to return to work more invigorated.

8 **Choose smarter fast food.** If coworkers invite you out for fast food, you don't have to decline on the basis of health considerations. Just choose wisely. Opt for a broiled chicken breast sandwich without the sauce or purchase a salad (store your own homemade or store-bought low-fat dressing in the break room fridge). At sit-down restaurants or the company cafeteria, opt for broth-based soup, fresh fruit cups, and grilled or steamed items. For more suggestions, see page 134.

9 **Create a sandwich-o-matic chart and stick it on your refrigerator.** This prevents the early morning haze from overcoming your better judgment and allowing you to leave the house without a packed lunch. In one category on your chart, list your bread options (whole wheat bread, pita, tortilla wrap, and so

on). In the next column, list your protein options, such as turkey breast, low-fat cheese or soy cheese, lean roast beef, hummus, or tuna or chicken salad. In another column, list vegetable toppings such as broccoli, sprouts, spinach, romaine, cucumber slices, tomato slices, roasted red peppers, and shredded carrots. Finally, in the last column, list your condiments, ranging from mustard to low-fat mayo to Italian dressing. You can also include a list of accompaniments such as cheese sticks, apples, oranges, yogurt, baby carrots, low-fat milk, and ready-made soup. Then, every morning (or, even better, the night before) pick one item from each column to pack. Voilà! A Stealth Health lunch!

10 **Mini-size your sandwich.** When purchasing sandwiches from a deli or company cafeteria, ask for a half portion. In one study, participants presented with a 12-inch sandwich ate the entire sandwich but felt just as satisfied afterward as when they ate an 8-inch sandwich. Apparently, seeing less translates into eating less.

11 **For a healthier lunch, eat a healthier breakfast.** Breakfasts composed of simple starches like doughnuts, white breads, or many popular breakfast cereals are quickly converted into sugar that floods your bloodstream and

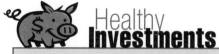

Healthy Investments

A Small Cooler and Cold Packs

Cold packs keep healthy food fresh until lunchtime, whether or not you have a refrigerator handy. A cooler and cold packs will be particularly useful if you have a job that keeps you on the road.

then goes away quickly. This leaves you craving fatty, high-calorie foods come lunch. Far better is to eat healthier breakfast foods that are slow to digest and thus leave you fuller longer. These include whole grains and lean proteins.

12 Exercise as you run errands.
If you need to run errands during your lunch break, get some exercise in at the same time. If possible, complete your errands as you power walk, hitting the bank, convenience store, and other locations on foot. The exercise will help refresh your mind and reduce the stress of the day.

13 Walk to the deli. If you must eat
out, walk to your destination. You'll burn some extra calories and refresh your mind at the same time. The short walk may also give you the willpower you need to order more healthfully.

14 Start a lunch bunch group. Eat
with other coworkers who are interested in weight control, health, and nutrition. Share foods for taste-testing, exchange tips and recipes, and once a week, have each member bring in one healthy contribution to the meal.

15 Improve your work performance with healthy food. When
Appleton Central High School in Wisconsin began serving more healthful food options and replaced soda-filled vending machines with juice, water, and energy drinks, students began behaving better and achieving more in the classroom. They stayed on task, were better able to concentrate, and paid better attention. If switching from fatty, sugary lunches produced that effect on high school students, just imagine what it can do for your mental outlook and motivation at work!

REMINDER

 Fast Results
These are bits of advice that deliver benefits particularly quickly—in some cases, immediately!

 Easy Gains
These are tips that give the biggest value for the least amount of effort.

 Super Effective
These are tips proven to be particularly effective through scientific research or widespread usage by experts.

Afternoon Doldrums

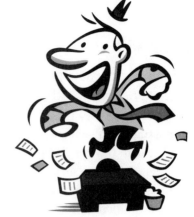

22 IDEAS TO LIFT YOUR SPIRITS AND YOUR ENERGY

If you're like many people, shortly after lunch, your head begins buzzing, your concentration plummets, your eyes droop, and the top of your desk begins to look as cozy as a feather mattress.

No one knows exactly why some people get the midday dips, but there are many plausible theories: the morning surge of hormones has petered out; you've used up a goodly part of your stored energy from last night's sleep; and perhaps most obviously, some degree of "brain tedium," i.e., boredom, has set in. The afternoon doldrums also may have something to do with what you ate for lunch. Not only does the midday meal divert blood from your brain to your gut, but, depending on what you ate, also bumps up levels of the soporific serotonin hormone.

While the midday doldrums are common, they're not inevitable. In fact, if your current daytime program includes such a post-lunch torpor, it's time to write a new program with the tips below.

Before Lunch...

1 **Head outside and sit in the daylight for 10 minutes.** Better still, have your lunch outside, and divide your break between eating and a walk. Here's why: Your office probably has about 500 luxes of light, which is equal to about 500 candles. That compares with 10,000 luxes at sunrise and 100,000 at noon on a July day. So when the afternoon doldrums hit, go outside and sit in the sunlight. It will help reset your chronological clock, kick down the amount of melatonin (the sleep hormone) your body produces during this circadian dip, and give you a valuable boost of beneficial vitamin D, reducing your risk of osteoporosis as well as various cancers.

2 **Take a brief midmorning break for tea, coffee, and/or a snack.** Use this time to relax and refocus, but more important, to consume a few calories that you might otherwise eat at lunchtime. Shrink lunch accordingly, which in turn will allow for a smaller, less stupefying midday meal.

3 **Snack all day long.** Simply snack on nutritious foods whenever you get hungry, rather than eating lunch per se. Then use your lunch break for some kind of exercise, whether it's in the company gym, walking around the campus, or running up and down the stairs.

51

During Lunch...

☆ 4 **Choose activating protein vs. energy-sapping carbs.** So a tuna salad without the bread is a better choice than a tuna sandwich. A green salad sprinkled with low-fat cheese, a hard-boiled egg, and some sliced turkey wins over a pasta salad. The change can really make a difference. When researchers compared men who ate a 1,000-calorie lunch with those who ate a 300-calorie lunch or skipped the meal altogether, they found that when given a chance to nap after lunch, nearly all the participants did so. But while the lunch-eaters slept an average of 90 minutes, those who skipped lunch slept for only 30 minutes. These were also high-carbohydrate lunches (carbs stimulate serotonin release, which increases sleepiness), which may have contributed to the napping. We're not suggesting you skip lunch altogether, but the combination of eating less (as noted in Tip 2) and eating fewer carbs should lead to less sleepiness.

After Lunch...

5 **Enjoy teatime.** The British have it right. Every day around midafternoon they have tea, getting over the doldrums with that little bit of a caffeine burst and a few quiet minutes. Now, while we're not suggesting scones and clotted cream, we do think you can do better than a Lipton's tea bag plunked in your unwashed coffee mug. Keep a selection of exotic flavored teas (preferably caffeinated) in your office and an aesthetically pleasing cup just for tea. When the doldrums hit, brew yourself a cup of tea and sit somewhere quiet (*not* your office) to sip and reflect. The meditative time will soothe your frenzied brain, while the caffeine will give you just enough of a kick start to get through the rest of your day.

6 **Make an "I was thinking of you" phone call.** To your wife, your kid, your siblings, your parents, a friend, a retired coworker. A five-minute keep-in-touch call will lift your spirits for hours and reinvigorate you to get your work done so you can go home a little early.

7 **Clean your desk off and clean out your e-mail in-box.** Both are relatively mindless tasks that don't require great gobs of concentration or clear thinking, and both will leave you feeling more energized because you'll have accomplished something visible as well as reduced energy-sapping clutter.

8 **Defer the work you most want to do to the time of day when you least want to work.** Get through the grunt work in the early a.m. so it's behind you, then stave off the midday doldrums by turning to the work you care most about or enjoy the most. Nothing stifles sleepiness like genuine enthusiasm.

9 **Have an afternoon snack designed to get the blood flowing.** That would *not* be a candy bar. The high glycemic index (i.e., jolts your blood sugar up) in the candy bar might give you a temporary boost, but once that jolt of sugar is gone, you'll sink faster than the stock market after an interest-rate hike. Instead, you want a snack that combines protein, fiber, and complex carbs (like whole grain crackers or raw veggies) to steadily raise your blood sugar levels and keep them up.

Snacks like:

- *Low-fat milk and high-fiber cereal.* Milk provides the protein as well as valuable fluid (tiredness is an early sign of dehydration), while the high-fiber cereal will curtail any sudden blood sugar rushes.
- *Peanut butter spread on whole wheat crackers.* Again, good source of protein in peanut butter, a bit of fat for staying power (healthy fat, as well), coupled with the fiber and complex carbs in the whole grain crackers.
- *Cut-up vegetables dipped into hummus.* These days, you can buy both these ingredients at any food store. Eaten together, you get the high fiber, antioxidants, and valuable vitamins of the vegetables, coupled with the fiber and protein of the hummus.
- *Low-sodium tomato or vegetable juice with soy nuts or peanuts.* The nuts provide a healthy dose of protein and monounsaturated fat, while the tomato juice provides not only the lycopene and other phytonutrients found in tomatoes, but energy-sustaining liquid as well.
- *A piece of string cheese and an apple.* Portable, easy, and a great pair. The cheese, with its fat and protein, cushions the fruit sugars from the apple, while the apple provides you with one of those all-important fruit servings for the day, along with a healthy dollop of antioxidants and fiber (make sure you eat the skin).

10 Go for a 10-minute walk and resist that candy bar.

When researchers at California State University in Long Beach compared study participants who ate a candy bar or who walked briskly for 10 minutes, they found the candy bar subjects felt tenser in the hour afterward, while those who walked not only had higher energy levels for one to two hours afterward, but reduced their tension.

Two-Second Quiz

Coffee or Tea?

Answer: *Tea.*
Black or green tea instead of java. These teas are jammed with heart-healthy antioxidants that provide more than just an energy-boosting punch; in addition to contributing to healthier arteries, they may also help prevent cancer.

11 Drink a cup of caffeinated coffee or tea.

The caffeine will perk you up; studies also find it will enhance your memory and make you more productive on tasks requiring concentration.

12 Put a drop of peppermint oil in your hand and briskly rub

your hands together, then rub them over your face (avoid your eyes). Peppermint is a known energy-enhancing scent.

13 Roll your shoulders forward, then backward,

timing each roll with a deep breath in and out. Repeat for 2 minutes.

14 Put on some high-energy music and dance for five minutes.

If you have an office, great. Just close the door. If not, bring a Walkman, head to the bathroom or an unused conference room, and let 'er rip! Get pumped, rather than pooped!

15 Consider a morsel of dark chocolate.

We're not encouraging overindulging, but dark chocolate at midday has some unique advantages. Unlike milk chocolate, it is truly a "healthful" food that is more in the category of nuts than candies, given the high levels of healthful fat and antioxidants it contains. Plus, it has abundant fiber and magnesium. Additionally, it provides a bit of caffeine, as well as a decadent feeling. Stick to one piece, though.

16 **Chew some "spicy" gum** such as Dentyne Wintermint Ice Chewing Gum—or MintABurst Mint Chewing gum. Strong minty flavors are stimulating, and the mere act of chewing is something of a tonic to a brain succumbing to lethargy. Plus, the act of chewing stimulates saliva, which helps clear out cavity and gum disease–causing bacteria from lunch. Just make sure to go sugarless.

17 **Plan group activities for midday.** If you often work on your own, try to cluster work involving others at the time of day when your concentration might otherwise be waning. We are social animals, and interactions always rev us up. Just make sure it's an interesting, interactive activity. Sitting in a room listening to someone else drone on and on will just send you snoozing.

18 **Do your filing.** It's a physical activity that gets you up from your desk, bending and stooping and pulling and stretching. Plus, it's something you can lose yourself in, and any activity that enables you to get into a "flow" will pull you through those doldrums as easily as an 18-wheeler could pull a MINI Cooper.

19 **Take 10 minutes for isometric exercises.** Isometric exercises involve nothing more than tensing a muscle and holding it. For instance, with your arm held out, tense your biceps and triceps at the same time and hold for 5 to 10 seconds. You can do this with your calf muscles, thigh muscles (front and back), chest, abdomen, buttocks, shoulders, and back. In

Do**Three**Things

To find a natural energy booster for the afternoon doldrums, we asked Chris D. Meletis, N.D., science officer and associate professor of natural pharmacology at the National College of Naturopathic Medicine, for his thoughts. While definitive scientific evidence of nutrient effects on daytime alertness is pretty thin, Dr. Meletis recommends the following based on his professional judgment.

1. **Chromium.** It is estimated that upward of 90 percent of Americans on the standard American diet don't get enough trace minerals like chromium, which is thought to be critical for maintaining proper blood sugar levels. Try adding a daily supplement of chromium picolinate, which may help balance blood sugar levels.

2. **Siberian ginseng.** If you have been more irritable and are having a harder time waking up and staying awake without having to use crutches like caffeine, then your adrenal glands may be talking to you. Try taking Siberian ginseng on a daily basis to replenish your energy.

3. **B-complex vitamins.** If you aren't remembering your dreams as well as you used to, or are generally feeling stressed out more often than usual, add a B-complex vitamin to help fuel your body to support peak performance.

As always, tell your health-care professional about any supplements you're taking, and follow package directions.

fact, if you wanted to, you could work a rotation, or cycle, of isometric exercises involving almost your entire body into your desk job every day. The total workout would be quite significant, despite never interrupting your work, and never breaking a sweat. Plus, you're not only toning your body, you're toning your mind.

All Day Long...

20 **Weave variety into your workday.** Tedium taxes the mind, and induces somnolence. Most studies suggest concentration for *anything* wanes after an hour, and is pretty near to pitiful at 90 minutes. So divide your tasks to maximize a balance between variety and productivity. For instance, if you have a large report to get out, work on it for 30 minutes, switch to something else for 30 minutes, then return to the report.

21 **Get up whenever reasonable and possible.** Just because you have an intercom and e-mail doesn't mean you always have to use them. Try darting down the hall or up the stairs even for simple questions or messages. Studies find that short bursts of even very modest activity burn calories, help tone muscles, and keep your mind brisk and alert.

22 **Keep a rosemary plant in your office.** Not only will sharing your space with a live, growing thing provide its own mood boost, but studies find the scent of rosemary to be energizing. Whenever you need a boost, just rub one of the sprigs between your fingers to release the fragrance into the air. Or, if you're really wiped out, clip off a sprig and rub it on your hands, face, and neck to saturate yourself in the scent.

At the Gym

17 IDEAS FOR HEALTHIER, EASIER WORKOUTS

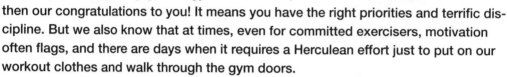

If you are one of the minority of grown-ups in America who regularly go to a gym for exercise, then our congratulations to you! It means you have the right priorities and terrific discipline. But we also know that at times, even for committed exercisers, motivation often flags, and there are days when it requires a Herculean effort just to put on our workout clothes and walk through the gym doors.

If you're lucky, the sights and sounds of exercise are all you need to motivate yourself to get moving. Other times, you still may not have the slightest urge to get started. For those days, this chapter is for you. Here are stealthy ways to get the most out of your workout.

1 **Avoid the mirrors.** Many fitness locations line exercise rooms with mirrors to allow you to watch your form as you work out. Yet a study of 58 women found that those who exercised in front of a mirror felt less calm and more fatigued after 30 minutes of working out than those who exercised without staring at their reflection. The national exercise chain, Curves, deliberately designs its small gyms without mirrors so women can concentrate on each other and the workout rather than on how they look. Other gyms are beginning to offer "reflection-free" zones. If yours doesn't, mention the idea— and the study—to the gym manager.

2 **Try using aromatherapy oils known to enhance energy,** such as rosemary. Mix them with water and store them in a squirt bottle in your gym bag. Give your gym clothing a few squirts before leaving the dressing room so you can smell the oil as you work out. If you're in the midst of a more meditative, slower-paced workout, such as Pilates or yoga, try lavender oil instead of rosemary.

3 **Create your own personal gym-mix tapes, CDs,** or digital recordings, and listen to them as you work out. Researchers from the University of Wisconsin-La Crosse found that people who listen to up-tempo music got significantly more out of their stationary bike workouts. They pedaled faster, produced more power, and their hearts beat faster than when they listened to slow-tempo music or sounds with no tempo. Overall, they worked between 5 and 15 percent harder while listening to the energizing beat. Although the type of music you choose is up to you, pick something with a fast beat that makes you want to break out in dance. You can custom-design your own exercise music to burn to a CD or

download to an MP3 player at Internet sites such as www.mywalkingmusic.com or www.workoutmusic.com.

4 **Turn off the tube when exercising.** It's tempting to try to lose yourself in television programming as you slog away on the treadmill or stationary bike. Yet a 1996 study found women worked out about 5 percent harder when they *weren't* watching TV than when they were. Although your favorite TV show may take your mind off your workout, it also causes you to lose touch with your effort level. You unconsciously slow down or use poor form as you get caught up in what you are watching. If television sets line the workout area, get on the equipment closest to the monitor tuned to C-Span. Sure you'll glance up at the monitor from time to time, but unless you're a complete political junkie, you probably won't get sucked in.

5 **Think of someone who irritates you.** Then step on the treadmill, stair stepper, stationary bike, or elliptical machine and sweat out your aggression as you run, climb, or cycle. You might even imagine that you are running an imaginary race against this person. You'll get in a better workout—and blast away anger and stress at the same time.

6 **Drink a bottle of water or juice** on your way to the gym. If you show up for your workout already dehydrated, you'll feel overly fatigued during your session, says Craig Horswill, Ph.D., principal scientist for the Gatorade Sports Science Institute in Barrington, Illinois. "Nearly half of all exercisers are starting their workouts at a real disadvantage—by arriving at the gym already dehydrated," he says. "When you're

Pick Your Video Wisely

In a study of 101 women completed at McMaster University in Ontario, Canada, exercise videos that featured super-skinny models with amazing muscles and revealing thongs made participants feel less confident about their fitness and less inclined to exercise in the future. Videos featuring an ultra-slender host surrounded by plumper, more normal-looking women reduced motivation even more. "We thought it would be okay if the fitness instructor was gorgeous and the others were normal looking," says study author Kathleen A. Martin Ginis, Ph.D., associate professor of health and exercise psychology at McMaster. "We found the exact opposite of what we thought." The researchers' hypothesis: Seeing a thin instructor surrounded by fleshier participants intensified the participants' awareness of the thinness of the instructor.

To choose a motivating exercise video or class, Ginis suggests looking for videos or classes with a teacher you can trust, who has a fitness background, and who must exercise to look great. In other words, videos created by personal trainers and exercise physiologists, or classes taught by them, will more likely motivate you than those hosted by supermodels and actresses, she says.

dehydrated, you can't work as hard, you don't feel as good, and your mental function is going to be compromised. Consequently, you're not going to get as much out of your workout."

7 **Think you can and you will.** So simple, yet so often ignored, positive thinking can help you power your way through a workout. In a study of 41 adults ages 55 to 92, exercisers who thought positively were more likely to stay active than those whose minds often uttered those

two evil words: "I can't." Whenever you find yourself making excuses, mentally put those self-defeating thoughts in a locked cabinet in your brain and replace them with positive messages such as, "I feel great" or "Bring it on."

8 **Work out with a friend.** If you're feeling stale and are thinking of skipping your gym workouts, ask a friend to meet you for a gym date. As you walk or run on the treadmill, you can share stories of your day. Thirty minutes will go by before you know it. You can also encourage each other to work a bit harder. Your friend can also help you find the courage to approach unfamiliar gym equipment, as it's easier to laugh off your foibles when you have a trusted companion nearby.

9 **Set a short-term workout goal.** We all know that goals help motivate you to work harder, and that the best exercise programs include measurable goals to achieve weeks or months down the road. Sometimes, though, when your motivation is drooping, a goal for what to achieve over the next 30 minutes is really what you need. So pick something achievable: Maintain a sweat for 20 minutes, or cover two miles on the treadmill, or give just your arms a really good strength workout. A target like that gives you focus to get through on even the tough days.

10 **Whenever you feel like you're just spinning your wheels,** hire a trainer. In just one session a trainer can open your eyes to a whole new world of workouts, helping you to squeeze just a little more motivation and juice out of yourself. (See "What to Look For in a Trainer," page 59.)

11 **Work out during the least crowded hours.** You'll squeeze in a more effective workout in less time if you hit the gym during the slowest period of the day, often midafternoon. You won't want to wait on line for equipment or feel hassled in the locker room.

12 **Change your routine every 3 to 4 weeks.** This will keep your body guessing—improving your results—and fuel your motivation. In the weight room, alternate exercises and modify the *way* you lift weights. If you usually do two sets of 15 reps, complete one set of about 15 reps, then increase the weight for another set of 8 reps. On cardio equipment, switch from the treadmill to the stair stepper or the stair stepper to the elliptical trainer. Mix up your exercise classes as well, switching around from Pilates to aerobic dance to yoga to kickboxing.

Two-Second Quiz

Free Weights vs. Machines

Answer: *Free weights.*
With free weights, you can always work both sides of your body separately, eliminating muscle imbalances. Only some machines allow that. Also, you don't need a degree in astrophysics to figure out how to operate them or adjust them to your size and strength. Also, gym machines are generally designed for a male body. If you are short and slight, your body may be too small for the machine, no matter how you adjust it. Finally, if you prefer to work out at home, which most of us do, who can afford the money or space for a quality, multi-exercise workout machine? Dumbbells are inexpensive, small, and nicely portable.

13 Slow down. In one study of 147 people completed at the South Shore YMCA in Quincy, Massachusetts, participants who lifted slowly—taking at least 14 seconds to complete one repetition—gained more strength than participants who lifted at a rate of 7 seconds per repetition. Slower lifting may help increase strength because it prevents you from using momentum or cheating with improper technique.

14 Put your mind behind every move. Rather than daydreaming through your workouts, put as much mental emphasis on what you do at the gym as you do at work—or at least *should* do at work. For example, when doing a strength exercise, feel the muscle contract as you lift. This inner focus will help you to tune in to your technique. You'll fatigue your muscles faster because you'll make every movement count.

15 Invent a competition with the person on the next treadmill. So you're on the treadmill and you're bored and underachieving. Glance at the display on someone else's nearby treadmill. If you're walking at 3.5 miles per hour and he's chugging away at 4, see if you can increase your speed and *catch* him, as if it were a race. Although the man or woman on the nearby treadmill has no idea you're racing, he or she can still provide the motivation needed to boost your pace.

16 Wear the right shoes for the right class. When it comes to workout gear, you might get away with skimping on your clothing, but resist the urge to wear those ratty old sneakers you found in the back of your closet. Various fitness disciplines require specific types of footwear. Wearing the wrong shoes will not only make your workout feel harder, it could get you injured. Wear running shoes for running, walking shoes for walking, aerobics or cross-training shoes for aerobics, and hard-bottomed cycling shoes for spinning.

17 Watch an inspiring movie. If you just don't feel like working out, pop a movie like *Rocky* into your VCR or DVD. Watching your hero working hard to succeed can inspire you to apply that intense feeling during your next workout.

Running Errands

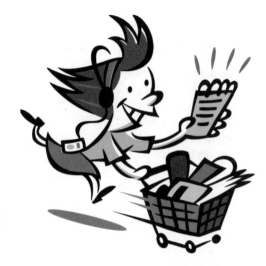

20 WAYS TO GET DONE QUICKER WHILE HAVING MORE FUN

Like death and taxes, there's no escaping errand running. Supermarket, drugstore, dry cleaner, library, post office. Pick up, drop off, wait for kids—or parents. If you're not careful, you can spend more than half of your leisure time with your butt glued to your car seat running errands—something only 10 percent of Americans say they enjoy, according to a study by Peter D. Hart Research Associates.

So what does any of that have to do with health? Plenty. All that errand running stresses you out and sucks you dry of energy. It also eats up hours better spent exercising, relaxing, cooking, having fun—the healthy stuff of life. So our goal here is to get you through your errands faster, easier, and with less stress. Just be sure to use the time you gain wisely!

1 **Group your errands.** This is a golden rule: Never run just one errand at a time. You'll save time, gas, energy, and stress hormones by grouping your errands into batches. If you have to drop a kid at piano practice, you can also swing by the bank and deposit the check, pop into the market for a gallon of milk, and pick up the dry cleaning.

2 **Run your errands in off hours.** In other words, *not* on weekends (which is when 92 percent of us run our errands). Instead, make sure your dry cleaner, bank, doctor, supermarket, etc., are near work so you can take care of these mundane tasks on your way into or out of work, or on your lunch hour. You'll avoid the jammed stores and byways on the weekends, and have those two days just for you and your family. One of the best times to grocery shop? After dinner, when the kids are in bed. One parent stays home and one goes to the store. You'll be in and out in half the time it normally takes with kids in tow.

3 **Create an errand center in your house.** This is where the library books that need to be returned, the dry cleaning that needs to be delivered, the packages that need to be mailed, all live. Everything in one place (ideally near the door you use most often) will make it easier to run "bulk" errands. Another option: Keep these things in your car, in the passenger seat. They'll be a visual reminder of all you need to do.

4 Keep an errand list with you at all times. This includes both the ordinary errands that must be done (dry cleaning, library, post office), but also those little things you keep forgetting (pick up socks for the six-year-old, make vet appointment for the dog, buy underwear for husband, find organic potting soil). Use a sturdy notebook that you carry with you at all times, and make sure the rest of your family knows where it is so they can add things to the list.

5 Buy in bulk. The less often you have to go shopping for mundane items like toilet paper, paper towels, dog food, cat litter, toothpaste, deodorant, tampons, etc., the less time you'll spend running errands. Storage space tight? Most of these items will hide under the bed quite nicely.

6 Always include a little fun. List all the things you find joyful. Maybe it's reading a novel, writing in your journal, or hitting a few golf balls on a beautiful spring afternoon. Now, plan to include one of these items in any extended errand run. Stash a novel in your purse as you head to the post office; you can read in line. Keep the clubs and plastic golf balls in your car— any vacant field you pass makes a perfect driving range. Carry your journal in your glove compartment—jot a few lines as you're waiting for the car to be washed.

7 Turn waiting time into *you* time. Anytime you're stuck in a line, shift the negative, glass-half-empty thinking ("Darn, I don't have time for this") into positive, glass-half-full thinking ("Ahhh! A few minutes of peace."). Close your eyes (yes, while you're standing there in line) and picture yourself in the most peaceful place you can imagine. It could

be a desert at sunrise, the vast ocean (and you in a lone canoe), or the middle of a massage in a luxurious spa. Let your mind go and take several long, deep breaths. Now how do you feel?

8 Offer to run errands for an elderly neighbor or a mother with young children. Studies find that helping others actually reduces our own stress hormones and makes us feel better.

9 Use the Internet for as many errands as possible. These days, you can bank online, order office supplies, buy garden perennials, shop for shoes, even grocery shop online. You can buy stamps at www.stamps.com, renew your library books online at your public library's Web site, arrange for a FedEx or UPS pickup from your house, even file your taxes electronically. The Internet, used smartly, can save you hours of time and immeasurable amounts of stress. Still worried about giving a credit card number over the Internet? If the Web site uses a secured server, then it is safer than giving your credit card over the phone and in some cases, using it at a store!

10 Keep an "errand bag" in the car at all times.
This includes such things as bills that need to be paid, stationery and envelopes for writing letters (yes, letters!), a variety of greeting cards (birthdays, graduation, "just thinking of you"), pens, an envelope of coupons, your calendar, magazines you haven't read, a good book. Then whenever you're sitting in a waiting room, stuck in traffic, waiting for a kid's too-long soccer practice to end, you're also completing other tasks on your list and/or catching up on your reading.

11 Keep your grocery list on the computer.
Most weeks, you're buying the same things anyway; having a master list on your computer makes it easy to add and subtract items. Organize the list in the same order as the store in which you shop. So, for instance, if the produce section is the first area you see, fruits and vegetables should be first on your list. Hit the print button, and off you go!

12 Keep a cooler and a basket in your trunk.
The cooler is to keep frozen and cold foods cold while you're running errands; the basket is to enable you to carry parcels into the house without making umpteen trips.

13 Learn to run errands with your kids and not go crazy.
There are few things more stressful than being stuck in traffic with ice cream melting in the trunk and a two-year-old melting down in the backseat. But today you're more likely than ever to be running your errands with kids, given government statistics showing that kids under five spend up to 65 minutes a day in cars. To cope:

- Run your errands at the right time of day for the kid. If you've got a toddler, that's morning, before naptime.
- Stock the car with snacks, juices, and toys. Keep a cooler up front with cool drinks and cut-up fruit that you can hand back to your toddler when he or she gets fussy. Keep the car stocked with a bag of toys that only come out when you're running errands.
- Keep an extra diaper bag in the car. This way, you don't have to worry about forgetting something, Make sure the bag is stocked with diapers, wipes, change of clothes, diaper medicines, crackers, even a couple of videos if you're lucky enough to have a DVD or VCR in your minivan.
- Combine errands for you with a treat for your child. It could be lunch out, an ice cream, or a side trip to the park.
- Don't forget your child during the errand running. So during grocery shopping, for instance, play patty-cake and peekaboo while your child is in the cart. Turn trips to the post office and dry cleaner into learning experiences. Many proprietors will even give you and your child a tour if it's not too busy.
- Play games while you're shopping. Give your school-age child a calculator and have him total up the cost of the groceries as you toss them into your cart. Let preschoolers put nonbreakable items into the cart. Toddlers can pick which color tissues to buy.
- Bring the right equipment for infants. That's a backpack type of carrier, or a front sling, both of which leave your hands free.
- Play a mind game with older kids to keep them disciplined and keep your mind focused and relaxed. One good game is "jotto." You each pick a word with five letters, no two the same, and have to

guess the other's word by stating five-letter words and being told how many letters match. Keeping track in your head is challenging, but fun.

14 Run your errands mindfully.
That is, rein in your racing mind and focus solely on the task at hand. Start by walking slowly and deliberately to and from your car to the stores. As you grocery shop, focus on the colors of the produce, the rich scents from the bakery, the abundant luxury that is an American grocery store. Pay attention to each step, each movement. By living mindfully in the moment—even while picking out brussels sprouts—you are performing what relaxation experts call walking meditation. Do errands this way and you'll find yourself far more calm and engaged, and at the end, less exhausted and frustrated.

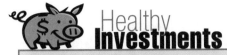

15 Buy yourself a treat. Your kids aren't the only ones who need a little motivation during errand running. So make sure you add one more item to your list—something nice for you. It could be flowers, a scented bath soap, an imported brand of beer, or a fancy cheese. Life is too short to limit it to Velveeta.

16 Use your time running errands to take a break from noise. Turn off your cell phone, your car radio, leave the MP3 player at home. Instead, as you drive from store to store, listen to the silence and let your own thoughts have a chance to come out. This quiet time will help recharge the energy that gets sapped by the overwhelming stimuli of daily life.

17 Keep several bottles of water in the freezer. When it's time to run errands in the summertime, grab one of

them to take with you. You'll have plenty of icy-cold water to drink throughout your errands.

18 Listen to inspirational tapes or books on tape in the car while running errands. It's a whole lot more relaxing than the commercials, the deejays, and the intensity of everyday radio.

19 Alternate tasks with your neighbors or kids' friends.
For instance, one week you do the grocery shopping for your neighbor; the next week, she does. Or she watches your kids while you run the errands for both families (or vice versa). Another option: Run errands *with* a friend. Not only will you benefit from the social support, but your kids will be much better behaved having a friend along.

20 If you're a dad, run errands with your kid. A University of California study finds that children who clean, cook, and run household errands with their fathers are better behaved and have more friends. An added bonus: The wives of these men find them more sexually attractive.

The Dinner Routine

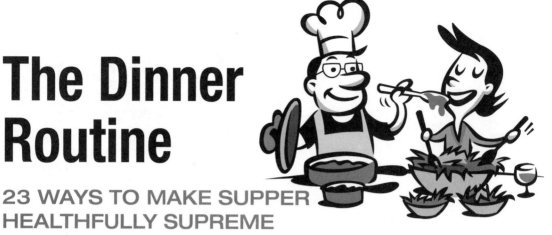

23 WAYS TO MAKE SUPPER HEALTHFULLY SUPREME

We are all busy. Whether it's working, caring for kids, running errands, going to school, getting exercise, volunteering, or some combination of the above, we are all busy. Which is why dinner has become such a challenge. Too tired or unprepared to cook after 10 or 12 hours of perpetual busy-ness, we take the easy path to eating: a pizza, a restaurant, a store-bought frozen meal, the fried chicken counter at the local grocery store. Yet such noncooking options add up to a whole lot of unhealthiness. First, prepared foods are filled with salt, sugar, and fat—a one-two-three punch against your heart and health. Then there's the shortage of vegetables, fiber, and vitamins. Then there are the portion sizes—huge—a fact we eventually display at our waistline and hind side.

There is a better way. Here are simple, realistic, stealthy tips to get you eating healthily at dinner again, mostly at home, mostly with your own cooking. (As for ideas for making your specific food choices healthier, look ahead to Part 3.)

1 **Keep your kitchen clean.** Families tend to congregate in the kitchen, bringing with them newspapers, mail, backpacks, school papers, toys, and a thousand other little this-and-thats. Don't allow it. Set a new policy: The kitchen is for cooking and eating only. Why? It's hard to get motivated about cooking if you have to clean up a mess first, not to mention what it does to your mood. The opposite also holds true: A clean, bright, inviting kitchen can be a wonderful oasis after a day of craziness.

2 **Speaking of which, make your kitchen a place you like to be.** Is there music playing? Do you have a glass of wine poured? Is the evening sun shining through the window? Are the knives sharp, the produce fresh, the pots good quality, the counters clutter-free? All of this contributes to your desire to make good food. If you can't honestly say you enjoy being in your kitchen, do what you need to do to change that.

3 **Enjoy the cooking process.** Sure, not everyone loves cooking. But there's no reason to not *like* doing it. If the thought of cooking brings dread, you need an attitude adjustment. Cooking is a pleasure, far easier than many non-cooks realize. For your health, your pleasure, your pocketbook, you should learn—or relearn—the pleasures of cooking. Make it

a project. Spend time with your friends and family while they cook so that you can absorb the methods and routines. Consider taking a class, or buy an introductory cookbook. Most of all, lose your fear. It is actually harder to be a bad cook than a good cook, particularly if you use good ingredients.

4 **Plan a week's worth of dinners.** Fewer than 30 percent of Americans know what they're having for dinner come 4 p.m. Yet planning ahead takes just a few minutes. Here's how. Every Friday night or Saturday morning, sit down with a pad of paper and your favorite cookbooks or cooking magazines. Think about what's in your freezer and fridge, what your family likes to eat, what your upcoming week entails. Then plan out the week's worth of menus (leave one night for pizza night). At the same time, write out your grocery list. Now post the list of menus on the kitchen refrigerator or bulletin board so it's the first thing you see when you get home. Voilà! No more thinking ahead. Just follow your own instructions. If you need help or inspiration, consider an online meal planner, such as the one at www.thewaytoeat.net (created by Dr. David Katz, this book's medical advisor).

5 **Delegate, delegate, delegate.** If you have kids older than 10 or another adult who gets home before you do, get them started on dinner. For example, you might ask your spouse to pick up ingredients on the way home, your teen to start chopping vegetables for the salad and fill the pasta pot with water, your preteen to gather needed ingredients for a given recipe and put them on the counter for you, preheat the oven, and set the table. Yes, they may think of it as a

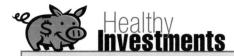

Healthy Investments

A Panini Machine

Panini are sandwiches grilled in a machine that looks like an oversized waffle maker and that presses all the ingredients together. Panini are quite delicious and turn an ordinary sandwich into a real treat. Panini machines are available widely. Keep whole grain bread on hand at all times (bread freezes well), and when you're in a bind for dinner, panini with various grilled veggies work beautifully.

chore, but if you build in a little opportunity for them to "create," (i.e., with place cards for dinner, fancy napkin foldings, their own recipes) it will make your kids more interested in nutritious food and trying new things.

6 **Stock your freezer with homemade meals.** Stews, soups, chili, and gumbo all freeze wonderfully. Figure out how much of a one-pot meal you need to feed your family for one dinner, and then buy plastic containers of that size. Make a pot of your family favorites on the weekend and you'll have four or five meals tucked in the freezer. A smart freezer is filled with plastic containers of several different homemade meals, each labeled with the contents and the date it was made.

7 **Go the next step with freezer food.** Side dishes also freeze well, particularly rices, pastas, and breads. For space, put the right portion amount in freezer bags and squeeze out the air before sealing.

8 **Go the next step with soup stock.** We are big advocates of soup for dinner. It's healthy, filling, delicious, and easy to make. If you keep

homemade chicken stock in the freezer, or cans of low-salt broth in the pantry, it often takes just a few minutes to whip together an impromptu vegetable soup. Use a quart of stock or low-sodium chicken broth as the base. Then just toss in a variety of chopped veggies such as spinach, carrots, corn, lima beans, green beans, and zucchini. Make sure to include chickpeas and other beans. They provide excellent protein, lots of fiber, an array of micronutrients, and are filling and satisfying at a relatively low cost in calories. To round out the meal, have some whole grain bread (dip it in olive oil rather than spreading it with butter) and a salad.

9 Or, make a pot of broth-based soup on Sundays, then start each meal during the week with a cup. Studies show watery foods such as soup tend to fill up the stomach, making you feel full quicker, despite being relatively low in calories. Having a healthy soup to start a meal also makes cooking the rest of the meal a little less demanding.

10 Include three old standbys on your weekly menu. No one expects you to come up with a new meal every night. Pick three low-fuss,

Two-Second**Quiz**

Bagged Lettuce or Head?

Answer: *Bagged.*
According to nutritionists, people are more inclined to use prewashed and prepared lettuce than their whole-head counterpart. The same goes for pre-chopped carrots, cauliflower, and other convenient raw vegetables.

nutritious recipes that you and the family enjoy, and, most important, that you can almost cook in your sleep. For example, you might designate Monday as pasta or casserole night, Tuesday as grilled fish night, and Wednesday as roasted chicken night. Include similar vegetable and grain side dishes as well. This eases the headache of grocery shopping—you'll need many of the same groceries from one week to the next.

11 Plan which night you will eat out—and stick to it. Rather than eating out whenever you lack the inspiration—or groceries—to cook at home, eat out on a designated night. This makes eating out what it should be—a treat. You'll enjoy your restaurant meals more and eat more healthfully throughout the week.

12 Try new recipes on weekends, when you have more time to cook. You'll enjoy the cooking process more when your mind feels rested and unfettered. Once you get the hang of the new recipe, incorporate it into your weeknight repertoire.

13 Eat together as a family at least three times a week. According to a national survey of more than 15,000 children ages 9 to 14, children who ate dinner at the table with other family members consumed more fruits and vegetables, fiber, calcium, and numerous other important nutrients than children who rarely or never ate dinner as a family. Those who ate with their families also consumed less saturated fat and fewer soft drinks. Hold a family meeting and pick nights and times that work for everyone. Make eating together at the table nonnegotiable.

14 Keep your grocery list and recipe list on the computer. That way, you can just rotate your weekly menus (along with the grocery list) every month or every two months. Thus, once you have, say, eight weeks of menus, you're set for the rest of the year!

15 Relax for 20 minutes before you eat. If you tend to skip breakfast, but gorge your way through dinner and then snack until bedtime, you may have a condition known as night eating syndrome. People who eat more than 50 percent of their calories after 6 p.m. tend to suffer from insomnia, gain weight more easily, and feel more stressed than people who spread their food intake throughout the day. One solution: relaxation. In a study of 20 people with night eating syndrome, a once daily progressive muscle relaxation session reduced stress, anxiety, fatigue, anger, and depression within eight days. Participants also felt hungrier in the morning and less ravenous at night. Although the name of the technique sounds complicated, progressive

muscle relaxation is actually very simple. Just sit in a chair or lie on your back. Then progressively tense and then relax various muscles in your body, starting at the top of your head and moving down your body and ending at your feet. Tense as you inhale. Slowly release as you exhale. When you hit your toes, it's time to eat!

16 Have your cocktail *after* dinner, not before. In a study conducted at the University of Liverpool in England, men who drank a glass of beer 30 minutes before a meal ate more during the meal than men who consumed a nonalcoholic beverage. They also ate more fatty, salty foods and felt hungrier after the meal than men who did not drink. Because alcohol stimulates appetite, sip on an alcoholic beverage after your meal rather than before, particularly if you are trying to lose weight.

17 To eat less at dinner, hold your afternoon snack to a small portion. When researchers at Pennsylvania State University in University Park offered study participants different-sized bags of potato chips as a midafternoon snack, participants ate the entire bag, regardless of size or calorie content. Those given smaller bags, however, felt just as satisfied after their snack as those who ate twice as many chips from a larger bag. Even more compelling, those who ate twice as many chips from the larger bags consumed an average of 150 calories more during dinner. If you need a midafternoon snack to get through the day, serve up a small portion and make it high in protein and fiber (such as a low-fat cheese stick and an apple). Your body digests protein more slowly than carbohydrates, keeping your appetite under control for a longer period of time.

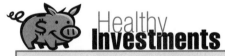

Healthy Investments

The George Foreman Grill

Although many infomercial appliances probably sit underneath your kitchen counter only to gather dust and cobwebs, the George Foreman grill may become the one appliance that occupies a permanent spot on your kitchen countertop. This device allows you to grill inside your house. A drip pan catches the grease, reducing the fat content of cooked meat and making cleanup a snap. The portable, indoor grill allows you the convenience of low-fat grilling during the winter months, when it's too cold to grill outdoors.

18 **Turn off the television during dinner.** A study of 548 students completed at the Harvard School of Public Health found that the more television and videos students watched, the fewer fruits and vegetables they ate. Researchers theorize that television programs and commercials depict unhealthy foods, causing people to reach more often for soft drinks and chips rather than fruits and vegetables. A separate study from the University of Minnesota found television watching during dinner reduced fruit and vegetable consumption during the meal.

19 **If your kids won't eat what you put on their plate,** bite your tongue. A study of 277 families completed at the University of Minnesota found that hassling children over their eating habits during dinner actually caused children—and their parents—to eat *less* nutritionally. Children and their parents consumed more fat during meals when they argued over eating behavior. The stress from the argument may have led to cravings for fatty comfort foods rather than an appetite for brussels sprouts and spinach.

20 **Instead of forcing kids to clean their plates,** enforce a one-bite rule. Encourage your children to take one bite out of all the foods on their plate. If, after one bite, they still don't want to eat their spinach or broccoli, let them push it aside. This technique encourages children to try new foods, but doesn't create a stressful eating experience. Involve young children in preparing any foods you want them to try. The sense of ownership will make them bolder.

21 **When out of ideas, serve ready-to-eat cereal.** This old bachelor standby provides a multivitamin's worth of vitamins and minerals, along with some protein in the milk and fiber, if you choose a high-fiber cereal. More important, serving cereal may help the entire family slim down. In a study completed at Purdue University in West Lafayette, Indiana, people who ate a bowl of cereal in place of either lunch or dinner consumed an average 640 fewer calories a day and lost an average of four pounds of fat during two weeks. A variation on the cereal theme is to make up a great big bowl of muesli for the whole family, mixing cut-up fruit with low-fat granola or muesli cereal with or without nuts, fat-free plain yogurt, and honey. If you are lucky enough to have leftovers, it's delicious the next day for the real breakfast.

22 **Have breakfast for dinner.** A great "breakfast" option for dinner is an omelet. Quick and easy to make, a great protein source, and relatively low in calories. Fill it with veggies instead of cheese, and you've got a complete meal in a frying pan!

23 **Use parts of last night's dinner for tonight's meal.** This allows you to cook once and eat twice. For example, if you have roasted chicken one night, use the leftovers to serve up chicken fajitas or chicken salad the next. Similarly, if you make grilled fish one night, try fish tacos the next. Prepare all key protein foods—chicken, turkey, fish, and so on—in larger-than-needed amounts so they will last two nights instead of one. Do the same with rice and other grain side dishes. Serve it up as a regular side dish one night and use the leftovers to make a casserole, stir-fry, or soup the next.

The After-Dinner Routine

27 IDEAS FOR HEALTHIER, MORE PLEASURABLE EVENINGS

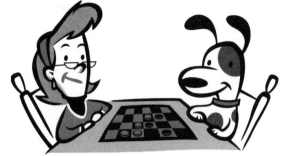

Dinner is finished, the dishes are done, and you're looking at a lovely three hours ahead of you before your body begins sending go-to-sleep signals. You could veg in front of the TV, as so many people do these days. Or you could pick one of the following to do and sneak a little health into your evening. We'll start off with pleasure-based ideas, and then shift into more practical ways to spend your evening time.

1 **Go for an after-dinner walk.** What better time for a hand-in-hand stroll through the neighborhood? To make it interesting, play a game of learning two new things about your neighbors on each walk, either through observation or conversation. It could be that the Smiths painted their living room red (something you spot through the window), or that the Bernsteins got a new car (which he proudly shows you). Playing this kind of "scavenger hunt" on your walk will make it go quicker, keep it more interesting. The best bonus, however: the health-promoting effects of the walk.

2 **Play a game with your partner or kids.** Try a board game, or work on a puzzle, or get up a rousing game of cards. Not only will it keep the television off, but it will make those brain cells move around a lot more than another episode of

Survivor. And the social bonding with your loved ones contributes mightily to emotional and physical health. Stumped for choices? Go back in time, from when you were a teenager—games like backgammon, dominoes, checkers, hearts, or chess. Crossword puzzles are great fun, as are visual, number, and logic puzzles that you can get cheaply in books and magazines. Have a dartboard, pool table, or Ping-Pong table? Go wear them out.

3 **Go up to your partner, put your arms around his/her waist,** and begin kissing the back of his/her neck. Hopefully, this will lead to something more. In addition to the obvious benefits of sex, you'll also be raising your heart rate, sending immune-boosting endorphins to your brain, and extending your life. One study found that sexually active men lived longer than those who had less

lovemaking. Sure, the study was in men, but it most likely applies to women too.

4 **Play with your dog or cat for 15 minutes.** Studies show significant stress reduction benefits from pets, particularly those that, like dogs and cats, can interact with you. Looking for ideas? Get an old sock and have your dog try to pull it out of your hand. Use a laser light to drive your cat slightly crazy (the laughing you'll do as you watch her try to "catch" the light will have its own health benefits). Teach your cat to "fetch" by tossing a crumpled piece of paper. Hide treats around the house and watch your dog go on his own treasure hunt. Don't have a pet? Get one!

5 **Do something totally mindless for 30 minutes.** It could be watching the junkiest show you can find on TV (and we'll leave that up to your own warped taste), holding a computer solitaire tournament with yourself, marinating in a steamy, scented bath, or just lying on the couch listening to a favorite piece of music and staring at the ceiling. The idea here is that your mind is disengaged, it is not focused on anything, it is allowed to run free in a kind of "active meditation."

6 **Slowly sip a glass of really good wine.** Now, the definition of "really good wine" is in the eyes of the beholder. If you're used to boxed Almadén, then a $15 bottle of merlot is just the ticket. If you're a moderate oenophile, you might reach for a $50 bottle of Bordeaux. The idea is that you savor this one glass. While you're identifying the fruits you taste and the elements in the bouquet, the wine will be providing significant heart-healthy antioxidants shown to reduce your risk of heart disease.

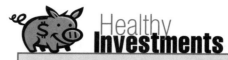

Healthy Investments

A Journal

Stop thinking of journals as a private place for teenage girls to write about their newest crushes. Every single adult—be it man or woman—can benefit by having a nice-quality notebook to record observations, thoughts, opinions, and reminders. At the front or the back of the journal, set aside pages for maintaining lists of books to read, music to buy, wine or beer that's been recommended, restaurants to try, even friends to call. While shopping for a journal, buy a nice pen to go with it. Keep them bedside so they're always ready for you at bedtime (and in the morning, when dreams and ideas are fresh). Don't feel compelled to write every night, but trust us: The more you write, the more you'll want to write in the future. You'll probably find that a private journal is an outstanding way to diffuse stress, clean your mind, and organize your thoughts.

7 **Get lost in a book.** Or a magazine or newspaper. Rekindle your love of reading. It's so much more rewarding for you than watching television. And it's much healthier, because it keeps your brain highly active and engaged.

8 **Savor a piece of dark gourmet chocolate.** Ounce for ounce, chocolate contains more healthy antioxidants, which repair damage to cells and prevent cholesterol from oxidizing (making it stickier), than any of the other antioxidant champs, including tea, blueberries, and grape juice. Plus, it's well known for its ability to soothe a troubled mind. It only takes one piece to provide the perfect post-dinner sweetness we often crave without a lot of fat or calories. Keep the chocolate dark—it has the most antioxidants—and plain. You don't need the extra sugar and calories from caramel, nougat, and other goodies.

9 On a dark, clear night, go outside and lie down in your backyard (or on the roof of your apartment building) and stare at the stars. Feel the immensity of the world as you view the heavens. Think about any problems you've been wrestling with and put them into context with the trillions of stars that are up there, only a few of which you can see tonight. If you find you enjoy this, consider learning about the stars with a star atlas.

10 Take a walk when the moon is full. The magic and mysticism of a moonlit night will energize you and provide an unexpected burst of positive thinking.

11 Go to sleep at 8 p.m. We're all horribly sleep-deprived in this country. So every now and again, pretend you're six years old, put on flannel pajamas, get into bed at 8 p.m. and turn out the light.

12 Give yourself a pedicure. Fill a basin with warm water and a few drops of peppermint oil. Soak until the water cools, then pumice away the rough skin on the soles of your feet. Massage a scented lotion all over your feet, inhaling the lovely scent and feeling your feet soften with every stroke. Trim your toenails and push back your cuticles and, if you desire, polish your toenails in some hot color you'd never dare wear on your fingernails. If you can, convince your partner to give you a foot massage.

13 Ask your partner, or even an older child or a friend, to wash your hair for you. Having your hair washed and your scalp massaged is an unexpected luxury that will help wash away the stress of the day and prepare you for bed.

14 Put a Glenn Miller CD (or whatever music you prefer dancing to) on the stereo and dance for 20 minutes. Jazz and cheek-to-cheek dancing not your thing? Fine, slip some high-energy rock music into the CD and pretend you're in a mosh pit. Either way, you'll get 20 minutes of physical activity and, if you're doing the mosh pit thing, you'll burn as many calories as if you were jogging. An added bonus: improved coordination and, if you do a lot of dips, some good stretches. Plus, this is a great way for younger parents to engage their kids in physical activity—the whole family can cut a rug, dancing energetically until just one is left standing.

15 Make a yogurt smoothie for dessert. Toss a frozen banana, a pint of plain or vanilla yogurt, a handful of blueberries, and a teaspoon of honey into the blender along with a cup of crushed ice. Blend the mixture until it is thick and smooth. The combination of the antioxidants in the blueberries, the potassium in the banana, and the live bacteria in the yogurt just gave you a health boost that no vitamin could match. Specific conditions you have just helped protect yourself against: Urinary tract infection (blueberries), high blood pressure (banana), and yeast infection or irritable bowel syndrome (yogurt).

16 Sip a cup of goldenseal tea. The herb, often found in over-the-counter remedies mixed with echinacea, may boost your immune system, preventing colds and other infections.

17 Plan a vacation. Whether or not you're actually going to take it doesn't matter. Get on the Internet or pull out some travel magazines and begin planning your fantasy vacation. Check out airline costs, pick a hotel, virtually (but not really) book a snazzy red convertible to drive while you're there. Write down all the details and print out any pictures you find. Then file them into a vacation journal. Over the course of a year, "book" one vacation a month, each time in a different location and for a different purpose (i.e., a golf vacation, a family vacation, an adventure vacation, a spa vacation). Taking this fantasy trip will provide a pleasant way to unwind before bed—and may ensure some really great dreams.

18 Set a timer and write in your journal for 10 minutes. Many people eschew keeping a journal because they can't stand the sense of responsibility it brings to write in it every night. But if you know you only have 10 minutes, suddenly what seemed like a chore takes less time than washing the dishes. Not sure what to write? Try just listing what you did that day. Write five things that made you smile that day. Write five things that made you angry—and why they made you angry. Numerous studies attest to the stress-busting power of regular journaling. Plus, it's just so much fun to leaf back through your journal and see what you were doing a year before. It provides a way of marking your life in a world in which our lives stream by faster than cars on the German autobahn.

19 Do some writing. Go one better than a journal: Compose a letter to a friend, or some e-mails, or a missive to your political representatives, or something

creative. Writing is wonderful brain activity, and who isn't better off learning how to better express themselves?

20 Write down your entire to-do list for the next day. It only takes five minutes, yet the peace of mind it provides is priceless. Now, instead of running a to-do list over and over in your mind—which makes your responsibilities morph into gargantuan proportions—you can enjoy the rest of your evening and have a better shot at falling asleep easily.

21 Pack your (or your kids') lunch for tomorrow, lay out your clothes, check your briefcase, and make sure the kids' school stuff is by the front door. The health benefits are clear: This will avoid the spike in stress hormones the following morning that comes from rushing around like a stockbroker on Black Monday while simultaneously screaming at your kids, ripping your pantyhose, and spilling juice on your silk shirt.

22 Once a week, hold a "chore free" night. Order in pizza and eat on paper plates, leave any dishes unwashed, forget the laundry, don't even wipe the counters. Tell the kids they're on their own for homework, arrange rides for them to soccer practice or piano. This is your night to be as lazy (or productive in other ways) as you like. Maybe you have a hobby like painting, woodworking, or scrapbooking that you never seem to have the time to get to. This is your night for you. Don't let anything—especially your own guilt—get in the way of this evening. If your life is just too crazy to pull it off once a week, make it every other week, or once a month. But make it sometime.

23 Have a cooking fest. Tonight you're going to cook meals for the next two weeks to stock your freezer. Try easy-to-double recipes like lasagna, meatballs (make 'em with turkey to reduce the heart-clogging saturated fat), lentil soup, roast chicken, and eggplant casserole.

24 Change into nightclothes and slippers early in the evening. Even before dinner. It will help separate the "daytime you" from the "evening you," and be a constant reminder throughout the evening to relax and unwind.

25 Write a "done" list. This is a list of everything you've accomplished today. It's guaranteed to give you a sense of accomplishment and take some of the stress you feel about your to-do list off your shoulders.

 26 Clean out one cupboard or closet in your house. This chore takes no more than 30 minutes, and leaves you with a sense of accomplishment at day's end, yet without any added stress because the task is simple and unchallenging, yet satisfying.

27 Do your weekend shopping and chores. Why buy your groceries or buy clothes when everyone else is doing it? Make Saturday a fun day, not an errand and shopping day. Stores are much emptier and shopping less stressful on weekday evenings.

REMINDER

 Fast Results
These are bits of advice that deliver benefits particularly quickly—in some cases, immediately!

 Easy Gains
These are tips that give the biggest value for the least amount of effort.

Super Effective
These are tips proven to be particularly effective through scientific research or widespread usage by experts.

Cleaning

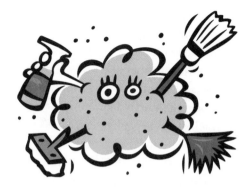

14 TIPS FOR HEALTH-FRIENDLY CLEANING

You may not realize it, but your house is hazardous to your health. Insect droppings, dust mites, bacteria-laden sponges, spoiled food—all can contribute to a plethora of health problems ranging from allergies and asthma to gastrointestinal upsets. In fact, germ guru Charles P. Gerga, Ph.D., a professor of microbiology at the University of Arizona in Tucson who studies so-called home hygiene, says you're more likely to get sick going home than nearly anywhere else in your life (except maybe hospitals).

What's scarier is that the cure for a dirty home can be worse than the problem as we attack germs with enough toxic chemicals to make the EPA shudder. Green Seal, a nonprofit environmental standards organization, estimates that cleaning products contribute approximately 8 percent of total nonvehicular emissions of volatile organic compounds, or VOCs. These can cause eye, nose, and lung irritation, as well as rashes, headaches, nausea, asthma, and, in some cases, cancer.

There is a solution. We talked to some of the leading "green" cleaners in the country about how to clean your house to minimize health threats to you, your family, and the environment. Here's what they recommend:

1 Clean in an organized manner.

There's no point in mopping the floor only to then dust the ceiling fan and deposit a gray film over everything again. To clean well—and that means to clean healthily—you need to clean efficiently. That means avoiding going back and forth around a room. Instead, work using a systematic approach. Think in terms of left to right, top to bottom. Begin with ceilings and walls, and work your way down to windows and furniture, finishing with the floors.

2 Clean the things you'd never think to clean.

For instance, your mattress is a magnet for allergy-causing dust mites. Washing the mattress cover in very hot water (140°F or more) every month, and wiping down the top of the mattress with hot water, can go a long way toward reducing morning stuffiness. Other never-thought-they-needed-to-be-cleaned areas:

▶ **Telephone receivers.** Dr. Gerba found significant numbers of illness-causing bacteria and viruses on telephone receivers, which could easily be spread to your lower lip and then, with a quick lick, into your mouth.

▶ **Indoor garbage cans.** Particularly those in the kitchen and bathroom. Emptying them isn't the same as cleaning them. Regularly scrub them to make sure germs aren't germinating.

- **Shower curtains.** They get wet most every day, and they often stay wet, making them a perfect home for mold.
- **Automatic dishwashers.** Take a close look at the edges of the door on your dishwasher. Many are breeding grounds for mold and mildew. The same is true of the rubber cushioning that surrounds some refrigerator doors.
- **The fireplace.** A clogged chimney is not only unhealthy, it can kill you if it ignites or, in the case of a gas fireplace, becomes blocked, sending dangerous carbon monoxide fumes into the house.
- **HVAC filters.** These filters are designed to filter allergy-causing dust from the air, but if they're clogged, they're more harmful than helpful.

3 **Dust with worn-out wool socks or a corner of an old wool blanket** or sweater. Wool creates static when rubbed on a surface, says Kim Carlson, who gives earth-friendly advice on the air for the NBC affiliate in Minneapolis/St. Paul. One wipe can keep your furniture dust-free without polishes or sprays.

Two-Second Quiz

Vinegar or Bleach?

Answer: *Vinegar.*
Health-conscious cleaners consider vinegar their number one ally. Studies find a straight 5% solution of vinegar kills 99 percent of bacteria, 82 percent of mold, and 80 percent of viruses. Chlorine bleach does a great job too. But it is irritating to the lungs and eyes and contains trace amounts of organochlorines—extremely persistent and toxic chemical compounds known to cause cancer in animals, among other serious health problems.

4 **Polish silver with toothpaste.** Some silver polishes contain petroleum distillates, ammonia, or other hazardous ingredients. Instead, Carlson recommends dabbing on toothpaste with your finger or rubbing it on with a cloth. Rinse with warm water and polish with a soft cloth. For larger trays and bowls, use a baking soda paste (baking soda mixed with water) on a wet sponge.

5 **Open your drains the nontoxic way.** Chemical drain cleaners (also called drain openers) are extremely corrosive and dangerous, containing such toxic ingredients as lye or sulfuric acid. Even the vapors are harmful. Instead, pour a pot of boiling water or toss a handful of baking soda followed by ½ cup vinegar down the drain weekly. Also effective, particularly in preventing clogs, are many brands of enzymatic cleaners, such as Nature's Miracle (used to clean up pet "accidents"), found in pet stores. Live enzymes "eat" the bacterial matter that clings to the drains.

6 **Clean your windows the Stealth Health way.** Mary Findley, veteran Oregon cleaning expert and president of Mary Moppins Cleaning System, recommends this homemade solution: Add ⅓ cup distilled white vinegar and a spoonful of dishwasher detergent, or ¼ cup rubbing alcohol, to a quart of distilled water. If you're using the latter recipe and your windows streak, don't blame the cleaner. You've probably got a wax buildup from the commercial products you were using before. Switch to the vinegar and dishwasher detergent formula. And don't forget these tools and tips:

- Use a sponge wand to soak the window in suds, rather than a spray bottle. Wet the windows thoroughly and let the solution do its work for about five minutes.

- Avoid cleaning your windows on sunny days or in bright sunlight. The sun dries the solution too quickly, which can result in streaks.
- Use a black rubber squeegee to dry the window. Make sure every iota of water comes off; otherwise, you're leaving dirt on the window.
- Use paper towels to dry the squeegee after each pass.
- For serious dirt, try an oversized razor blade wet with soapy water.

> ### How to Check Toxicity
>
> Don't believe us about the toxicity of many commercial cleaners? Check the Household Products Database—part of the Specialized Information Services of the National Library of Medicine—a vast compendium of common household products that includes the potential health effects. Just go to http://hpd.nlm.nih.gov and click on the category of the product you're interested in.

7 Forget Formula 409; make this fabulous all-purpose cleaner.

Fill a spray bottle nearly full with water and add a good squirt of Ivory liquid dishwashing detergent, says Findley. Shake just a bit. That's all you need. For some disinfecting oomph for the kitchen and bathroom, add ¼ cup rubbing alcohol. This is safe to use on Corian counters, sinks and showers, tile and marble.

8 Sanitize your toilet bowl safely.

Pity poor Dr. Gerba. He spends his days swiping cotton swabs over every conceivable household surface, then peering at the results under a microscope and identifying the germs and other icky things he finds there. You can only imagine what he finds in the bathroom.

- To clean the toilet safely, turn to your vinegar, says Findley. Fill a spray bottle with straight white vinegar. Pour a capful of vinegar into the toilet, then spray the sides of the bowl. Also, sprinkle baking soda in the toilet, wait 15 minutes, and scrub with a bit of baking soda sprinkled on the brush. Once a month pour one cup vinegar into the toilet and leave overnight. The vinegar dissolves any alkali buildup to prevent hard-water rings in the toilet. Whenever you leave for vacation,

pour a cup of vinegar into the toilet to prevent buildup while you are gone.
- To disinfect the toilet completely, wipe all surfaces with a cloth soaked in rubbing alcohol or with some of the alcohol-based hand cleaner available in stores.

9 Clean your kitchen floor the easy way.

Don't try to disinfect it, says Findley. "Unless you disinfect your feet, disinfecting your floors serves no purpose." Instead, use these homemade floor cleaners:

- **Hardwood and laminated floors.** One-quarter cup white vinegar per quart of water. Use only 100 percent cotton terry towels on hardwood floors and don't use self-wringing or microfiber mops. Microfiber is made from 80-85 percent polyester, which is plastic. Plastic scratches and will eventually scratch the sealant off the floor.
- **Marble, tile, and granite floors.** Just use very hot water. Cleaners of any kind will pit these floors.
- **Linoleum floors.** Hot water with just a bit of Ivory liquid dish soap if needed.

10 Clean out your washing machine and dryer.

You'd think they would be clean, right? Wrong. In a study of 50 homes in Tucson and

50 in Tampa Bay, Florida, Dr. Gerba found high levels of coliform bacteria, an indicator of unsanitary conditions, and diarrhea-causing *Escherichia coli* in home washing machines. When researchers washed sterile cloths in non-bleach laundry detergent, they found that 40 percent emerged contaminated with *E. coli* bacteria—with enough extra to contaminate the next load. The greatest risk from the germs comes when transferring wet laundry with your bare hands to the dryer. The solution? Try using rubber gloves when doing your wash, and add a cupful of hydrogen peroxide to your loads instead of bleach. Also, for germ control, wash your clothes on the hottest water setting.

 11 Disinfect your cutting board. In his research, Gerba found 200 times more fecal bacteria on the average cutting board in the home than on the toilet seat. To get it clean, run it through the dishwasher, spray it with straight 5% vinegar and let it set overnight, microwave it on high for 30 seconds, or swab it with alcohol to disinfect it if you don't want to use bleach.

12 Microwave your kitchen sponges for 30 seconds every day. Gerba found that the common household sponge may contain 320 million opportunistic bacterial pathogens, enough of which could be transferred from the sponge to your hand to your eyes or mouth to make you sick.

13 Make your own. In addition to the cleaning recipes above, Findley provides the following recommendations for homemade, environmentally and health-friendly products. She also recommends keeping a box of borax around for

---

Grocery List for Healthy Cleaning

You can get just about everything you need for healthy cleaning at the grocery store without ever wandering down the commercial cleaning aisle. Here's a shopping list from cleaning expert Mary Findley:

- 1 gallon white vinegar
- 1 bottle rubbing alcohol
- 1 large box baking soda
- 1 gallon distilled water
- Ivory liquid dishwashing detergent
- An oxygen-based cleaning product like Bio-Ox (www.bio-ox.com)
- Nature's Miracle (found at most pet stores or in the pet aisle)
- Foaming shaving cream
- Hydrogen peroxide (in the first-aid aisle)

Also pick up three or four spray bottles. Use each bottle for the make-your-own cleaning products listed above.

---

extra-tough cleaning jobs. Borax is a natural product made of sodium, boron, oxygen, and water and is unbeatable for tough cleaning jobs, as a bleach substitute, or mixed with water for a disinfectant. Dr. Gerba suggests rubbing alcohol as another good natural disinfectant. Just don't light any matches around it.

- **Tub and tile cleaner.** Two to three capfuls of Bio-Ox or other oxygen-based natural cleanser mixed with 1 quart water.
- **Furniture polish.** Mix olive oil and vinegar together for an excellent cleaner and polish.
- **Oven cleaner.** Mix Bio-Ox and baking soda together into a paste. First scrape off as much residue as you can with a scouring pad, then scrub with the Bio-Ox mixture.

- **Air freshener.** To remove kitchen odors, boil a 50/50 solution of white vinegar and water for several minutes. One capful of Bio-Ox mixed in a quart of water also makes an excellent room freshener.
- **Mildew remover.** Mix equal parts of water and hydrogen peroxide (20% strength).
- **Laundry whitener.** Use hydrogen peroxide rather than bleach. Soak your dingy white clothes for 30 minutes in the washer with ½ cup 20% peroxide, then launder as usual. This removes the graying caused by chlorine bleach.
- **Stain remover.** Most stains can be removed with Bio-Ox. Here are four other methods:

1. **Grease and paint stains.** Spray a bit of foaming shaving cream on the stain, then wipe up.

2. **Red Dye #40 that comes from pet food, punch, Popsicles, etc.** Spray hydrogen peroxide on the stain, then blot up.

3. **Underarm stains on clothes.** Spray hydrogen peroxide on underarm stains in shirts 30 minutes before laundering.

4. **Mold remover.** Spray with a 5% solution of white vinegar (undiluted). Let sit.

14 **"Shampoo" your rug safely.** Instead of commercial brands, just sprinkle dry cornstarch or baking soda on the carpet before vacuuming. The powders help remove deep dirt, and the baking soda helps remove odors.

The Sleep Routine

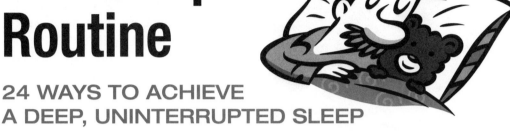

24 WAYS TO ACHIEVE A DEEP, UNINTERRUPTED SLEEP

Blessed sleep—the holy grail of health. Did you know, for instance, that a chronic lack of sleep may lead to insulin resistance, a risk factor for diabetes? Lack of sleep can send your blood sugar levels skyrocketing, contribute to weight gain, lead to depression, and cause brain damage.

That's just the warm-up. Sleep deprivation can alter your levels of thyroid and stress hormones, potentially affecting everything from your memory to your immune system, heart, and metabolism.

Of course, lack of sleep can kill you instantly—as when you run your car off the road because you've dozed at the wheel (an estimated 71,000 people are injured in fall-asleep crashes each year). In fact, studies find that if you've been awake through the night, it's as if you had a performance impairment equal to .10 percent blood alcohol content, more than enough to get you arrested for drunk driving in most states.

Given the evidence, you'd think we'd all be hitting the pillow as soon as the sun dropped below the horizon. Ha! Today Americans get 25 percent less sleep than they did a century ago. Nearly 4 out of 10 don't get the minimum 7 hours of sleep necessary for optimal health and daytime functioning, while 15 percent get less than 6 hours most nights.

Plus, 7 out of 10 Americans experience frequent sleep problems. The most common one? Old-fashioned insomnia, defined as having continued trouble falling asleep, staying asleep during the night, or waking up unrefreshed in the morning.

Since we're all in agreement that a good night's sleep is one of the best things you can do for your health and mood, pick three of these tips to follow each night until you get the night's sleep you so desperately crave.

1 Create a transition routine. This is something you do every night before bed. It could be as simple as letting the cat out, turning out the lights, turning down the heat, washing your face, and brushing your teeth. Or it could be a series of yoga or meditation exercises.

Regardless, it should be consistent to the point that you do it without even thinking about it. As you begin to move into your "nightly routine," your mind will get the signal that it's time to chill out and tune down, dialing down stress hormones and physiologically preparing you for sleep.

Two-Second**Quiz**

Pajamas or Underwear?

Answer: *Pajamas.*
Warm skin helps slow your blood's circulation down, cooling your internal temperature and generally contributing to a deeper sleep. Just don't overdo it. Your body goes through a few cool-warm cycles as a night passes, and so you want pajamas, sheets, and covers that keep you comfortable through these changes.

2 **Figure out your body cycle.** Ever find that you get really sleepy at 10 p.m., that the sleepiness passes, and that by the time the late news comes on, you're wide-awake? Some experts believe sleepiness comes in cycles. Push past a period of sleepiness and you likely won't be able to fall asleep very easily for a while. If you've noticed these kinds of rhythms in your own body clock, use them to your advantage. When sleepiness comes, get to bed. Otherwise, it might be a long time until you are ready to fall asleep again.

3 **Sprinkle just-washed sheets and pillowcases with lavender water** and iron them before making up your bed. The scent is scientifically proven to promote relaxation, and the repetition and mindlessness of ironing will soothe you. Or, instead of ironing your sheets, do the next best thing: Put lavender water in a perfume atomizer and spray above your bed just before climbing in.

4 **Hide your clock under your bed or on the bottom shelf** of your night stand, where its glow won't disturb you. That way, if you do wake in the middle of the night or have problems sleeping, you won't fret over how late it is and how much sleep you're missing.

5 **Switch your pillow.** If you're constantly pounding it, turning it over and upside down, the poor pillow deserves a break. Find a fresh new pillow from the linen closet, put a sweet-smelling case on it, and try again.

6 **Choose the right pillow.** One Swedish study found that neck pillows, which resemble a rectangle with a depression in the middle, can actually enhance the quality of your sleep as well as reduce neck pain. The ideal neck pillow should be soft and not too high, should provide neck support, and should be allergy tested and washable, researchers found. A pillow with two supporting cores received the best rating from the 55 people who participated in the study. Another study found that water-filled pillows provided the best night's sleep when compared to participants' usual pillows or a roll pillow. Yet another study found that a pillow filled with a special "cool" material composed of sodium sulfate and ceramic fiber provided a much better night's sleep than one filled with polyester. The reason, the researchers suggest, is that the cooler pillow kept the subjects' head cooler during the night, improving their sleep. While you may not be able to find a sodium sulfate-filled pillow, you can buy a pillow made of natural fibers, which are better at releasing heat than polyester.

Other pillow tips: if you're subject to allergies or find you're often stuffed up when you awake in the morning, try a hypoallergenic pillow. And experiment with the pillow's thickness. While a thick, fluffy pillow might sound appealing, it might be too thick for you, leading to neck strain. Try a thin pillow.

7 **Switch to heavier curtains over the windows, and use them.** Even the barely noticeable ambient light from streetlights, a full moon, or your neighbor's house can interfere with the circadian rhythm changes you need to fall asleep.

8 **Clean your bedroom and paint it a soothing sage green.** Or some other soothing color. First, the more clutter in your bedroom, the more distractions in the way of a good night's sleep. The smooth, clean surfaces act as a balm to your brain, helping to smooth out your own worries and mental to-do lists. The soothing color provides a visual reminder of sleep, relaxing you as you lie in bed reading or preparing for sleep.

9 **Move your bed away from any outside walls.** This will help cut down on noise, which a Spanish study found could be a significant factor in insomnia. If the noise is still bothering you, try a white noise machine, or just turn on a floor fan.

10 **Tuck a hot-water bottle between your feet or wear a pair of ski socks to bed.** The science is a little complicated, but warm feet help your body's internal temperature get to the optimal level for sleep. Essentially, you sleep best when your core temperature drops. By warming your feet, you make sure blood flows well through your legs, allowing your trunk to cool.

11 **Kick your dog or cat out of your bedroom.** A 2002 research study found that one in five pet owners sleep with their pets (and we're not talking gold-

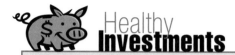

Healthy Investments

A Good Mattress

When ARC Consulting surveyed 400 adults for the Better Sleep Council, they found that 8 in 10 thought a bad mattress could cause sleep problems. Ironically, nearly half said they had a "bad" or "very bad" mattress they were trying to sleep on. You need a new mattress if:

- Yours is 10 years or older

- The topography of your mattress resembles a mountain range, with all its peaks, valleys, and slopes

- You wake up feeling sore or stiff, despite not being physically active the day before

Although no one mattress works best for everybody, there are some guidelines to follow. Make sure you buy one that's larger than you think you will need, especially if you sleep with someone else. Other key considerations:

- **Firmness.** This is strictly an individual decision. But make sure you try out any mattress in the store. Lie on it. Roll over. Get into your typical sleeping position. *Consumer Reports* found that firmer mattresses don't resist permanent body sagging any better than softer mattresses; that thicker mattresses sag more than thinner ones; and that the more padding there is, the greater the possibility the mattress will sag.

- **Frame.** Make sure you get a sturdy, quality frame, one with at least 10 slats and a fifth leg as a center support.

- **Maintenance.** Make sure you turn your mattress over and upside down at least every three months.

fish here). The study also found that dogs and cats created one of the biggest impediments to a good night's sleep since the discovery of caffeine. One reason? The study found that 21 percent of the dogs and 7 percent of the cats snored!

12 **Sleep alone.** Sure you love your spouse or partner, but studies find one of the greatest disruptors of sleep is that loved one dreaming away next to you. He might snore, she might kick or cry out, whatever. In fact, one study found that 86 percent of women surveyed said their husbands snored, and half had their sleep interrupted by it. Men have it a bit easier; just 57 percent said their wives snored, while just 15 percent found their sleep bothered by it. If you absolutely will not kick your partner out (or head to the guest room yourself), then consider these anti-snoring tips:

▶ Get him (or her) to stop smoking. Cigarette smoking contributes to snoring.
▶ Feed him (or her) a light meal for dinner and nix any alcohol, which can add to the snoring.
▶ Buy some earplugs and use them!
▶ Play soft music to drown out the snoring.
▶ Present your lover with a gift-wrapped box of Breathe Right strips, which work by pulling the nostrils open wider. A Swedish study found they significantly reduced snoring.
▶ Make an appointment for your sleeping partner at a sleep center. If nothing you do improves his or her snoring, your bedmate might be a candidate for a sleep test called polysomnography to see if sleep apnea is the cause. Better to help your partner—and yourself—than to exile the poor sonorous soul!

13 Take a combination supplement with 600 mg calcium and 300 mg magnesium before bed. Not only will you be providing your bones with a healthy dose of minerals, but magnesium is a natural sedative. Additionally, calcium helps regulate muscle movements. Too little of either can lead

DoThreeThings

If you can only do three things, do these to get a good night's sleep, says Helene A. Emsellem, M.D., director of the Center for Sleep & Wake Disorders in Chevy Chase, Maryland, and an associate clinical professor of neurology at George Washington University Medical Center in Washington, D.C.

1. Allow one hour before bedtime for a relaxing activity. Watching the news or answering e-mails does not count! Better choices are reading or listening to soft music. As for sex...well, some people say it just wakes them up and they have trouble sleeping afterward. So factor this into the timing of your bedtime routine.

2. If your mind is relaxed but your body is tense, do some low-intensity stretches and exercises to relax your muscles, especially those in your upper body, neck, and shoulders. Before you get into bed, use light weights (3 to 5 pounds for women, 5 to 10 pounds for men) to calmly exercise these muscles. Do one set of 8 to 10 repetitions of a basic exercise for each upper body muscle. We call this "automassage."

3. Allow at least three hours between dinner and bedtime. The brain does not sleep well on a full stomach. If you know that you have a busy day planned the following day, have your big meal at lunchtime and a lighter meal as early as possible in the evening. If you find you are still hungry before bedtime, try one of the many protein-enriched power bars (without chocolate) for your bedtime snack.

to leg cramps, and even a slight deficiency of magnesium can leave you lying there with a racing mind.

14 **Eat a handful of walnuts before bed.** Walnuts are a good source of tryptophan, a sleep-enhancing amino acid.

15 Munch a banana before bed. It's a great natural source of melatonin, the sleep hormone, as well as tryptophan. The time-honored tradition, of course, is warm milk, also a good source of tryptophan.

16 Drink water before bed, not fruit juice. One study found it took participants an extra 20 to 30 minutes to fall asleep after drinking a cup of fruit juice, most likely because of the high sugar content in juice.

17 Take antacids right after dinner, not before bed. Antacids contain aluminum, which appears to interfere with your sleep.

18 Listen to a book on tape while you fall asleep. Just as a bedtime story soothed and relaxed us when we were children, a calming book on tape (try poetry or a biography, stay away from horror novels) can have the same effect with us grown-ups.

19 Simmer three to four large lettuce leaves in a cup of water for 15 minutes. Remove from heat, add two sprigs of mint, and sip just before you go to bed. Lettuce contains a sleep-inducing substance called lactucarium, which affects the brain similarly to opium. Unlike opium, of course, you won't run the risk of addiction!

20 Give yourself a massage. Slowly move the tips of your fingers around your eyes in a slow, circular motion. After a minute, move down to your mouth, then to your neck and the back of your head. Continue down your body until you find you're so relaxed you're ready to drop off to sleep. Another option: alternate massage nights with your significant other. You get Monday, Wednesday and Friday. Your significant other gets Tuesday, Thursday and Saturday. You do each other on Sundays.

21 Take a hot bath 90 to 120 minutes before bedtime. A research study published in the journal *Sleep* found that women with insomnia who took a hot bath during this window of time (water temperature approximately 105°F), slept much better that night. The bath increased their core body temperature, which then abruptly dropped once they got out of the bath, readying them for sleep.

22 Use eucalyptus for a muscle rub. The strongly scented herb provides a soothing feeling and relaxing scent. You can find eucalyptus oil to mix into a carrier oil, or even a eucalyptus-scented cream.

23 Spend 10 minutes journaling the day's events or feelings after tucking yourself into bed. This "data dump" will help turn off the repeating tape of our day that often plays in our minds, keeping us from falling asleep.

24 Keep a notepad at your bedside along with a gentle night-light and pen. Then, if you wake in the middle of the night and your mind starts going, you can quickly transfer the to-do list to the page, returning to sleep knowing you "caught" those thoughts.

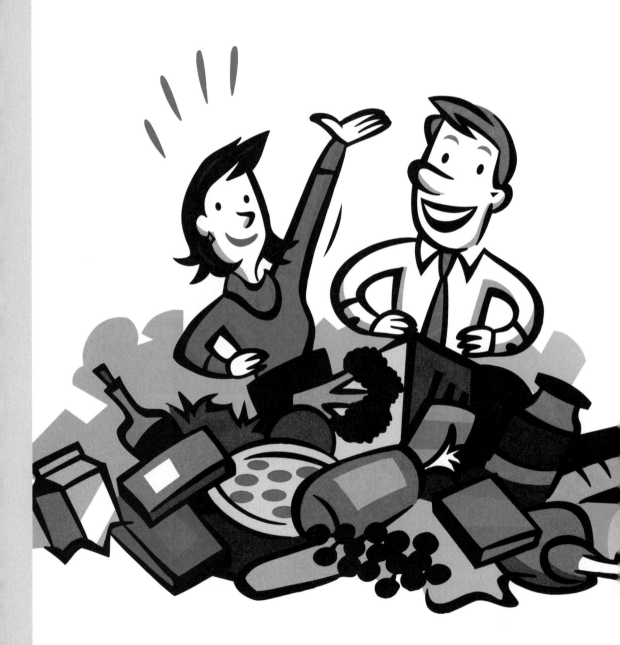

PART TWO

Stealth Healthy COOKING

Probably the easiest and most effective way to improve your health is with food. Learn the best tricks for eating the right stuff—and avoiding the bad.

Food Shopping
25 Tips for Your Grocery List

Sneaking In Vegetables
29 Ways to Get Your Fill

Sneaking In Fruits
25 Ways to Get Yours

Sneaking In Fiber
29 Ways to Plant More
"Good Carbs" Into Your Diet

**Cutting Back on
"Bad" Carbs**
16 Ways to Make
Low-Carb Healthy

Cutting Down on Sugar
23 Ways to Get Rid
of the Sweet Stuff

**Cutting Back
on Bad Fats**
35 Ways to Get Lean
the Right Way

Cutting Back on Salt
22 Ways to Eat Well Without It

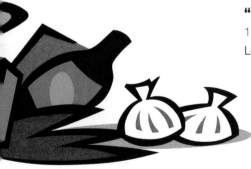

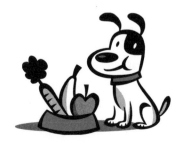

Food Shopping

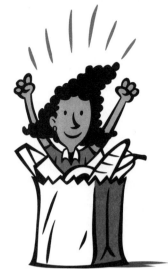

25 TIPS FOR YOUR GROCERY LIST

The typical American consumer hits the grocery store at least twice a week, spending an average of $25 each trip. And the average supermarket stocks over 40,000 items. Why, then, does it feel like we never have anything to eat at home? Maybe we're not attacking the grocery shopping with the right attitude, or list. Follow the advice below to make sure you not only have a well-stocked pantry for healthful eating, but are buying the right products at the right time in the right way.

You'll notice, by the way, that many of the tips below have you looking at a food product's nutrition label and ingredients list for information. If you haven't become expert at this, time to study up. Go straight to the source—the U.S. Food and Drug Administration—via the Internet at www.fda.gov, put "nutrition facts" into the search line, then click on "go" for a full menu of food-labeling information.

1 Rule number one: Buy fresh food! There is no simpler, no easier, no plainer measure of the healthiness of your food than whether it comes in boxes and cans or is fresh from the farm or the fields. If more than half your groceries are prepared foods, then you need to evolve your cooking and eating habits back to the healthy side by picking up more fresh vegetables, fruits, seafood, juices, and dairy.

2 Shop the perimeter of the store. That's where all the fresh foods are. The less you find yourself in the central aisles of the grocery store, the healthier your shopping trip will be. Make it a habit—work the perimeter of the store for the bulk of your groceries, then dip into the aisles for staples that you know you need.

3 Think of the departments (dairy, produce, meat, and so on) as separate stores within the supermarket. You wouldn't shop at every store at a mall the same way, would you? You know better than to idly browse through a jewelry store, don't you? So apply the same approach to the grocery store. Target the sections that are safe to browse through—the produce section, primarily—and steer clear of the dangerous sections (the candy, ice cream, and potato chip aisles).

4 Shop with a list. Organize your shopping list based on the tip above—that is, by the sections of the store. This will have you out of the supermarket at the speed of light. If you're a woman, consider getting your husband or son to do the food shopping, says Joan Salge Blake, R.D., clinical assistant professor of nutrition at Boston University's Sargent College. The latest survey from the Food Marketing Institute shows that compared to women, men are more likely to buy only what's on the grocery list. But shopping with a list has benefits beyond speed and spending. By lashing yourself to the discipline of a well-planned shopping list, you can resist the seductive call of aisle upon aisle of junk food, thereby saving your home, your family, and yourself from an overload of empty calories.

5 Food-shop with a full stomach.
We're sure you've heard this one before, but it's worth repeating. Walking through the grocery store with your tummy growling can make you vulnerable to buying anything that isn't moving, says Blake. If you can't arrange to shop shortly after a meal, be sure to eat an apple and drink a large glass of water before heading into the store.

6 Buy a few days before ripe.
There's no point in trying to buy fresh vegetables and fruits for your family if the bananas turn brown and the peaches mushy two days after you get them home. Buy fruit that's still a day or two behind ripeness. It will still be hard to the touch; bananas will be green. Feel carefully for bruises on apples, check expiration dates on bagged produce, and stay away from potatoes or onions that have started to sprout. If the produce on the shelves looks a bit beyond its peak, don't walk away; ask to speak to the produce manager. Chances are, there's a fresh shipment in the back just waiting to be put out on store shelves. For a real taste treat, if you're going to eat them within the next couple of days, pick up a bunch of vine-ripened tomatoes. There's just no comparison.

7 Buy in season.
Sure, it's tempting to buy strawberries in December, and once in a while that's fine. But fresh fruit and vegetables are best when purchased in season, meaning they've come from relatively close to home. They often cost less, are tastier, and have less risk of pathogens such as *E. coli*.

8 Buy organic whenever possible.
Sure, it costs a few dollars more. But a study in the *Journal of Agricultural and Food Chemistry* found that organically grown fruits and vegetables contain higher levels

Two-Second**Quiz**

Paper or Plastic?

Answer: *Paper.*
The debate over which bag is better for the environment is a long one, and there is no widely accepted answer. While plastic can be recycled, it's not as easy as recycling paper. And plastic production and processing require the use of toxic chemicals. Plus, plastic bags often don't degrade, because most of the garbage generated in this country is landfilled, i.e., buried beneath mounds of dirt. Plastic only decomposes when air and sunlight are present, and even then, it takes a long time. The negative side of paper bags is that they are made with manufacturing techniques that require pollution of water and air. But they are increasingly made from reprocessed materials, are more easily recycled, break down easier, and often have more uses around the house. But your best bet, if you're interested in protecting the environment, is to use cloth or string bags that can be reused again and again.

of cancer-fighting antioxidants than conventionally produced foods. However, if organic is too pricey for you, don't worry; organic or not, fruits and veggies are key to a healthy larder.

9 **Buy frozen.** Frozen fruits and vegetables are often flash frozen at the source, locking in nutrients in a way fresh or canned can't compete with. Stock your freezer with bags of frozen vegetables and fruits. You can toss the veggies into soups and stews, microwave them for a side dish with dinners, or thaw them at room temperature and dip them into low-fat salad dressing for snacks. Use the fruits for desserts, smoothies, and as ice cream and yogurt toppings.

10 **Stock up on canned tomato products.** Here's one major exception to the "fresher is better" rule. Studies find that tomato sauces and crushed and stewed tomatoes have higher amounts of the antioxidant lycopene than fresh, because they're concentrated. Canned tomatoes are a godsend when it comes to quick dinners in the kitchen. Warm up a can with some crushed garlic for a chunky pasta sauce; pour a can over chicken breasts and simmer in the crock pot; add to stews and sauces for flavor and extra nutrients.

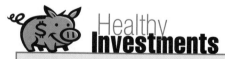

Healthy Investments

A Cheese Knife

A good cheese knife allows you to cut paper-thin slices of your favorite hard cheeses, says Joan Salge Blake, R.D., clinical assistant professor of nutrition at Boston University's Sargent College. You'll use less cheese (meaning less saturated fat and calories) and still get the flavor you desire.

11 **Stock up on canned beans.** Although they may have a bit more sodium than we like, that's easy enough to get rid of with a good rinse in the sink. Beans can be mixed with brown rice, added to soups and stews, pureed with onions and garlic into hummus for dipping, or served over pasta for a traditional pasta e fagioli. In fact, all the hype about pasta raising blood sugar really comes down to this: What are you putting on your pasta? The soluble fiber in beans lowers blood sugar and insulin, making the combination of pasta and beans a healthful—as well as delicious—dish.

12 **Spend some time in the condiment aisle.** With the following basic ingredients you have the underpinnings for wonderful sauces, low-fat marinades, and low-salt flavorings. These delightful flavorings enable you to stay away from the less-healthy condiment items, such as mayonnaise, butter, stick margarine, creamy salad dressings, and so on: flavored ketchups and barbecue sauces (look for sugar-free varieties), horseradish, mustards, flavored vinegars, extra-virgin olive oil, jarred bruschetta and pesto sauces (luscious spooned atop salmon and baked), capers, jarred olives, sun-dried tomatoes, jarred spaghetti sauce, anchovies, roasted red peppers, Worcestershire sauce, chili sauce, hot pepper sauce, soy sauce, sesame oil, walnut oil, teriyaki sauce, jarred salsas, and various kinds of marmalades.

13 **Try some of the new whole grain alternatives.** Today you can find wonderful whole grain pastas and couscous, instant brown rice that cooks up in 10 minutes instead of the old 50, even whole grain crackers. Hodgson Mills

makes a delicious whole wheat pasta with flaxseeds. It really tastes great, and you can scarcely do any better when it comes to nutrition. While you're at it, pick up a bag of whole wheat flour to replace the white stuff in your canister.

14 Choose prepared foods with short ingredient lists. We don't expect you to cut out prepared foods entirely. Just remember: The shorter the ingredient list, the healthier the food usually is. Of course, if the ingredients are sugar and butter, put the item back on the shelf.

15 Reject foods and drinks made with corn syrup. Corn syrup is a calorie-dense, nutritionally empty sweetener perhaps even worse than refined sugar (see page 113 for more on corn syrup). A shocking number of foods and drinks are thick with it, including such apparently healthy foods as fruit juices, pre-made spaghetti sauces, and even bread. Some experts argue that corn syrup is one of the main causes of America's obesity problem. If a food has corn syrup in its first four ingredients, then it lacks the whole-someness and healthiness you want.

16 Look for fiber. You want at least 1 to 2 grams of fiber for every 100 calories you consume.

17 If partially hydrogenated oil, or trans fats are listed on the label, step away from the box and nobody will get hurt.

18 Pick up a jar of dried shiitake mushrooms. They may look weird, but toss them in some hot water for half an hour and you have a meaty, healthy

Two-Second Quiz

Cash or Credit?

Answer: *Cash.*
You'll almost certainly spend less for your groceries if you pay with cash. In one study, researchers asked several hundred families to do all their grocery buying with cash for three months, then, for the next three months, to use only a credit card. When the families used credit cards, they spent between 20 and 30 percent more.

addition to soups, stews, and sauces, not to mention a unique filling for tarts and omelets. Plus, they keep forever.

19 Whenever you find yourself reaching for a package of ground meat, switch over to the poultry section instead and pick up ground turkey, ground chicken, or soy crumbles. Works just as well as ground beef for meatballs, meat loaf, or chili. This little substitution can cut more than 30 percent of the calories and at least half of the fat and saturated fat in a three-ounce serving, says Blake. When it's smothered in a zesty tomato sauce or fla-vored with seasonings, you'll never be able to tell the difference. If you're feeling a little gun-shy about abandoning the beef, use half turkey and half lean beef, or half soy crumbles and half beef.

20 Choose strong cheeses. Instead of American, cheddar, or Swiss, pick up feta, fresh Parmigiano-Reggiano, or a soft goat cheese. These strongly fla-vored cheeses will satisfy your yen for cheese without damaging your waistline, says Blake.

21 Buy macadamia nut oil. It has more good-for-you monounsaturated fats than any other oil in the world and a higher smoke point than olive oil, so there's no trans fatty acid formation when you cook. It makes any dish you make heart-healthier, says Fred Pescatore, M.D., author of *The Hamptons Diet*.

22 Confirm that a wheat bread is whole wheat. Some of the folks selling bread are trying to pull the wool (or is it wheat chaff?) over your eyes. Sure, a wheat bread is made from wheat. But if the first ingredient is refined wheat flour, then it's made from the same wheat as white bread—which means, stripped of fiber and nutrients, and in some cases, dyed brown for a fake healthy appearance. What you're really looking for are the words "*whole* wheat." That's the stuff with minimum refining and maximum beneficial nutrients.

23 Buy plain yogurt and flavor it at home. Pre-flavored yogurts have oodles of sugars that destroy any healthy benefits they once had. If you add a teaspoon of all-fruit jam at home, it'll still taste yummy, you'll consume far fewer useless calories, and you'll save lots of money.

24 Buy healthy add-ins for plain cereals. These include raisins, fresh berries, dried berries, almond slivers, pumpkin seeds, sesame sticks, and bananas. The best breakfast-cereal strategy is to buy unsweetened cereals and then add in your favorite flavors. That helps you bypass all the empty sugary calories—and lets you enjoy the cereal more. For ease, keep a wide-mouth, well-sealed jar on your counter with shelf-stable ingredients for quick mix-ins. Keep a scoop and ziplock

---

The Basics of Food Labeling

The FDA sets the rules on what food manufacturers can put on their labels, providing very specific definitions for everything from the word "healthy" to the description "low fat." Here's what it all means:

Healthy. The food is low in fat (especially saturated fat and trans fat, which have been linked to heart disease) and has limited amounts of cholesterol and sodium.

Free (for example, sugar-free). The food contains only tiny amounts of fat, saturated fat, sodium, sugar, cholesterol, or calories per serving.

Good source. One serving provides 10-19 percent of your total daily needs for a specific nutrient.

Low sodium. One serving has 140 mg of sodium or less.

Low cholesterol. One serving has 20 mg of cholesterol or less and 2 grams or less of saturated fat.

Low fat. One serving contains 3 grams of fat or less.

Reduced (for example, reduced fat). One serving has 25 percent less fat, saturated fat, sodium, sugar, cholesterol, or calories per serving than the regular version of the food.

Light (or lite). One serving has 50 percent less fat or one-third fewer calories than the regular version of the food.

One caveat on the label-reading thing: Serving sizes are not standardized. So check how much is in a serving for whichever prepared food you're eating.

---

bags handy, and you've got a handy, nutritious meal or snack for home or on the go.

25 Read juice labels carefully. Orange juice, although quite healthy, often has 20 grams of sugar in the average 8-ounce glass. Instead, try guava juice. It has three times more vitamin C, and is loaded with potassium (a great blood pressure regulator) and beta-carotene.

Sneaking In Vegetables

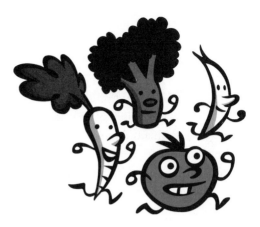

29 WAYS TO GET YOUR FILL

The average American is lucky to get two servings of vegetables a day. Nutrition experts would have us eating five to seven helpings a day. This pretty much captures America's health problems in a nutshell. If we ate more vegetables and fewer processed foods, we'd lose weight, clean our arteries, balance our blood sugar, and shut down a large number of hospitals. But getting from two servings a day to seven doesn't come without planning or effort. We're here to help. Here's the Stealth Health *painless* way to sneak more veggies into your daily diet.

1 Serve raw vegetables at every meal. Nearly everyone likes carrot sticks, celery sticks, cucumber slices, string beans, cherry tomatoes, and/or green pepper strips. They're healthy, they have virtually no calories, they have a satisfying crunch, and they can substantially cut your consumption of the more calorie-dense main course. So make it a practice: A plate of raw vegetables in the center of the table, no matter what the meal is.

2 Take advantage of prepared veggies. We usually don't espouse prepared foods. They're usually more expensive and high in artificial flavorings, sugars, and sodium. But when it comes to prepared veggies—bagged salads, prewashed spinach, peeled and diced butternut squash, washed and chopped kale—we're all for it. Numerous consumer studies find that we're more likely to use bagged salads and other produce. In fact, the introduction of bagged, prewashed spinach in the late 1990s is touted as the main reason spinach consumption increased 16.3 percent in the United States between 1999 and 2001.

3 Sneak vegetables into breakfast and lunch. One reason we don't get enough vegetables is that many of us consider them merely a side dish to dinner. If you really want to increase your vegetable consumption, you have no choice but to eat them at other meals. How?

- Make salad a part of your everyday lunch.
- Make egg scrambles a regular breakfast, using a scrambled egg to hold together sautéed vegetables such as peppers, mushrooms, zucchini, asparagus, or onions.
- Eat leftover veggies from last night's dinner with breakfast or lunch.
- Cherry tomatoes, cucumbers, carrots, and celery, *all the time.*

• Make vegetable sandwiches, using almost any vegetable that won't roll out of the bread.

4 Start each dinner with a mixed green salad before you serve the main course. Not only will it help you eat more veggies, but by filling your stomach first with a nutrient-rich, low-calorie salad, there'll be just a bit less room for the higher-calorie items that follow.

5 Once a week, have an entrée salad. A salade niçoise is a good example: mixed greens, steamed green beans, boiled potatoes, sliced hard-boiled egg, and tuna drizzled with vinaigrette. Serve with crusty whole grain bread. Bon appétit!

6 Fill your spaghetti sauce with vegetables. We typically take a jar of low-sodium prepared sauce and add in string beans, peas, corn, bell peppers, mushrooms, tomatoes and more. Like it chunky? Cut them in big pieces. Don't want to know they're there? Shred or puree them with a bit of sauce in the blender, then add.

7 Order your weekly pizza with extra veggies. Instead of the same old pepperoni and onions, do your health and digestion a favor and ask for artichoke hearts, broccoli, hot peppers, and other exotic vegetables many pizza joints stock these days for their gourmet pies.

8 Puree into soup. Potatoes, carrots, winter squash, cauliflower, and broccoli—just about any cooked (or leftover) vegetable can be made into a creamy, comforting soup. Here's a simple recipe:

In a medium saucepan, sauté 1 cup finely chopped onion in 1 tablespoon vegetable oil until tender. Combine the onion in a blender or food processor with cooked vegetables and puree until smooth. Return puree to saucepan and thin with broth or low-fat milk. Simmer and season to taste.

9 Add a bit of sweetness to your veggies. A study conducted at the State University of New York found that students like broccoli and cauliflower more when the vegetables had a 5 percent sugar solution added to them (basically, just a bit of sugar dissolved in water).

10 Follow the golden rule: Half of your dinner plate should be vegetables. That leaves a quarter of the plate for a healthy starch and a quarter for lean meat or fish. This is the perfectly balanced dinner, says Joan Salge Blake, R.D., clinical assistant professor of nutrition at Boston University's Sargent College.

11 Build a sandwich that has more lettuce and tomato than meat. Stack the meat filler in the sandwich to no higher than the thickness of a standard slice of bread. Then pile on low-calorie

slices of lettuce and tomatoes to the combined height of both slices of bread. Presto: Your sandwich tower has the height of the Empire State Building yet the svelteness of the Eiffel Tower, says Blake.

12 **Have a veggie burger for lunch once a week** topped with a sliced tomato and lettuce. Honestly, they taste better than you imagine.

13 **Open a can of low-sodium soup** and add a bag of precut broccoli and carrots, either fresh or frozen. Voilà! You have a superfast and easy lunch or dinner entrée, ready to be flavored with your preferred spices, herbs, or hot sauce. As the soup simmers, it will simultaneously cook the veggies, boosting the nutritional value and fiber, say the nutrition twins, Tammy Lakatos Shames, R.D., and Lyssie Lakatos, R.D. The two are the authors of *Fire Up Your Metabolism: 9 Proven Principles for Burning Fat and Losing Weight Forever.*

14 **Move your veggies to the top shelf of the refrigerator.** As long as they are bagged properly, they'll last as well as if in a vegetable crisper. More important, now they'll be visible and

Healthy Investments

A Vegetable Grater

Grating vegetables like carrots, cabbage, celery, cucumber, and so on, adds volume to your meals, meaning you eat fewer calories while eating more food. Plus, grating helps you "hide" your veggies in casseroles, meat loaves, and other dishes.

enticing, say the nutrition twins. In particular, keep fast-to-eat vegetables like baby carrots, precut red and green pepper strips, broccoli florets, tomatoes, and cucumbers as accessible as possible.

15 **Eat vegetables like fruit.** Half a cucumber, a whole tomato, a stalk of celery, or a long, fresh carrot are as pleasant to munch on as an apple. It may not seem typical, but who cares? A whole vegetable makes a terrific snack.

16 **Have a V8.** Although higher in sodium, vegetable juices do provide the nutrition of a vegetable serving. Throw a six-ounce can of vegetable juice or tomato juice into your tote in the morning; many come in low-sodium forms, says Mary Gregg, R.D., director of Human Care Services for NutriSystem, Inc.

17 **Always start with mirepoix.** This blend of onions, celery, carrots, parsley, and bay leaves, pronounced "meer-pwah," is a great way to sneak veggies into nearly every entrée you prepare. Sauté a cup (or more) of the mixture (which you can buy already cut up and prepared in some groceries) in two tablespoons of olive oil, then use as a starter for sauces, stews, and soups.

18 **Serve chili, soup, stew, pastas, or rice in a scooped-out tomato** or green pepper. Then make sure you finish the "bowl."

19 **Add chopped kale or other hearty greens** to your next soup or stew. Just a couple of minutes is all that's needed to steam the greens down to tenderness and add quantities of potassium,

fiber, and calcium to your soup, says Lisa C. Andrews, R.D., a clinical dietitian for the VA Medical Center in Cincinnati.

20 Use low-sodium vegetable juice as the base for soups instead of chicken or beef broth.

21 Go vegetarian one day a week. You can do this by merely substituting the meat serving with a vegetable serving (suggestion: make it a crunchy, strong-flavored vegetable like broccoli). Or you can dabble in the world of vegetarian cooking, in which recipes are developed specifically to make a filling, robust meal out of vegetables and whole grains. For those times, you should get yourself a good vegetarian cookbook. The Moosewood Restaurant cookbook series is popular, and for good reason. Other good options include: *Cooking Vegetarian: Healthy, Delicious, and Easy Vegetarian Cuisine* by Vesanto Melina and Joseph Forest, and *Becoming Vegetarian: The Complete Guide to Adopting a Healthy Vegetarian Diet* by Vesanto Melina et al.

22 Use salsa liberally. First, make sure you have a large batch filled with vegetables. One good approach: Add chopped yellow squash and zucchini to store-bought salsa. Then put salsa on everything: baked potatoes, rice, chicken breasts, sandwiches, eggs, steak, even bread. Salsa shouldn't be just for chips. It's too tasty and healthy not to be used all the time.

23 Throw shredded carrots and cabbage into your next soup, salad, or casserole. These coleslaw ingredients add flavor, color, and lots of vitamins and minerals, says Andrews.

The Cooking Corner

Vegetables are easier to cook than chicken, burgers, or pork chops. But they do require a little more creativity. Here are four mini-recipes to show what we mean:

- Add grated carrots, chopped squash, and steamed spinach to a pound of ground beef or turkey, then shape into patties and grill for your own version of a veggie burger.

- Toss the strands from a cooked spaghetti squash with olive oil, fresh parsley, and Parmesan cheese. This makes a wonderful replacement for mashed potatoes or white rice as a side dish, suggests Jorj Morgan, author of *At Home in the Kitchen: The Art of Preparing the Foods You Love to Eat.*

- Substitute sweet potatoes topped with a splash of maple syrup and a sprinkle of low-fat granola for mashed potatoes. This way, you'll get extra helpings of beta-carotene and vitamins B and C, plus six grams of fiber.

- Stuff eggplant with tomatoes, lay slices of Parmesan cheese over them, drizzle with olive oil, wrap in aluminum foil, then bake or grill until softened. Voilà! A wonderful grilled "sandwich."

24 Roast your vegetables. Here is one of the great side dishes, easy to make, delicious to eat, and amazingly healthy. Plus, it tastes surprisingly sweet, and lasts well as a leftover, meaning you can make large batches and serve throughout the week. Cut hearty root vegetables like parsnips, turnips, rutabagas, carrots, and onions into inch-thick chunks and arrange in a single layer on a cookie sheet. Drizzle with olive oil and sprinkle with kosher or sea salt, freshly ground pepper, and fresh or dried herbs. Roast in a 450°F oven until soft, about 45 minutes, turning once. That's it!

25 **Use vegetables as sauces.** How about pureed roasted red peppers seasoned with herbs and a bit of lemon juice, then drizzled over fish? Or puree butternut or acorn squash with carrots, grated ginger, and bit of brown sugar for a yummy topping for chicken or turkey. Cooked vegetables are easily converted into sauces. It just takes a little ingenuity and a blender.

26 **Nix the bitterness of healthy veggies with a sprinkle of salt.** Of course, we're going to be talking about how to reduce the sodium in your diet later, but the chemical reality is that salt helps neutralize bitterness. For an added kick, try capers, olives, or mashed anchovies instead of salt.

27 **Grill your vegetables.** If you only use your grill for meats, you've been missing out! Peppers, zucchini, asparagus, onions, eggplant—even tomatoes—all taste amazingly good when grilled. Generally, all you need to do is coat them with olive oil and throw them on. Turn every few minutes and remove when they start to soften. Or skewer chunks of veggies on a bamboo or metal skewer and turn frequently. You can also buy grilling baskets that keep the veggies from falling through the slats in the grill.

28 **Go exotic.** Every week, try one exotic vegetable, the kind that will stump the grocery store cashier. Here are some to try, and ways to try them:

- **Belgian endive.** This type of lettuce has a mild, slightly bitter flavor, and is packed with fiber, iron, and potassium. Use it in salads and instead of crackers with vegetable dips.
- **Jicama (HEE-kah-mah).** Known as the Mexican potato, jicama is a root tuber (like potatoes). Buy it smooth and firm with unblemished roots. Serve it peeled, cold, and raw in thin slices or strips, either straight up with a dip or in salads or coleslaw. Or throw it into soups, stews, or stir-fries. It works great as a substitute for water chestnuts.
- **Bok choy.** An Oriental cabbage, bok choy is excellent chopped and stir-fried in a bit of peanut oil and soy sauce. Or throw it into soup just before serving.
- **Chayote (chi-OH-tay) squash.** A summer squash native to Latin America, chayote squash is also known as vegetable pear because of its shape and color. It has a mild taste, like zucchini, with a slightly citrus tang. You don't have to peel it, and the seeds inside are edible. Just cut into cubes, add 1 cup water, cover, and microwave for about 8 minutes.
- **Kohlrabi.** A member of the turnip family, it is often called a cabbage turnip. It's sweeter, juicier, crisper, and more delicate in flavor than a turnip. The cooked leaves have a kale/collard flavor. Trim and

Two-Second**Quiz**

Fresh or Powdered Garlic?

Answer: *Fresh.*
Technically the jury is still out. The man conducting the be-all-and-end-all trial that should determine whether fresh garlic has greater health benefits than powdered, Christopher Gardner, Ph.D., of Stanford University Medical Center, hasn't published his results yet. But, he notes, the active ingredient in garlic is allicin, which can easily be destroyed if you futz with it too much. Indications suggest that fresh is best.

pare the bulb to remove all traces of the fibrous underlayer just beneath the skin, then eat raw, boil, steam, microwave, or sauté, or add to potato casseroles.

▸ **Fennel.** Also known as sweet anise, fennel has a sweet, mild licorice flavor. The feathery fronds can be used as an herb, like dill weed, to flavor soups and stews. The broad, bulbous base is treated like a vegetable and can be eaten raw, or sliced and diced for stews, soups, and stuffing.

▸ **Spaghetti squash.** Also called vegetable spaghetti, this oval-shaped yellow squash is a relative newcomer and a novel one: When cooked, the flesh of the squash can be pulled apart to form slender strands that resemble spaghetti.

29 Use canned pumpkin for dessert.
Just sprinkle it with cinnamon, and mix in two packets of Splenda. Even if you eat the whole can, this dessert is only 140 calories and packs a healthy 9 grams of fiber. For ½ cup you get 40 calories and 3.5 grams of fiber, not to mention tons of beta-carotene.

Counting to Nine

Hearing you need to get nine or more servings of fruits and vegetables can be daunting. But consider the definition of a serving, below (from the National Cancer Institute). All varieties of fruits and vegetables—fresh, frozen, canned, dried, and 100 percent juice—count. Measure out some of these in your kitchen so you can see how reasonable a serving size is!

- One medium-size fruit (such as apple, orange, banana, pear)

- ½ cup raw, cooked, canned, or frozen fruits or vegetables

- ¾ cup (6 ounces) 100 percent fruit or vegetable juice

- ½ cup cut-up fruit

- ½ cup cooked or canned legumes (beans and peas)

- 1 cup raw, leafy vegetables (such as lettuce and spinach)

- ¼ cup dried fruit (such as raisins, apricots, and mangoes)

REMINDER

 Fast Results
These are bits of advice that deliver benefits particularly quickly—in some cases, immediately!

 Easy Gains
These are tips that give the biggest value for the least amount of effort.

 Super Effective
These are tips proven to be particularly effective through scientific research or widespread usage by experts.

Sneaking In Fruits

25 WAYS TO GET YOURS

You've no doubt heard tell of the global economy. Well, you need look no farther than your local supermarket to see it in action. There grapes from South America meet kiwis from New Zealand and pineapples from Hawaii—in February. Today's produce section is definitely *not* your grandmother's fruit stand. And with all this variety, fresh fruit in season every season, there's no excuse not to stock up.

You know the drill—for optimal health you're supposed to get four or five servings of fruit *a day*. It needn't be overwhelming; not with these clever Stealth Health tips.

1 Make it a rule: Every breakfast includes a piece of fruit. It's the perfect morning food, filled with natural, complex sugars for slow-release energy, fiber, and nutrients galore. Cantaloupe, an orange, berries—all are perfect with whole wheat toast, cereal, or an egg.

2 Make another rule: Fruit for dessert at least three nights per week. A slice of watermelon, a peach, a bowl of blueberries—they're the perfect ending to a meal, and are so much healthier than cookies or cake. Like your desserts fancier? How does chocolate-covered strawberries, poached pears in red wine, peach and blueberry crisp, or frozen fresh raspberry yogurt sound? They count too.

3 Every Monday, start your week with a fruit slushie. Add one cup fresh fruit, ½ cup fruit juice, and one cup ice to a blender and liquefy. That's two servings of fruit before 8 a.m.! If you'd prefer a creamier smoothie, toss in ½ cup plain nonfat yogurt.

4 Substitute fruit sorbet for ice cream. One scoop (¼ cup) contains up to one serving of fruit, says Carolyn Lammersfeld, R.D., who leads the nutrition team at Cancer Treatment Centers of America at Midwestern Regional Medical Center in Chicago. To whip up your own, try freezing peaches packed in their own juice for 24 hours, then submerge the can in hot water for one minute. Cut the fruit into chunks and puree until smooth.

5 Or substitute frozen fruit bars for ice cream. Buy pure-fruit versions that don't add extra corn syrup or sugar. Feel free to have one every single day.

6 Keep a fruit bowl filled wherever you spend the most time. This could be at work, near your home computer, or even in the television room.

And keep five to eight pieces of fresh fruit in it at all times, such as bananas, oranges, apples, grapes, or plums. Most fruit is fine left at room temperature for three or four days. But if it's out and staring at you, it's not likely to last that long. A piece of fruit makes a perfect snack—as often as four times per day.

7 **Get your fruits dried.** Dried fruits are very portable and have a long shelf life. Take them to work, on shopping trips, or even on vacation. Raisins and prunes are classic choices. Also try dried cranberries and blueberries, which are extremely high in phytonutrients, or dried apricots, which are chock-full of beta-carotene, says Mary Gregg, R.D., director of Human Care Services for NutriSystem, Inc. Other options include dates, figs, dried peaches, dried pears, and dried bananas.

8 **Bring fruit with you anytime you plan on driving your car** for more than an hour. Once you are on the highway and cruising along, an apple or a nectarine tastes great and helps break the tedium.

9 **Keep an apple in your pocket whenever you go for long walks.** It will be your reward for getting to the midpoint of your walk.

10 **Substitute prune puree for oil in baking.** This works particularly well for brownies, says Lammersfeld. You can also try applesauce.

11 **Make Monday red day.** And eat only red fruits. Tuesday should be orange day, and so on. Here are some ideas from Peggy Hughes, author of *30 Days to a Healthier Family*.

Two-Second Quiz

Strawberries or Blueberries?

Answer: *Blueberries.*
Of course, both are great for you. Eat lots of both! But when you compare the nutrients in an equal amount of each, blueberries have a slight edge. Blueberries are particularly rich with fiber—four times that in strawberries—more natural sugars, much more vitamin E, and some unique micronutrients good for memory.

Monday. Red. Apples, cherries, cranberries, red grapes, plums, strawberries.
Tuesday. Orange. Apricots, cantaloupes, kumquats, nectarines, oranges, papaya, peaches.
Wednesday. Yellow or white. Bananas, yellow apples, grapefruit, mangoes, pineapple.
Thursday. Blue or violet. Blackberries, black raspberries, grapes, plums, figs.
Friday. Green. Limes, pears, kiwi.

12 **Mix fruits in with your salad.** A sprinkle of raisins, some cut-up strawberries, a diced apple, or some sliced kiwi all make great additions to the typical tossed salad.

13 **Puree fresh or canned fruits** (peaches, pear, mangoes, apricots, etc.) and use as an ice cream or pancake topping, suggest the nutrition twins, Tammy Lakatos Shames, R.D., and Lyssie Lakatos, R.D. The two are the authors of *Fire Up Your Metabolism: 9 Proven Principles for Burning Fat and Losing Weight Forever.*

14 Toss fresh or frozen berries onto cereal, salads, or ice cream. They're also great stirred into yogurt or pancake and muffin mixes.

15 Freeze banana slices or grapes for a refreshing summer snack.

 16 Every time you want a candy bar, have a small box of raisins instead. Raisins are sweet and healthy, and small boxes are just the right amount to fulfill a yen for a sweet treat.

17 Add fresh fruits like strawberries, blueberries, and bananas to pancake or waffle batter. Or dice over frozen pancakes or waffles.

18 Get your fruit in bread and cake once a week. How about applesauce cake, banana bread, strawberry, apple, or blueberry pie? Pineapple upside-down cake, anyone?

19 Use orange juice as a base for cooking whole grains.

20 Spice up store-bought salsas with fruit. Or make your own fruit-based salsas with pineapple, mango, or papayas. Mix with onions, ginger, a bit of garlic, some mint and/or cilantro, sprinkle on a few hot pepper flakes for fire, and chill.

21 Add diced kiwi, sliced grapes, or chopped apple to chicken, tuna, and turkey salads.

22 Keep cut-up melon in a container in the fridge. Use as a first course before dinner; wrap with prosciutto for an appetizer; mix with

In**Perspective**

Deconstructing Antioxidants

The reason fruits (and vegetables) are so important to your overall health is that they are major purveyors of antioxidants. Antioxidant molecules are like the missile defense system of your body, preventing damage from molecular bombs called free radicals. It works like this: In order to breathe, move, or eat, your body's cells convert food and oxygen into energy. This chemical reaction releases harmful byproducts, the free radicals we mentioned. Basically, they're highly reactive forms of oxygen that are missing an electron. Desperate for that missing electron, they steal them from normal cells, damaging the healthy cell and its DNA in the process. This damage eventually contributes to any number of major health problems, including heart disease, memory loss, and cancer.

Antioxidants, however, interfere with this process by giving free radicals one of their own electrons to stabilize them. Or they combine with free radicals to form different, more stable compounds. There are also antioxidant enzymes that help free radicals react with other chemicals to produce safe, instead of toxic, substances. Antioxidants, for instance, help prevent "bad" LDL cholesterol from becoming stickier and forming plaque.

This is the reason the health establishment is so insistent on people eating more fresh produce: It provides around-the-clock defenses against free-radical damage to your arteries.

cottage cheese for breakfast; have a small bowl for a snack; even consider pureeing for a quick sauce over fish.

23 Shred (yes, we said shred) fresh fruit over plain yogurt. Use the large holes of a boxlike grater.

24 Use all-fruit jam on toast, bagels, waffles, or other breakfast foods. You can also mix it into nonfat cottage cheese or yogurt, or melt it in the microwave and use in place of syrup on pancakes and ice cream.

25 Every week, buy one exotic fruit you've never tried. It could be something as relatively common as a mango, or as unique as a lychee. Here are some tips on what these fruits are and how to enjoy them:

▸ **Asian pear.** Also called an Oriental, Chinese, salad, or apple pear, this firm pear is meant to be eaten immediately when it's hard. It's sweet, crunchy, and amazingly juicy.

▸ **Cherimoya.** Also called a custard apple, this large tropical fruit tastes like a combination of pineapple, papaya, and banana. Purchase fruit that's firm, heavy for its size, and without skin blemishes or brown splotches. Let soften at room temperature, then refrigerate, wrapped, up to four days. To serve, cut in half, remove seeds, and spoon the fruit from the shell.

▸ **Guava.** Sweet and fragrant with bright pink, white, yellow, or red flesh. Buy when it is just soft enough to press, and refrigerate for up to a week in a plastic or paper bag. To use, cut in half and scoop out the flesh for salads, or peel and slice. Try cooking and pureeing slightly under-ripe guava as a sauce for meat or fish.

▸ **Kiwi.** This fruit never took off until they changed the name from Chinese gooseberry to kiwifruit. Now it's one of the most popular of the exotics. With a flavor that's a cross between strawberries and melon, kiwis are ready to eat when they're slightly soft to the touch. Peel and chop, or cut in half and scoop out the flesh with a grapefruit spoon.

▸ **Lychee.** Once, lychee trees were found only in southern China, but the popularity of this tropical fruit has caused its spread (it is now widely raised in Florida). The lychee fruit is about 1½ inches in size, oval, with a bumpy red skin. Peel off the inedible skin and you get a white, translucent flesh similar to a grape, but sweeter, surrounding a cherrylike pit. Eat 'em like large grapes, one after another. They're available only for a few months a year, but buy a pound next spring and discover why Asians call lychees the king of fruits.

▸ **Mango.** One of the most commonly eaten fruits in the world, along with bananas. The flavor is a combination of peach and pineapple, but spicier and more fragrant (it is sometimes called the tropical peach).

▸ **Papaya.** Soft, juicy, and silky-smooth flesh with delicate, sweet flavor. The center of the papaya is filled with small, round, black, peppery-tasting seeds,

Two-Second**Quiz**

Fresh Fruit or Dried?

Answer: *Fresh.*

The higher water content (most fresh fruits are more than 80 percent water) means a larger volume, making the fruit more filling and satisfying with fewer calories. But for convenience and shelf life, use dried fruit as your backup plan.

which can be eaten but usually aren't. Peel, then slice into wedges or cut into chunks, or slice in half, remove seeds, and scoop out the flesh with a spoon. Unripe papayas can be peeled, seeded, and cooked as a vegetable, and you can grind the seeds like pepper for adding to sauces or salads.

Passion fruit. Passion fruit has golden flesh with tiny, edible black seeds and a sweet-tart taste. When ripe, it has wrinkled, dimpled, deep purple skin. To serve, cut in half and scoop out the pulp with a spoon.

▸ **Persimmon.** Delicate in flavor and firm in texture, persimmons can be eaten like an apple, sliced and peeled, and are great in salads.

▸ **Pomegranate.** Available in the fall, it's the seeds of this crimson fruit that you eat. Each tiny, edible seed is surrounded by translucent, brilliant red pulp that has a sparkling sweet-tart flavor. Choose fruit

Two-Second**Quiz**

Fruit Juice or Fruit?

Answer: *Fruit.*
Get the real thing. Not only are most fruit juices loaded with sugar, they've been stripped of an important element in fruit—fiber.

that feels heavy for its size with bright color and blemish-free skin. They can be refrigerated up to a month, while the seeds can be frozen for three months. To serve, cut the fruit in half and pry out the seeds. Use them to top ice cream, sprinkle into salads, or simply as a snack.

▸ **Quince.** Tastes like a cross between an apple and a pear, with a dry, hard, yellowish-white flesh that has a tart flavor. Better cooked than raw. Quinces keep up to two months wrapped and refrigerated, and are primarily used for jams, jellies, and preserves.

▸ **Star fruit.** Although they look exotic, most star fruits today come from south Florida. Slice them crosswise for perfect five-pointed star-shaped sections as a garnish or for fruit salads. Star fruit's flavor combines the best of plums, pineapples, and lemons.

▸ **Tamarillo.** This subtropical fruit is sometimes called a tree tomato, but the comparison ends there. Native to South America, this egg-shaped fruit has a glossy outer skin that hides crimson fruit that turns golden when cooked or heated. The orange-yellow flesh, studded with a swirl of edible dark red seeds, has the texture of a plum and is slightly tart. To peel tamarillos, plunge into boiling water for about 30 seconds, then slip off the skins. Cut crosswise into slices.

Rating Fruits and Vegetables

So of the hundreds of fruits out there, which ones give you the biggest bang for your buck? Why, the ones with the highest ORAC scores, of course. ORAC stands for oxygen radical absorbance capacity, a fancy way of saying, "Which fruits and vegetables pack the greatest antioxidant punch?" The good people at the Agricultural Research Service's Human Nutrition Research Center on Aging at Tufts University in Boston figured it out. Here are the top 10:

1. Prunes	**6.** Raspberries
2. Raisins	**7.** Plums
3. Blueberries	**8.** Oranges
4. Blackberries	**9.** Red grapes
5. Strawberries	**10.** Cherries

Sneaking In Fiber

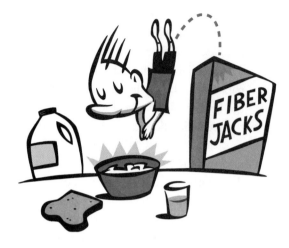

29 WAYS TO PLANT MORE "GOOD CARBS" INTO YOUR DIET

In the lexicon of weight loss, the term "good carbs" refers to complex carbohydrates. These are foods like whole grains, nuts, beans, and seeds that are composed largely of complex sugar molecules that require lots of time and energy to digest into the simple sugars your body needs for fuel. Virtually every weight-loss program—be it Atkins, South Beach, Weight Watchers, or Dr. Dean Ornish's—welcomes complex carbs as part of a healthy, lean, long-term diet.

One of the biggest benefits of foods rich in complex carbs is that they also contain large amounts of fiber. Fiber, in basic terms, is the indigestible parts of plant foods. It is the husk on the grain of wheat, the thin strands in celery, the crunch in the apple, the casings on edible seeds. Fiber protects you from heart disease, cancer, and digestive problems. Depending on the type of fiber (yes, there are more than one!), it lowers cholesterol, helps with weight control, and regulates blood sugar. Bottom line: This is one nutrient you don't want to miss. Yet the average American gets just 12-15 grams of fiber a day—far below the recommended 25-30 grams. And that was before so many of us started cutting carbs for weight loss—and cutting fiber in the bargain.

In the next two chapters, we'll talk about "bad carbs" and how to remove them from your diet. But if you increase your consumption of high-fiber complex carbs, you'll have already done most of the work—and you'll have done one of the most beneficial things you can do for your health. Here's how to sneak "good carbs" and extra fiber into your daily diet with a minimum of effort.

1 **Eat cereal every day for breakfast.** Ideally, aim for a whole grain, unsweetened cereal with at least 4 grams of fiber a serving. Just eating any cereal might be enough, however. A University of California study found that cereal eaters tend to eat more fiber and less fat than non-cereal eaters. Healthy, high-fiber cereals you might want to consider include Kellogg's All-Bran Original, Kashi GOLEAN, and Kellogg's Raisin Bran.

2 **Eat two apples every day.** Not just to keep the doctor away, but because apples are a good source of pectin, a soluble fiber that contributes to a feeling of fullness and digests slowly. A 1997 study published in the *Journal of the American*

College of Nutrition found that 5 grams of pectin was enough to leave people feeling satisfied for up to four hours.

3 Make a yogurt mix every Wednesday for breakfast. Take one container of yogurt and mix in ⅓ cup All-Bran cereal, 1 tablespoon ground flaxseeds, and 5 large, diced strawberries for a whopping 12.2 grams of fiber—nearly half your daily allowance!

4 Make baby carrots and broccoli florets dipped into low-fat ranch dressing your afternoon snack three days a week. You'll fill up the empty afternoon space in your tummy while getting about 5 grams of fiber in each cup of veggies.

5 Keep a container of gorp in your car and office for the munchies. Mix together peanuts, raisins, a high-fiber cereal like All-Bran, and some chocolate-covered soy nuts. Allow yourself one handful for a sweet, yet high-fiber, snack.

6 Switch to whole grain crackers. You'd never think a tiny cracker can make a difference, but one regular whole wheat cracker has ½ gram of fiber. Ten crackers give you 5 grams of fiber. So next time, spread your peanut butter on whole grain crackers (look for brands that proclaim they're trans-fat-free) instead of bread for a different taste treat.

7 Mix your regular cereal with the high-test stuff. Okay, we'll be honest. We wouldn't want to face an entire bowl of All-Bran either. But just ⅓ cup packs a walloping 8.5 grams of fiber. Mix it with an equal amount of Apple Cinnamon Cheerios and you'll barely know it's there (but you will be

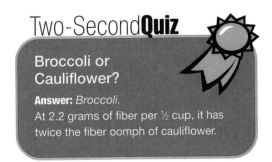

Two-Second Quiz

Broccoli or Cauliflower?

Answer: *Broccoli.*
At 2.2 grams of fiber per ½ cup, it has twice the fiber oomph of cauliflower.

one-third of the way to your daily fiber intake). Check out the Nature's Path brands, which offer several truly delicious, high-fiber choices.

8 Add kidney beans or chickpeas to your next salad. A quarter cup adds an additional 5 grams of dietary fiber, notes Lisa Andrews, R.D., a nutritionist at the VA Medical Center in Cincinnati.

9 Make sure that the first ingredient in whole grain products has the word "whole" in it, as in "whole wheat," or "whole grain." If it says multi-grain, seven-grain, nutra-grain, cracked wheat, stone-ground wheat, unbromated wheat or enriched wheat, it's not whole wheat, and thus is lacking some of the vitamins and minerals, not to mention fiber, of whole grains.

10 Every week, try one "exotic" grain. How about amaranth, bulgur, or wheatberries? Most are as simple to fix as rice, yet packed with fiber and flavor. Mix in some steamed carrots and broccoli, toss with olive oil and a bit of Parmesan or feta cheese, maybe throw in a can of tuna or a couple of ounces of cut-up chicken, and you've got dinner. Or serve as a side dish to chicken or fish. Make sure all grains you try are whole grains.

11 Once a week, make pearl barley (which doesn't require any soaking before cooking) as a side dish. One cup sports 10 grams of fiber, nearly half your daily allotment.

12 Sneak in oatmeal. Use regular oatmeal in place of bread crumbs for meat loaf and meatballs, sprinkle it atop casseroles and ice cream, bake it into cookies and muffins, and add it to homemade breads and cakes.

13 Use whole wheat bread to make your lunchtime sandwich every day. Even Subway and other such sandwich shops offer whole wheat options for lunchtime munching. If you want to gradually break into the whole wheat club, use whole wheat bread as the bottom slice of your sandwich and regular bread as the top layer, suggests Joan Salge Blake, R.D., clinical assistant professor of nutrition at Boston University's Sargent College. Eventually, make the whole switch to whole grains.

14 Every week, switch from a white food to a brown food. So instead of instant white rice, you switch to instant brown rice. Instead of regular pasta, you switch to whole wheat pasta. Similarly, whole wheat pitas instead of regular, whole wheat burritos instead of corn, whole wheat couscous instead of regular. Within two months, you should be eating only whole grains, and should have increased your daily fiber consumption by an easy 10 grams without radically changing your diet!

15 Spread your sandwich with ½ cup hummus. Bam! You just got 7.5 grams of fiber in a tasty package. Lay some spinach leaves and a tomato slice atop for another couple of grams.

16 Make beans a part of at least one meal a day. They're packed with fiber (15 grams in just a cup of black beans) and, since they come canned, so easy to use. Just rinse before using to remove excess sodium. Here are some Stealth Healthy tips for getting your beans:

▶ Puree a can of cannelloni beans for a tasty dip. Add 2 cloves garlic and a tablespoon each of lemon juice and olive oil to the blender. Use as a dip for veggies and whole grain crackers.

▶ Spread nonfat refried beans on a whole wheat burrito and sprinkle with chopped chicken and shredded cheese.

▶ Use ½ cup black beans and salsa as a filling for your morning omelet.

▶ Make a bean salad with canned black beans, fresh or frozen corn kernels, chopped cilantro, chopped onion, and chopped tomato. Drizzle with olive oil and a dash of vinegar, salt, and pepper.

▶ Make your own special chili pizza. Top a prepared (whole wheat) pizza crust with some kidney beans, shredded cheese, and ground turkey cooked with chili flavorings.

Do**Three**Things

From Fred Pescatore, M.D., author of *The Hamptons Diet*, comes this list of the best ways to get more fiber in your diet:

1. Eat more fruits and vegetables. They're the healthiest fiber sources around.

2. Start each day with a bowl of whole-grain cereal.

3. Switch to a whole grain bread.

▶ Start serving edamame (soybeans) as a side dish. You'll get 4 grams of fiber in ⅔ cup of the sweet legumes, not to mention the cancer-fighting phytonutrients inherent in soy.

17 Add pureed cauliflower to mashed potatoes. You won't taste a difference, but you will get some extra fiber, say the nutrition twins, Tammy Lakatos Shames, R.D., and Lyssie Lakatos, R.D. The two are the authors of *Fire Up Your Metabolism: 9 Proven Principles for Burning Fat and Losing Weight Forever.*

18 Have a beet salad for dinner. These bright red veggies have virtually no fat, no cholesterol, no sodium, quite a bit of potassium, and 2 grams of fiber. Try roasting whole, peeled beets for 45 minutes, chilling, then dicing into a summer salad.

In Perspective

The Weight-Loss Wars

For nearly two decades, there has been a war among both consumers and doctors regarding the best approach to weight loss: a low-carb diet or a low-fat diet. On a popular basis, the winner is clear: Low-carb diets such as Atkins, South Beach, and the Zone have won the hearts of weight-minded Americans. But the medical establishment remains vehement about the low-fat message. Can't they all just get along?

Well, yes. As is often the case, research has caught up with all the claims, and proved that there are strengths and weaknesses to both approaches. Today the war is near its end, and a truce is emerging that brings the best science from both sides to form what is likely to be the standard weight-loss message for the next several years—and beyond, we hope.

The message is that excess animal fat in your diet is indeed bad for your health and your weight. But certain fats, particularly plant-based ones like olive oil, are necessary for good health and nutrition. Likewise, excessive amounts of simple carbohydrates are bad for your health too. They are converted too easily into blood sugar, and cause all types of metabolic havoc when you eat them regularly. Much better are unrefined, whole grain foods that take longer to digest and contain more nutrients and fiber.

Put it all together, and you get a sensible diet rich with complex carbohydrates and lean, healthy meats and seafood. Plus loads and loads of vegetables. We can all live with that, can't we?

Problem is, the low-carb movement is so strong that the pendulum may be swinging too far in its favor. Recall what happened a decade ago: The low-fat movement was so prevalent that the marketplace became flooded with low-fat snacks and alternatives. The problem was these products were loaded with calorie-dense carbs, and people consumed huge amounts of them. The result: Many people kept gaining weight.

That is the big fear today of the low-carb diet craze—that people will think they can eat unlimited low-carb snacks and meals. And currently, the marketplace is suddenly overrun with low-carb products and outlandish claims of weight-loss success using them.

At the end of the day, weight loss is about eating moderate amounts of healthy foods. What we've confirmed most recently is that simple carbs are more unhealthy than we thought. Respond *sensibly* to that finding, and you are on your way to a lifetime of healthier weight and diet.

19 **Make rice pudding for dessert tonight.** Only instead of white rice, use brown to, as Emeril would say, "kick it up a notch."

20 **Snack on popcorn.** The microwave variety works just fine, but we prefer air-popped popcorn without the oil. Each cup of popcorn delivers 1.2 grams of fiber.

21 **Switch to whole wheat flour when baking.** You can start by going half and half, eventually using only whole wheat flour for all your cooking needs.

22 **Throw some flaxseeds, wheat germ, or other high-fiber** add-ins into batter. They add crunch to your cookies, muffins, and breads—and loads of fiber.

23 **Eat the skin of your baked and sweet potatoes.** Eating baked potatoes with the skin instead of mashed ups the fiber at least 3 grams (depending on the size of the potato).

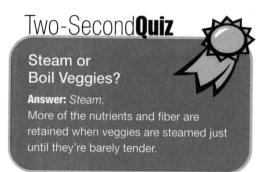

Two-SecondQuiz

Steam or Boil Veggies?

Answer: *Steam.*
More of the nutrients and fiber are retained when veggies are steamed just until they're barely tender.

24 **Start every dinner with a mixed green salad.** Not only will it add fiber, but with a low-calorie vinaigrette dressing, it will partially fill you up with very few calories, and thus offers great benefits in weight loss/control.

25 **Always add lettuce and tomato slices** rather than cheese to sandwiches. Not only do they add fiber, but they also reduce calories.

26 **Use beans or lentils as the main protein source for dinner** once or twice a week. A classic dish such as pasta e fagioli works well.

27 **Make your fiber sources suit the seasons.** A cold lentil salad, or corn and black bean salad in summer (or maybe a salade niçoise), then vegetarian chili in winter.

28 **Snack on dried fruit every day.** Tasty, chewy, satisfying, easy to eat on the go—and loaded with fiber. Try dried apricots, dates, figs, peaches, pears, and bananas.

29 **Drink your fiber.** Make your own smoothies by blending whole fruits (cut out the big seeds). If everything in the fruit goes into your glass, you'll get the fiber from the peel, often missing from fruit juice.

Don't Forget To...

Drink plenty of water. You need water to help the fiber pass through your digestive system without getting, ahem, stuck. So as you're increasing the fiber in your diet, also increase the amount of water or other unsweetened beverage you're getting. Also, don't up your fiber load all at once. That's just going to overwhelm your system, leading to gas, bloating, and constipation. Instead, start slowly. Try one tip a week for the first couple of weeks, then two, then three. By week four or five, you should be up to the full 25-30 grams—or more.

Cutting Back on "Bad" Carbs

16 WAYS TO MAKE LOW-CARB HEALTHY

Thanks to the popularity of low-carb diets, nearly half of Americans say they are watching the amount of carbohydrates they eat. If you're among them, we're providing these 16 tips so your carb control is stealthy, healthy, and wise!

Bear in mind that there is a huge difference between Cheese Doodles and oatmeal. Both might be categorized as carbs, but their benefits are on opposite ends of the health spectrum. In the last chapter, we detailed the benefits of "good carbs." Now it's time to explain what a "bad carb" is. Here's the simplest answer: white flour, refined sugar, and white rice. More broadly, any food made primarily of a carb that has been processed in such a way as to strip out ingredients that hinder quick and easy cooking. Why are refined carbs a problem? Easy: They digest so quickly that they cause blood sugar surges that lead to weight gain and other health troubles.

In the next chapter we show you ways to reduce the amount of sugar you eat. Here we'll give you other ways to avoid troublesome carbs while still getting the fuel you need for good health. Carb-counting meets common sense, right this way...

1 **Tell the waiter to hold the bread.** At almost every restaurant, your meal starts with a basket of rolls, breads, and crackers made from white flour. If it's not put on the table, you won't eat any. Or, if you really need something to nibble on, ask if they have whole wheat varieties.

2 **At Chinese restaurants, ask for brown rice,** and limit how much you eat to one cup. In fact, some Chinese restaurants have started offering to swap a vegetable for the rice in their combo dinners, knowing that many people are on low-carb diets. At home, always cook brown rice instead of white. Brown rice hasn't been processed and still has its high-fiber nutrients.

3 **Instead of bread, use eggplant slices** to make a delicious sandwich. Broil two thick slices of eggplant until brown, then add mozzarella and tomato, olive oil and basil to one slice, suggests Nicole Glassman, owner of Mindful Health in New York City. Top with the other slice of eggplant and broil again until the cheese melts.

4 **Wrap your food in lettuce leaves.** Yes, skip the bun, tortillas, and bread slices and instead make a sandwich inside lettuce leaves. Glassman suggests going Mexican with a sprinkle of cheddar cheese, salsa, and chicken; Asian with sesame seeds, peanuts, bean sprouts, cut up green beans,

Mustard or Ketchup?

Answer: *Mustard.*
Most ketchups have nearly the sugar content of a candy bar. Some mustards have added sugar, too, but most don't, so finding one without added sugar shouldn't be a problem.

and shrimp with a touch of soy sauce; or deli style with turkey, cheese, and mustard.

5 Buy old-fashioned snacks in kid-size bags.

Truth is, pretzels, tortilla chips, potato chips, and cookies are mostly bad carbs, made primarily of refined flour, sugar, salt, and/or oil. You want to remove as many of these foods from your daily eating as you can. But if you can't live without them, buy them in small bags—1 ounce is a typical "lunch box" size—and limit yourself to just one bag a day.

6 Break yourself of your old spaghetti habits.

Almost everyone loves a big bowl of pasta, topped with a rich tomato sauce. The tomato sauce couldn't be better for you; the spaghetti, however, is pure carbohydrate. While spaghetti is fine to eat every now and then, for those sensitive to carbs or wishing to cut back on their noodle intake, here are some alternatives to the usual spaghetti dinner:

▸ Here's the easiest choice: Switch to whole wheat pasta. It is denser than traditional pasta, with a firm, al dente texture similar to what you'd get in Italy.
▸ Grill vegetables such as eggplant, zucchini, bell peppers, and onion and slice them into long, thin pieces. Mix up and pour your spaghetti sauce over the vegetables for a delicious and immensely healthy meal.

▸ Substitute spaghetti squash for the pasta. Boil or microwave the squash until soft, then scoop out the seeds and pull the strands of squash from the shell with a fork. Top with your favorite sauce and a grating of real Parmesan.
▸ Try healthy whole grains as a replacement for pasta. Spaghetti sauce goes better than you'd expect on brown rice, barley, chickpeas, and such.

7 Cut up 1-ounce portions of cheese and divvy up 1-ounce portions of nuts

into tiny snack bags. Now you have a handy snack at the ready.

8 Eat potatoes boiled with the skin on.

The effect of potatoes on blood sugar depends on how the potatoes are prepared. No need to unspud yourself completely! Also, new potatoes tend to have fewer simple carbs than other types of potatoes.

9 Eat lightly of the new low-carb products.

More than 1,000 low-carb products were introduced in 2003, but the FDA has yet to publish any guidelines as to what "low carb" really means. Instead, many new "low carb" foods are to carb-cutting what "low fat" cookies were to fat-cutting: just a new way of pitching foods high in calories and low in nutrient value. In fact, *Consumer Reports* found that many packaged low-carb foods are actually higher in calories than their regular counterparts. For instance, a serving of Keto's low-carb Rocky Road ice cream has 270 calories, almost double the calories found in many regular ice creams and twice as much fat.

10 Think lightly of the new net-carb measurements.

Many of the low-carb weight-loss programs are trying to get their followers to use "net carbs" as the measurement of choice for the appropriateness of a carb food in their diet. This is a measurement of the "bad carbs" left in a food after you adjust for those carb ingredients that don't immediately affect blood sugar. The folks at Atkins Nutritionals say the proper way to measure net carbs is to subtract fiber (as well as sugar alcohols and glycerin, when applicable) from the total carbs listed on the nutrition facts panel of a product. But that's just their version, and that's the problem. "Net carbs" is not a regulated or standardized measurement—manufacturers can define it how they want, and say what they want on product packaging. And there is no science to say that tracking net carbs offers any unique weight-loss benefit.

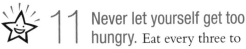 **11** **Never let yourself get too hungry.** Eat every three to five waking hours, and eat only until you're satisfied but not stuffed. You should never reach the point where you feel ravenous. Not only is that a recipe for overeating, but your body will want sugary, quick-to-digest "bad carbs" to quickly satiate your need for fuel.

12 **Instead of eggs and bacon, try low-carb versions of cereals.** For example, the Nature's Path cereal line offers all the benefits of whole grains without the "problem" carbs found in added sugar. Another option is low-carb, high-fiber muffins and breads (spread with no-sugar-added jams or nut butter).

 In**Perspective**

Glycemic Index vs. Glycemic Load

The glycemic index (GI) is a measure of how much, and how fast, the sugar in a food raises the level of sugar in your blood. A high or fast rise in blood sugar leads to high blood insulin levels, contributing to weight-control problems and possibly even increasing your risk of diabetes over time. So, in theory at least, a high glycemic index is a bad thing.

But the measure has very important limitations. For one thing, it is based on comparing foods directly to one another to determine which raise blood sugar more. These comparisons are based on an equivalent "dose" of sugar in each food

in an effort to be fair. To make the dose of sugar in carrots equivalent to the dose of sugar in ice cream, however, calls for the comparison of a tiny dish of ice cream to a bushel of carrots. Of course, the carrots will have the higher glycemic index.

Another limitation of the GI is that it is based on the effects of just one food, eaten alone. In real life, of course, the foods we eat interact with each other to determine blood sugar levels. High-fiber cereal at breakfast, for example, will blunt the rise in blood sugar from eating high GI foods at lunch.

A newer measure, called the glycemic load, accounts

for both how fast the sugar in a food is converted to blood sugar and the dose of sugar in the food. Whereas the glycemic index of soda is similar to that of carrots, the glycemic load of the soda is fully 10 times higher than that of carrots.

Should you worry about the glycemic index or load of the foods you eat? That's one for your doctor to answer. If you have diabetes or are prone to blood sugar swings and weight gain, being aware of the impact of food on your blood sugar is important. But for most of us, a healthy diet probably precludes the need to track these measurements.

13 At the movies, skip the popcorn. Popcorn isn't a bad food—we suggest it in the fiber chapter, in fact. But it does happen to be a simple carb with little other nutritional value and, when bought at the theater, is often drowning in salt and fat as well. Better movie snacks are small bags of nuts or seeds and fresh or dried fruit. Just sneak them into the theater in your purse or a backpack.

14 Mix up a sweet dessert. Combine nonfat cream, unsweetened cocoa, sugar substitute, and ice in a blender. Or mix mascarpone and sugar substitute with whipped cream and a hint of lemon zest.

15 Make your own quickie low-carb pizza. Lightly toast a whole grain, low-carb tortilla and top with chopped tomatoes and shredded, part-skim, mozzarella cheese. Season with salt

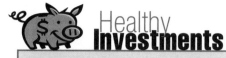

Healthy Investments

An Egg Slicer

Eggs are an ideal source of protein, low in calories and saturated fat. For a great lunch treat, use an egg slicer to slice and dice hard-boiled eggs for egg salad. Mix in some low-fat mayonnaise, chopped celery, and salt and pepper to taste. Serve on lettuce leaves.

and pepper and return to the toaster oven until cheese is melted and bubbling.

16 Make french fries with turnips. Missing those fries with that bunless burger? Heimowitz suggests cutting turnips into sticks and tossing with olive oil and salt. Bake at 425°F for 30 minutes, turning frequently. Voilà! A crisp side dish with none of the fat of frying and far fewer carbs than from potatoes.

Cutting the Carbs Without Hitting Your Pocketbook

When food marketing expert Phil Lempert of the Supermarket Guru Web site analyzed grocery bills for one person following the first phases of the Atkins and South Beach diets, (the two most popular low-carb diets) he found that the cost of observing strictly the portion size and ingredients in a week-long program totaled $99.89 on Atkins and $91.28 on South Beach. In contrast, the Food Marketing Institute finds that the average one-person household spends about $59 a week on groceries.

For easy ways to stay low-carb without breaking the bank, follow these recommendations from Lempert:

- Replace salmon and other more expensive fishes with chicken breast or tofu.

- Always buy frozen fish rather than fresh (most fresh fish has been previously frozen anyway). There is little nutritional or taste difference, but you will see a price savings.

- Buy frozen berries, including blueberries, strawberries, and raspberries. They're almost always less expensive than fresh (except

maybe during peak growing season for your area).

- Instead of Canadian or other bacons, choose lean boiled ham. It could cost half as much.

- Replace mixed green salads with any dark leafy green (mustard, kale, spinach). Buy whole heads of greens rather than bagged and washed greens, which could cost up to 20 percent more.

- Replace extra virgin olive oil on salads and in recipes with canola oil.

Cutting Down on Sugar

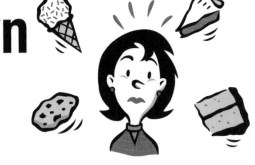

23 WAYS TO GET RID OF THE SWEET STUFF

America is a country drowning in sugar. In fact, the amount of sugar we eat and drink every year has soared nearly 30 percent since 1983 and is likely a major contributor to the soaring rates of overweight and obesity in this country. Even worse, since sugary foods often replace more healthy foods, nutrition experts say the influx of sweets indirectly contributes to diseases like osteoporosis, heart disease, and cancer—all of which are directly affected by what we eat.

Although the USDA recommends we get no more than 10 teaspoons of sugar a day, the average American downs about 34 teaspoons—more than three times as much. In this third chapter on carbohydrates, we show you ways to get your sugar consumption down to healthy levels. But beware: Uncovering all the sugar in your diet isn't easy. Sugar often hides under several pseudonyms and turns up in even the most innocuous foods (like bread, crackers, salad dressing, ketchup, and mustard). But with the following Stealth Health tips, you should be able to have your cake and eat it too.

1 **Cut down slowly.** Forget going cold turkey. Therein lies failure. Instead, if you normally have two candy bars a day, cut to one a day. Then next week, one every other day. The following week, one every three days, until you're down to just one a week. If you normally take 2 teaspoons of sugar in your coffee, use the same routine, cutting down to 1½ teaspoons for a week, then 1, then ½. Eventually, get to the point where you're using artificial sweetener if you still need the sweet taste. The more sugar you eat, the more you'll crave. So cutting down slowly is the best way to tame a sweet tooth gone wild.

2 **Go half and half.** Mix half a regular soda with half a diet soda. Half a carton of sweetened yogurt with half a carton of plain yogurt. Half a cup of regular juice with half a cup of seltzer. Do this for two weeks, then cut back to one-quarter sweetened to three-quarters unsweetened. Continue until you're only drinking the unsweetened version.

3 **Grant yourself a daily sugar "quota," and use it** on foods where it matters most. For most of us, that means desserts. Don't waste it on dressings,

spreads, breakfast cereals, and soda. Not only will this reduce your sugar intake in a day, but it will help you lose your sweet tooth. Sugar is incredibly addictive: The more you eat, the more addictive it becomes and the more it takes to satisfy you. The opposite is also true: Train your taste buds to become accustomed to less and you'll be satisfied with less.

4 Establish rules about dessert. For instance, only have dessert after dinner, never lunch. Only eat dessert on odd days of the month, or only on weekends, or only at restaurants. If you have a long tradition of daily desserts, then make it your rule to have raw fruit at least half the time.

5 Similarly, establish rules about ice cream. A half gallon of ice cream in the freezer is temptation defined. A rule we recommend: No ice cream kept at home. Ice cream should always be a treat worth traveling for.

6 Instead of downing sugary-sweet drinks like lemonade, make your own "sun tea." Steep decaffeinated tea bags in water and set the pitcher in the sun for a couple of hours. Add lemon, lots of ice and sugar substitute for a carb-free summer quaff.

7 Buy dietetic condiments at the grocery store. Given that 1 tablespoon ketchup can contain about ½ teaspoon sugar, buying sugar-free condiments can make a big dent in your sugar consumption. Most condiments and other packaged foods for people with diabetes are made without sugar or with sugar substitutes.

8 Remember these code words found on ingredient lists. The only way to know if the processed food you're buying contains sugar is to know its many aliases or other forms. Here are the common ones: brown sugar, corn syrup, dextrin, dextrose, fructose, fruit juice concentrate, high-fructose corn syrup, galactose, glucose, honey, hydrogenated starch, invert sugar maltose, lactose, mannitol, maple syrup, molasses, polyols, raw sugar, sorghum, sucrose, sorbitol, turbinado sugar, and xylitol.

9 Look for hidden sources of sugar. Cough syrups, chewing gum, mints, tomato sauce, baked beans, and lunch meats often contain sugar. Even some prescription medications contain sugar. For a week, be particularly vigilant and scan every possible food label. You likely won't forget what you'll find.

10 If you must eat sweets, eat them with meals. The other foods will help increase salivary flow, thus clearing the sugary foods from your mouth faster and helping prevent cavities. Of course, this does nothing for the calories you're imbibing and won't affect your weight, but at least you'll have a healthier mouth.

Two-Second**Quiz**

Apple or Sugar-Free Applesauce?

Answer: *Apple.*
You'll get all the nutrients of the applesauce, but you'll also get the added fiber kick from the skin of the apple, which is removed before making applesauce.

11 Try all-fruit spread. Sweet as sugar, but without the added sugar, all-fruit spreads are wonderful not just on toast, but melted into hot tea, mixed into cottage cheese and plain yogurt, and drizzled onto pancakes and waffles instead of syrup (heat for 10 seconds in the microwave to make it syrupy).

12 Substitute applesauce or pureed prunes for half the sugar in recipes. You can also use them in place of the recipe's fat.

13 Nix the sports bars and drinks. They're loaded with the "s" word! Same with many protein powders.

14 Try xylitol. A great sugar alternative, it's safe for those with diabetes and it actually improves the quality of your teeth. Plus, it has fiber-like health benefits.

15 Get your chocolate in small doses. Dip fresh strawberries into nonfat chocolate sauce, scatter chocolate sprinkles over your plain yogurt, or eat a mini-piece of dark chocolate—freeze it so it lasts longer in your mouth. Think rich and decadent but in tiny portions.

16 Choose the right breakfast cereal. Many of them are loaded with sugar. You want one with less than 8 grams sugar per serving or, preferably,

In Perspective

Corn Syrup

Ask someone what he thinks of when he hears the word "sweet," and chances are he'll respond "sugar." But since its arrival in the marketplace in 1966, the real story in the sweetness world has been corn syrup, to the point that newspapers and magazines are now declaring this alternative sweetener the number one evil in our diets. Today the average American consumes more than 62 pounds of corn syrup a year.

High-fructose corn syrup is generally cheaper and easier to refine than granulated sugar. So, increasingly, processed food companies have been switching to corn syrup to add sweetness to

their products. It is most used in soft drinks and juices. That would have been the end of the story, except for recent research results that suggest that the human body processes corn syrup differently from sugar.

According to the studies, when the body processes sugar, it triggers the production of a chemical that signals fullness to your brain, and also prevents the release of a chemical that signals hunger. But when scientists monitored how the body processes corn syrup, the worst-case scenario seemed to have occurred: The hunger chemical wasn't affected, and the fullness chemical

was suppressed. In short, corn syrup, in theory, makes you hungrier.

Is this true? Doctors are debating the point. Many believe that the issue is merely that calories consumed as liquid are less filling than calories from solid food, independent of the form of the calories.

Whatever the case, corn syrup is a big issue for anyone trying to eat healthily. It is ubiquitous, and it is a huge source of empty calories that mess with your body's chemistry. So fight back, starting with bottled drinks. If corn syrup is one of the first four ingredients in a drink, put it back.

Brown Sugar or White Sugar?

Answer: *Neither.*
They're both sugar. Neither has any nutritional benefit or is any better than the other. Here's a case where the brown color does *not* imply a healthier version.

unsweetened altogether (steel-cut oatmeal anyone?). Use diced fruit to sweeten your cereal.

17 **Don't skip meals.** Too busy to eat? When you go without breakfast, lunch, or dinner, your blood sugar levels drop, propelling you toward high-sugar (often convenience) foods to quell your cravings.

18 **Seek out substitutes.** With Equal, Splenda, Nutrasweet, and the natural sweetener stevia now easily available, you can still get the sweetness of sugar without the calories.

19 **Don't add sugar to foods.** Many everyday recipes—including those for vegetables, soups, casseroles, and sauces—call for sugar to add sweetness. In most cases, it's just not needed. So if you're making biscuits, for instance, you probably can skip the sugar. Likewise, make your

own barbecue sauce with fresh ingredients, which will cut out the extra sugar in the ketchup.

20 **Watch out for mixed alcohol drinks.** Have you ever stopped to think about the sugar quotient of a cosmopolitan? How about a margarita or mai tai? Drink mixes and many alcoholic beverages are absolutely thick with sugar. Stick with beer, wine, or if you prefer spirits, mix only with unsweetened seltzer or drink it straight. Of course, seltzer water with lime will also do just fine.

21 **Go for a walk when you crave sweetness.** Studies find that athletes' preference for sweetened foods declines after exercise. Instead, they prefer salty foods.

22 **Go fat-free if you must have sweets.** Studies find that many sweet foods, such as doughnuts, muffins, ice cream, and so on, are also high in fat, more than doubling the calorie load. When you do indulge in sweets, go fat-free so you get the calories from the taste you want—but not from the fat.

23 **If you're having a hard time cutting back on sodas or juices,** try having a glass of iced water or soda water every *other* time you reach for a drink.

Cutting Back on Bad Fats

35 WAYS TO GET LEAN THE RIGHT WAY

We've come a long way nutritionally from the days when all fat was bad. Today researchers and doctors recognize that there's no reason to tar every fat with the same brush. Instead, they've now identified the "good" fats (monounsaturated and polyunsaturated) and the "bad" fats (saturated and trans fats).

The good news is that we can now eat certain fats and still be perfectly healthy. And let's be honest—fats often taste rich and wonderful. The downside? To make smart choices, you have to be conscious now of four types of fats. But there's an easy way to figure this out. Basically, if a fat is a solid when at room temperature, chances are it's a bad fat. That would include most animal fats, butter, shortening, and some nut oils. Good fats are usually in fish and plant oils. Remember that, and you are well on your way to choosing the right fats.

Of course, even good fats have their limits. All fats provide your body with 9 calories per gram, more than twice as much as proteins or carbohydrates. And in the end, weight gain and weight loss are about calories. For good health and weight, keep your total fat intake to 30 percent of calories or less, and keep saturated fat intake to less than 10 percent of calories in a day or less. Trans fats? Try to keep them to zero. Here is a slew of ways to follow all of these important health rules:

1 **We'll start with the easiest: Choose low-fat products over regular.** Do not accept the argument that low-fat versions don't taste as good. It's not true! Low-fat versions may not taste the way you or your family is *used to,* but after a week or two of using the new version, you'll stop noticing the subtle decline in richness. Here are the places to start:

- *Milk:* You need not jump all the way to no-fat; 1% milk is perfectly healthy, but still has that rich milk flavor. Use 2% as a stepping-stone from whole milk, but don't stop there—35 percent of the calories still come from fat in 2% milk.
- *Ice cream:* Most "light" versions taste as rich and creamy as the full-fat versions. We particularly like the Breyer's line of light ice creams.
- *Yogurt:* Given that most people eat their yogurt flavored, it is hard to notice the difference between regular and low- or no-fat versions.

- *Ground beef:* Don't think that buying fatty ground beef and pouring off the grease makes it fine. Much of the fat is bound in with the meat. Good quality, 90-percent-or-more ground sirloin is leaner and healthier for you.
- *Cheese:* Particularly mozzarella cheese for pizza. Low-fat versions still have all the taste and texture you so desire.

2 **Keep your spreads soft.** That means choosing soft margarines, and leaving your butter out of the refrigerator. The softer the spread, the less you'll use on your toast or bagel, thus the fewer saturated fats you'll get. Also, remember this: The softer the margarine is at room temperature, the lower the amount of trans fats it contains.

3 **Choose sat-fat-free spreads.** It's amazing what manufacturers can come up with when they put their minds to it. Today you can find butter-like spreads in your refrigerated sections that are low or even free of all saturated and

In**Perspective**

The Ins and Outs of Fat

Confused about fat? Don't be. It's really quite simple. There are three naturally occurring types of fat: monounsaturated, polyunsaturated, and saturated. A fourth type of fat—"trans fats"—is man-made. Here's what you need to know about each one, minus all the science.

- **Monounsaturated fat.** These fats should take the lead in your diet (at least, as far as fat is concerned). They star in the so-called Mediterranean diet, proven to lower cholesterol and reduce the risk of heart disease. A primary source of mono fats is olive oil. Other good sources include canola oil, seeds and nuts, and avocados.

- **Polyunsaturated fat.** This form of fat is prevalent in vegetable oils, nuts, fish, and some leafy green vegetables. There are two main types of the "polys": omega-6s, which we tend to get plenty of through corn and other vegetable oils, and omega-3s, found primarily in fish and certain seeds, which we rarely get enough of. Focus on increasing the amount of omega-3 fatty acids in your diet while reducing the amount of omega-6s and you'll get the right ratio of polys.

- **Saturated fat.** This form of fat is found in the highest amounts in animal products, as well as palm and coconut oil. You'll know a fat is heavy on the saturated side if it's solid at room temperature, like shortening or lard. Saturated fat raises levels of "bad" LDL cholesterol, and can increase your risk of heart disease. In fact, switching just 5 percent of your overall calories from saturated to unsaturated fats could slash your risk of a fatal heart attack as much as 42 percent.

- **Trans fats.** Trans fats are polyunsaturated fats gone bad. They don't exist in nature, but are created when polyunsaturated fats are whipped with hydrogen to make them solid at room temperature. They not only increase LDL levels, but they can decrease HDL levels. They've been implicated in heart disease and breast cancer. When it comes to trans fat, no level is safe. Yet they're everywhere you find processed foods, including nearly all crackers, cookies, baked goods, snacks, and other packaged foods. The good news is, these days you can find trans-fat-free options in nearly every food category; you just have to look for them.

trans fats, and that actually taste good. Good brands to try include Benecol (which will also help lower your cholesterol when used regularly), Canoleo, Earth Balance Natural Buttery Spread, and Blue Bonnet. All except Blue Bonnet are trans-fat-free; Blue Bonnet has 0.5 mg trans fat per serving.

4 **Buy a pretty bottle, fill it with olive oil, then top it with a liquor stop.** You know, the kind you use to pour out shots of liquor. Now keep the bottle on your counter in plain view and use it for everything short of frying (olive oil burns at high temperatures). Olive oil is the best oil to use because it contains high amounts of monounsaturated fats and low amounts of saturated fats (all oils contain a mixture of the three: mono, poly, and saturated; the key is the ratio), isn't too strongly flavored, and is affordable. Buy the deepest green, extra virgin olive oil you can find—the darker the color, the greater the amount of phytonutrients, potent little plant-based cancer fighters.

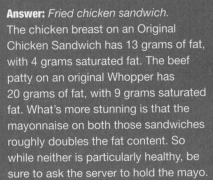

Two-Second**Quiz**

Burger King Fried Chicken Sandwich or Whopper?

Answer: *Fried chicken sandwich.* The chicken breast on an Original Chicken Sandwich has 13 grams of fat, with 4 grams saturated fat. The beef patty on an original Whopper has 20 grams of fat, with 9 grams saturated fat. What's more stunning is that the mayonnaise on both those sandwiches roughly doubles the fat content. So while neither is particularly healthy, be sure to ask the server to hold the mayo.

5 **If you can't go without your butter, mix it with olive oil.** Let a stick of butter soften at room temperature, suggests Barbara Morris, R.Ph., a pharmacist, speaker, and anti-aging expert and author. Beat the butter smooth, then slowly beat in ¼ or ½ cup olive oil. You've just significantly cut the amount of saturated fat while adding loads of healthy monounsaturated fat.

6 **Eat the right meats.** Sure, meat is one of the primary forms of saturated fat. But meat—whether red or white—is also an excellent source of protein and trace minerals like zinc and iron. The key is choosing the right meats. For instance, of the 19 cuts of beef that meet the USDA's labeling guidelines for lean, 12 have only 1 more gram of saturated fat on average than a comparable 3-ounce cooked serving of skinless chicken. The best choices include top sirloin beef, with 2.4 grams saturated fat, and chuck pot roast, with 3 grams saturated fat.

7 **Don't be taken in by the "other white meat" slogan.** Put simply, lean chicken is much less fatty than lean pork. A 3-ounce serving of broiled chicken breast (no skin) provides 140 calories, 27 from fat, and only one-third of that fat is saturated. The same serving of roasted lean pork loin delivers 275 calories, 189 of them from fat, half of which is saturated. To top it off, the chicken has 6 more grams of protein than the pork.

8 **Once a week, eat an exotic meat in place of beef or pork.** We're talking emu, bison (buffalo), venison, wild boar, or ostrich. All have less than 1 gram of saturated fat per 3-ounce serving, are super rich with protein, and taste extremely good.

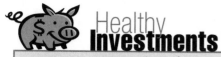

Healthy Investments

A Nonstick Pan

In the old days, you needed lots of butter and oil in order to keep your meats and veggies from sticking to the pan. A nonstick pan eliminates all that. Hint: Make sure the pan is hot before adding the oil. This creates a barrier between the pan and the food, eliminating any possibility of sticking. Another great option: a panini maker for grilled sandwiches.

9 Rinse ground meat under hot water after cooking. This rinses away a good deal of the fat.

10 Find ways to cook your steak with other ingredients. The goal: Stop putting whole slabs of steak in front of you. Instead, slice the raw beef and sauté with peppers and onions, fajita style. Or cook steak pieces in a wok with lots of vegetables (pepper steak, beef and broccoli). Or top a crunchy, robust salad with steak slices. Or make shish kebab with steak cubes and veggies. Why? You almost always eat less meat when you prepare it as part of a nicely integrated dish. Hold off on the whole steak for very special occasions.

11 Be wary, though, of recipes that allow starches and veggies to absorb fat. Many classic winter dishes have potatoes, carrots, turnips, and other vegetables roasting slowly with chicken, beef, lamb, or pork. Delicious, sure. But all those foods are soaking up a whole lot of fat that's dripped off the meat. It's a little more effort, but either find ways to cook the vegetables separately, or wait until you've skimmed the fat from the meat juices before adding in the vegetables.

12 Follow a simple rule: If you can plainly see fat on your food, remove it. Here's what we mean:

- If there is fat on the meat, trim it off.
- If there is skin on the chicken, remove it.
- If there is oil pooling on the top of the pizza, sop it up with a paper towel.
- If there is dressing pooled at the bottom of your salad, pour it off.
- If there's a pool of juice under a cooked meat (and it's not a sauce), drain it.
- If there's fat at the top of a bowl of stew or soup, skim it.

13 Cook your flavor into breads, pancakes, muffins, and other carb-based foods so you don't need to add butter. For example, add herbs to breads; blueberries to pancakes; nuts and bananas to muffins. Grain-filled foods are often the ones that you most want to butter, but if you make them more flavorful, you get around the urge.

14 Put salsa on your baked potato, not butter or sour cream. You not only skip the fat, but add in a healthy, low-cal serving of vegetables.

15 Mist your fat. Use a nonfat spray like PAM to coat pans and foods. You can even make a butter-free grilled cheese sandwich by spraying both sides of the bread and the pan with PAM. You'll get the same crunchy, delectable flavor without the fat. You can also buy a contraption called the Misto, which enables you to mist your olive oil, thus using far less than if you poured it.

16 Sauté foods in broth, wine, even juice. These are just a few of the alternatives to filling the bottom of your cookware with calorie-dense oils.

17 Buy the right whole grain crackers. We want you to eat whole grains, but when it comes to crackers, even these supposedly healthy nibbles are often packed with trans fats. Some good ones that either have little or no trans fats include: Ak-Mak 100% Whole Wheat Crackers, Finn Crisp, GG Scandinavian Bran Crispbread, Kavli Whole Grain Crispbread, Wasa, and Kashi TLC.

18 Watch out for trans fats in unexpected places. That would be peanut butter, graham crackers, energy bars, frozen pizza, cereal, and frozen waffles. Even foods you might think of as health foods—such as granola—often carry large amounts of trans fats.

19 Use nonfat evaporated milk in place of cream for cream-based soups and other recipes.

20 Put soups and stews in the refrigerator overnight. Voilà! The next morning you can just skim the congealed fat off the top.

21 Shred your cheese. You'll use less on pasta dishes, sandwiches, etc., if it's shredded than if it's sliced.

22 Use peanut butter in place of butter. Yes, peanut butter is high in fat (21-27 grams per 3 tablespoons) but most of the fat is monounsaturated. Look for sugar- and salt-free peanut butter for an even healthier spread. Also try natural peanut butters, which won't have any trans fats. Stir before eating, as they tend to separate.

23 Order pizza without the fat. Sausage and pepperoni are very high in fats. Whole-milk mozzarella cheese is also high in fat. And excessive olive oil adds too many calories from fat. The answer? As mentioned, mop up the excess grease on the top of the pizza, order vegetables on top, ask for low-fat cheese, and on occasion, order a cheeseless tomato pizza. The *Harvard Women's Health Watch* newsletter notes that a vegetable pizza can have 25 percent fewer calories and about 50 percent less fat and saturated fat than a meat pizza.

24 Stick to mustard, steak sauce, ketchup, and other non-creamy condiments in place of mayonnaise and tartar sauce. Mayonnaise is particularly dense with fat. You should avoid it at all costs. That means making your coleslaw, pasta salads, potato salads, and tuna salads with healthier choices.

25 Puree a cooked potato and an onion to thicken soups instead of cream.

26 Use avocados in place of butter and cream. There's a reason these green fruits are called butterfruit in Mexico—they mash up into the same creamy texture as butter. Try them in soups as a thickening agent, and in mashed potatoes to provide a creamier texture as well as an added taste treat. Interestingly, avocados and olives are the only two fruits high in fat—yet both are rich in heart-healthy monounsaturated fat.

27 Eat a high-fiber cereal for breakfast. So, you're asking, what's cereal got to do with your fat intake? Plenty. Fiber fills you up and seems to reduce your interest in fatty foods. Researchers from the University of Mississippi found that men who ate two daily servings of cereal, each containing 7 grams fiber, reduced their average total fat intake from 91 to 82 grams a day, and their saturated fat intake to less than 10 percent of calories.

28 Substitute soy for meat or cheese at least once a week.
Soy cheese, soy burgers, and soy crumbles (like ground meat) are a great way to cut the saturated fat while retaining some semblance of the original food. Okay, soy products may not be gourmet, but you can certainly handle a switch once a week!

29 Try soy milk on your cereal.
These days, you can even get flavored soy milks. Just make sure to look for brands with added calcium. You can also substitute soy milk in baking and other recipes.

30 Look for the keywords on labels.
Although manufacturers aren't required to begin listing the amount of trans fats in their products until 2006, you can still suss out the bad stuff with a bit of careful label reading. You're looking for the words "partially hydrogenated" or "hydrogenated." If you see that, step away from the food and nobody will get hurt!

31 Do the math yourself.
Even before manufacturers begin listing trans fats on their labels, you can figure out the amount. Simply add the amount of polyunsaturated and monounsaturated fats to the saturated fat. Subtract the sum from the total fat listed on the label. The remainder is trans fat.

32 Take manufacturer labeling with a grain of, ahem, fat.
By 2006, when the government's mandated labeling of trans fats goes into effect, manufacturers will be able to tout their

Two-Second Quiz

Green Olives or Black Olives?
Answer: *Green olives.*
Green olives haven't ripened fully, so they contain roughly half the fat levels that they would have achieved had they ripened and blackened.

products as "trans-free." Some already do. Take their claims with skepticism. Federal rules allow this claim as long as the product has less than 0.5 grams of the nasty fat. But if you eat several servings a day of foods with these tiny amounts of trans fats, you could be getting 5 or more grams a day!

33 Be fast-food savvy.
The amount of fat in a fast-food restaurant meal can be stunning. The french fries, the burgers, the "special sauces" made from mayonnaise, the fried this-and-that, even the salads swimming in oily or creamy dressings may be your worst dietary enemy. Our recommendation: Go to the Web site of each of the fast-food chains you frequent, and take 15 minutes to look at the nutritional analyses of the foods you prefer. After the shock wears away, make a commitment to healthier choices—or much smaller portions.

34 Keep a jar of homemade salad dressing in the fridge.
Bottled dressings are a veritable fount of trans fats. For a good recipe, see page 125.

35 Puree silken tofu.
Works great as a substitute for mayonnaise in recipes, or to blend with frozen fruit and sweetener for a yogurt-like snack. Also try layering it with granola for a parfait.

Cutting Back on Salt

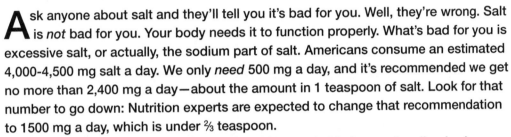

22 WAYS TO EAT WELL WITHOUT IT

Ask anyone about salt and they'll tell you it's bad for you. Well, they're wrong. Salt is *not* bad for you. Your body needs it to function properly. What's bad for you is excessive salt, or actually, the sodium part of salt. Americans consume an estimated 4,000-4,500 mg salt a day. We only *need* 500 mg a day, and it's recommended we get no more than 2,400 mg a day—about the amount in 1 teaspoon of salt. Look for that number to go down: Nutrition experts are expected to change that recommendation to 1500 mg a day, which is under ⅔ teaspoon.

Why lower the sodium recommendation? You probably know of sodium's close connection with high blood pressure. But studies also find high sodium intake can lead to heart and kidney problems, as well as osteoporosis and other bone disorders.

Surprising fact: Only 25 percent of your daily supply of salt comes from the salt-shaker. Most of the rest comes from processed and packaged foods. Manufacturers add loads of sodium to food, both for flavor and to keep it fresh. Even non-salty foods like cereal are loaded with sodium. So the best way to do battle against salt is to cut back on packaged or prepared foods. In addition, try these Stealth Healthy tips for making your food taste great without all that shaking going on.

1 **Stock up on lemon pepper.** This seasoning adds wonderful flavor, not sodium, to your vegetables, meats, and starches. Use it freely as a salt substitute.

2 **Mix low-sodium foods with regular foods** to start you on the path of less sodium intake. Mix no-salt peanuts with regular peanuts, unsalted peanut butter with regular peanut butter, or lite salt with regular salt, suggests Lila Ojeda, R.D., a bionutritionist at Oregon Health Sciences University. Slowly increase the amount of the salt-free product as you decrease the amount of the real thing until you're eating only the salt-free version.

3 **Pick chips over pretzels—but only if salt is the main issue** in your diet. Pretzels can have four times the salt per serving as potato or tortilla chips. But that's because chips get much of their flavor from being cooked in oil, making them much fattier and higher in calories. Pretzels are baked and contain far less fat, so much of their flavor comes from the salt. The better choice for a crunchy snack: baked potato or tortilla chips, which

are relatively low in both fat and sodium. (An even better choice would be an apple or a carrot.)

4 Skip artificial flavorings in chips. That is, say no to barbecue flavor, ranch style, or those sour-cream-and-onion potato chip varieties. Also say no to those fancy flavored corn chips. Those extra flavorings are largely extra salt, and typically double the amount of sodium in a serving.

5 Switch to kosher salt. Because it's coarser, there's less per unit volume. So 1 teaspoon kosher salt has nearly half the sodium of 1 teaspoon table salt. Plus, it's got none of the additives (anticaking agents, whiteners, and iodine).

6 Keep your table salt in a small bowl, and use a tiny spoon or a pinch of your fingers to season your food. You'll find that you use far less of it. Cover it with a snug lid or some plastic wrap to keep it dry (and make it less accessible).

7 Put a big X on your calendar for six weeks from today. Unlike our preference for sugar, which we're born with, salt is an acquired taste, learned from habit. So it takes time to "unlearn" your preference—about six weeks, to be exact. Slowly reduce your intake of salt between

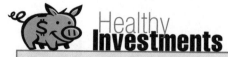

Healthy Investments

Garlic Peeler and Garlic Crusher

These two gadgets make using fresh garlic not only easy, but fun. A garlic peeler—really, a small plastic tube—takes the work and mess out of peeling garlic. Just put a whole garlic clove inside the tube and roll it back and forth, pressing firmly. Voilà! A naked clove, ready for your garlic crusher.

now and then, focusing on food categories where the salt will be missed the least, such as cereals, breads, and dessert items. As long as you know you aren't going to stop wanting salty food overnight, you won't get discouraged.

8 Look out for non-salt sources of sodium. Here's what to watch out for on food labels: sodium, Na, monosodium glutamate or MSG, sodium citrate, baking soda, baking powder, and sodium bicarbonate. They're all forms of—you guessed it!—sodium.

9 Say no to sports drinks. Research does indicate that endurance athletes need higher levels of sodium and far more to drink than everyday folk. Drinks like Gatorade deliver on both—they are rich in salt, which not only provides needed sodium but also stokes continued thirst. For the rest of us, the extra salt provides no benefit at all. Even if you exercise regularly, unless you are testing your body's physical limits for extended periods, water should do fine to quench your thirst.

10 Replace salt in the saltshaker with a salt-free mixture. This way you can still use the shaker, but hold off on the salt, says Jennifer

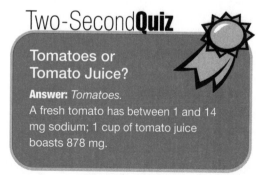

Two-Second Quiz

Tomatoes or Tomato Juice?

Answer: *Tomatoes.*
A fresh tomato has between 1 and 14 mg sodium; 1 cup of tomato juice boasts 878 mg.

Leslie, R.D., a clinical dietitian at the Clarian Heart Failure Clinic in Indianapolis. Mix garlic powder, black pepper, onion powder, and oregano together. Grind the mix fine enough for it to come out the shaker's holes, or buy a Parmesan cheese shaker from a kitchen supply store. Another fun mixture is garlic, onion and chili powder, cumin, dried oregano, and a touch of red pepper flakes.

12 Rinse off canned veggies and beans under running water before cooking. This gets rid of much of the extra sodium.

13 Watch out for salty condiments and nibbles. Capers, pickles, and olives are packed with salt. In fact, the pickling and brining processes used to make foods like these primarily involves soaking them in a solution dense with salt.

11 Use low-sodium alternatives of prepared foods. Read the label and make sure it says the product contains less than 500 mg sodium per serving. See the chart below for some comparisons between the high-test stuff and the low-test stuff. Even if you wind up adding your own salt to the low-sodium versions, you'll still end up with far less salt than if you bought the regular kind.

Instead Of	Sodium (mg)	Choose	Sodium (mg)
La Choy Soy Sauce (1 tablespoon)	1260	La Choy Lite Soy Sauce (1 tablespoon)	530
Del Monte Whole Leaf Spinach, canned (½ cup)	360	Fresh spinach, cooked (½ cup)	45
Nabisco Original Premium Saltines (5)	180	Nabisco Low Sodium Premium Saltines (5)	35
Pasta Roni, Herb & Butter (1 cup)	710	Ronzoni Bow Ties (1 cup)	0
Campbell's Classics Vegetable Beef Soup (½ cup)	810	Campbell's Healthy Request Vegetable Beef Soup (½ cup)	450
Ore-Ida Twice Baked Potato, Garlic Parmesan (1)	390	Baked potato (1)	4
Ragu Old World Style Flavored With Meat (½ cup)	800	Ragu Light Chunky Mushroom & Garlic Spaghetti Sauce (½ cup)	410
Post Raisin Bran (1 cup)	360	Kellogg's All-Bran (1 cup)	130
Stouffer's Chicken Parmigiana (1 package)	1,060	Healthy Choice Cheese Ravioli (1 package)	290
Oscar Meyer Deli-Style Brown Sugar Ham (2 ounces)	812	Boar's Head Deluxe Ham, Lower Sodium (2 ounces)	460

14 Skip meat that's been dried or cured. This includes beef jerky, salami, corned beef, prosciutto, ham, and dried sausages. Each is dense with salt, which was used to draw out the liquid and preserve the meat. Come lunchtime, go for the turkey instead. If you like meat snacks, turkey jerky has far less salt than beef.

15 Brush off visible salt. For instance, on salted bagels or pretzels.

16 Read food labels carefully. They will tell you the amount of sodium per serving. But the labels also give you up to three ways to put that sodium level in perspective. First, food labels often use descriptive phrases, regulated by the federal government. Here's what the phrases mean:

▸ **Sodium free:** Less than 5 mg/serving.
▸ **Low sodium:** 140 mg or less per serving; if the serving is 30 g or less or 2 tablespoons or less, per 50 g of the food.

Two-Second Quiz

Pork Chop or Ham?

Answer: *Pork chop.*
A 3-ounce serving of pork has 59 mg sodium; the same amount of ham has 1,114 mg. That's typical of the difference between raw meat and cured meat.

▸ **Very low sodium:** 35 mg or less per serving; if the serving is 30 g or less or 2 tablespoons or less, per 50 g of the food.
▸ **Reduced or less sodium:** At least 25 percent less per serving than the reference food.

Second, labels tell you sodium per serving as a percentage of the recommended Daily Value (DV) of the mineral (currently 2,400 milligrams for adult men and women). If a serving provides less than 5 percent of the DV, then the food is low in sodium. If it is between 10 and 19 percent, it is moderately high, and if it is over

---

The Problem With Processed

Manufacturers of processed foods load on the salt to help create big, attractive flavors. Here are examples of what happens to "real" food once manufacturers get their hands on it:

Natural Food	Sodium	Processed Food	Sodium
Baked potato	8 mg	Potato chips, about 4 ounces	600 mg
		Large order of french fries	350 mg
		Instant mashed potatoes	770 mg
		Potatoes au gratin	355 mg
Fresh ear of corn	15 mg	Corn chips 7-ounce bag	630 mg
		Cornflakes	230 mg
		Cheese popcorn	840 mg
Fresh broccoli	27 mg	Frozen broccoli and cheese sauce	330 mg
		Canned cream of broccoli soup	770 mg
Brown rice	5 mg	Rice and sauce	900 mg

From *The Way to Eat* by David Katz, M.D., and Maura Gonzalez, R.D. (Sourcebooks, 2002). Reprinted with permission.

20 percent, it is very high. Make sure you're choosing foods with less than 10 percent of the DV.

The third way is to see where the sodium-containing ingredient falls in the list of ingredients. The higher in the list, the more sodium the food contains.

17 Use the calories-to-salt formula. To meet, or at least approximate, the recommended salt intake requires taking in no more milligrams of sodium than calories. So if a food has fewer milligrams of sodium per serving than calories, you'll hit the target. If it has more sodium than calories, you'll have a much harder time remaining within the recommended daily limits.

18 When cooking, use the wine you drink, *not* cooking wine.
Cooking wine has gobs of added sodium.

19 Check your medications for sodium. You wouldn't think you'd find sodium in your drugs, but there they are! Particular culprits are antacids, cough medicines, pain relievers, and laxatives. If

Know Your Garlic

The hot, strong taste of fresh garlic gives food a zing no amount of salt can equal. Buy cloves in bulk and store in a cool, dark place. To get the most health benefits out of your garlic:

- Always peel it first. Otherwise, some of the disease-preventing compounds might not form.

- Give it a break after cutting or crushing it. Leave it there on the cutting board for about 10 minutes to allow the health-promoting compounds to form.

- To get rid of garlic breath, chew on fresh parsley, mint, or lemon or orange peels, and use lemon juice to get the odor off your hands.

you find high sodium levels, talk to your doctor about alternatives.

20 Make your own salt-free salad dressing. Mix 1 cup olive oil, ⅓ cup balsamic vinegar, 1 package Splenda, and 2 crushed garlic cloves in a bowl. Blend until emulsified. Keeps in the refrigerator for a month. Just remove an hour before serving so it can liquefy.

21 Substitute citrus juice like orange or lemon for salt in salad dressings.

22 Drink responsibly. Some beverages, like V8 juice, provide a whole day's supply of sodium in one serving!

Two-Second**Quiz**

Sparkling Water or Club Soda?

Answer: *Sparkling water.*
There's a reason soda and sodium sound similar. Soda is called that because it is based on the use of sodium bicarbonate to "carbonate" it; thus it should come as no surprise that "soda" is sodium-rich. With only 3 mg sodium, sparkling water beats club soda's 75 mg hands down.

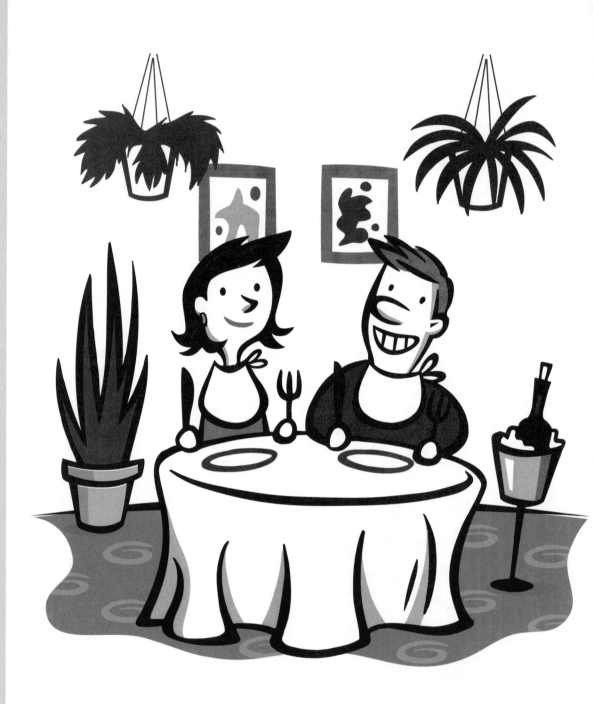

PART THREE

Stealth Healthy

DINING OUT

Being healthy in the kitchen is terrific. But for all-round healthy eating, you need to master what you eat when you're not at home. Here's our best advice.

Full-Service Restaurants
24 Ideas for Eating Well When Eating Out

Fast Food
23 Ways to Make the Right Choice

Take-Out Food
16 Ways to Make It as Healthy as Home Cooking

Coffee and Doughnut Shops
11 Ways to Get Out Healthy

Picnics
17 Ways to Go Beyond Fried Chicken and Potato Salad

Full-Service Restaurants

24 IDEAS FOR EATING WELL WHEN EATING OUT

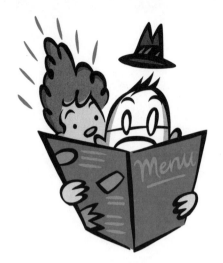

Suddenly it seems that chain restaurants like Applebee's, T.G.I. Friday's, Olive Garden, and Bennigan's are almost as ubiquitous as the Golden Arches. No surprise. There are nearly 200,000 "table side" restaurants in the United States today, a number that continues to grow. For many, they offer a reliable, pleasant alternative to cooking—plentiful servings, service with a smile, relatively good value for the dollar. But like fast-food outlets, these dining establishments can be ticking time bombs when it comes to nutritional health. Government surveys find that the food you typically eat when you're not home is nutritionally worse *in every way* than the food you eat at home.

The good news is that's changing. For instance, 7 out of 10 adults surveyed by the National Restaurant Association in 2003 said there are more nutritious foods available to them in such restaurants than there were five years ago. Nearly all the chains have added healthier options to their menus—if you know how to look for them. But whether you're dining out at a major national chain or a locally owned family restaurant, following a few of these Stealth Health tips can guarantee you a pleasant dinner (or lunch) out without busting your health goals.

1 **Above all else, be assertive.** Dining out is no time to be a meek consumer, notes Michael F. Jacobson, Ph.D., executive director of the Center for Science in the Public Interest (CSPI) and coauthor of the book *Restaurant Confidential.* "You need to be an assertive consumer by asking for changes on the menu," he says. For instance, if an item is fried, ask for it grilled. If it comes with french fries, ask for a side of veggies instead. Ask for a smaller portion of the meat and a larger portion of the salad; for salad instead of coleslaw; baked potato

instead of fried. "Just assume you can have the food prepared the way you want it," says Dr. Jacobson. "Very often, the restaurant will cooperate." Below, you'll find more specific requests.

2 **Ask your waiter to "triple the vegetables, please."** Often a side of vegetables in a restaurant is really like garnish—a carrot and a forkful of squash. When ordering, ask for three or four times the normal serving of veggies, and offer to pay extra. "I've never been charged," says dietitian Jeff Novick, R.D.,

director of nutrition at the Pritikin Longevity Center & Spa in Aventura, Florida. "And I've never been disappointed. I get full, not fat."

3 **Ask how the food was prepared; don't go by the menu.** For instance, cholesterol-free does *not* mean fat-free; the dish could still be filled with calorie-dense oil. Neither does "lite" necessarily mean light in calories or fat.

4 **Order from the "healthy, light, low fat" entrées** on the menu. Most chains will even list the calories and nutritional content of such foods. Applebee's, for instance, offers approved Weight Watchers options, Bennigan's has its Health Club entrées (which it will serve in half portions), and Ruby Tuesday lists the nutritional information for its entire menu.

5 **Beware of the low-carb options.** Restaurant chains have jumped on the low-carb bandwagon, offering numerous low-carb options on their menu. But low-carb doesn't mean low-cal. For instance, at Ruby Tuesday the Low-Carb New Orleans Seafood packs 710 calories and 42 grams of fat—ouch! A much better bet—the Low Carb Veggie Platter—leaves you with just 297 calories and 16 grams of fat.

6 **Ask the waiter to box half your entrée** before it ever gets to the table. Or split an entrée with your dining partner. A CSPI survey found that restaurants often serve two to three times more than food labels list as a serving.

7 **Try double appetizers.** If there is a nice selection of seafood- and vegetable-based appetizers, consider skipping the entrée and having two appetizers for

your meal. Often, that is more than enough food to fill you up.

8 **Order a salad before ordering anything else on the menu.** Scientists at Pennsylvania State University found that volunteers who ate a big veggie salad before the main course ate fewer calories overall than those who didn't have a first-course salad, notes Novick.

9 **But remember: Salads shouldn't be fatty.** This is a vegetable course—keep it tasty but healthy. That means avoiding anything in a creamy sauce (coleslaw, pasta salads, and potato salads), and skipping the bacon bits and fried noodles. Instead, load up on the raw vegetables, treat yourself to a few well-drained marinated vegetables (artichoke hearts, red peppers, or mushrooms), and for a change, add in some fruit or nuts. Indeed, fruits such as mango, kiwi, cantaloupe, and pear are often the secret ingredient in four-star salads.

10 **Watch the add-ons to vegetable salads.** Even salads that are mostly raw vegetables are a problem if they're loaded with cheese and meats. Take the

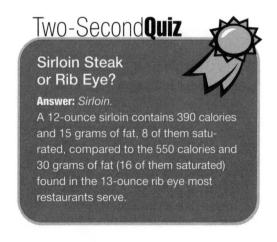

Two-Second**Quiz**

Sirloin Steak or Rib Eye?

Answer: *Sirloin.*
A 12-ounce sirloin contains 390 calories and 15 grams of fat, 8 of them saturated, compared to the 550 calories and 30 grams of fat (16 of them saturated) found in the 13-ounce rib eye most restaurants serve.

New England or Manhattan Clam Chowder?

Answer: *Manhattan.*
Not that we have anything against the Patriots, but the tomato-based version of this popular soup has much less fat than the cream-based version.

13 **Read between the lines.** Any menu description that uses the words creamy, breaded, crisp, sauced, or stuffed is likely loaded with hidden fats—much of it saturated or even trans fats. Other "beware of" words include: buttery, sautéed, pan-fried, au gratin, Thermidor, Newburg, Parmesan, cheese sauce, scalloped, and au lait, à la mode, or *au fromage* (with milk, ice cream, or cheese).

14 **Ask the waiter to skip the bread basket.** If you must have something to munch on while you wait for your order, ask for a plate of raw vegetables or some breadsticks.

15 **Skip the fancy drinks.** If you must order an alcoholic drink, forget the margaritas, piña coladas, and other exotic mixed drinks. They include sugary additions that only add calories. Opt instead for a glass of wine, a light beer, a vodka and tonic or a simple martini (without the chocolate liquor, sour green apple schnapps, or triple sec).

16 **Top a baked potato with veggies from the salad bar.** Or ask if they have salsa—the ultimate potato topper, both in terms of flavor and health. Just avoid the butter and sour cream.

17 **Order fish.** Just make sure it's not fried. When the CSPI evaluated food served at seafood chains and independent restaurants, researchers found low-fat and low-sodium options abounded. Plus, you can order seafood so many different ways—steamed, baked, broiled, sautéed, blackened, or grilled. Nix any sauces, or ask for them on the side.

typical Caesar salad in most restaurants (the one topped with chicken or shrimp as well as plenty of cheese and mayo in the dressing). Add in the fried croutons and the calories add up to a whopping 560, with 36 grams of fat, 6 of them saturated. Italian antipasto salads also are a health challenge, with all their salami, spicy ham, and cheese. Get the salad, but ask for vegetables only.

11 **Do the fork dip.** The best way to combine salad dressing with salad? Get your dressing on the side, in a small bowl. Dip your empty fork into the dressing, then skewer a forkful of salad. You'll be surprised at how this tastes just right, and how little dressing you'll use. Plus, your lettuce won't wilt and drown in a sea of oil.

12 **Check the menu before you leave home.** Most chains post their menus on their Web sites. For instance, Ruby Tuesday's Smart Eating menu tells you the restaurant only uses canola oil and even provides nutritional information on its salad bar. You can decide before you ever hit the hostess stand what you're going to order. Conversely, if you don't see anything that's healthy, pick another restaurant.

18 **Drink water throughout the meal.** It will slow you down, help you enjoy the food more, and let the message get to your brain that you're full—before your plate is empty.

19 **Always dress up to go out.** Even if it's just a regular family restaurant. If you view eating out as an event or a treat, rather than a way to get an everyday dinner, you won't eat out as often. And that's good from both a health and a cost standpoint.

20 **Skip the dessert.** You can always have some sorbet or even a small piece of chocolate at home. That is much better healthwise than the Triple Chocolate Meltdown or a mountain of ice cream topped by a second mountain of whipped cream.

Cuisine-Specific Advice

A perk of modern living is having so many restaurants to choose from. But with choice comes confusion. To help, here are tips for sensible eating at four of the most popular ethnic restaurant types.

21 **Stealth Healthy Chinese dining means you:**
- **Avoid the fried noodles.** If the waiter plops them down on the table, ask him to take them away. If you get a packet with your soup, hand them back. Each half-cup serving adds about 150 calories.
- **Order fewer dishes than there are people at the table.** Chinese entrées are designed for sharing, not for one person.

- **Start with soup to fill you up.**
- **Avoid fried appetizers.** This means no egg rolls or pupu platters. Get your dumplings steamed, not fried.
- **Opt for steamed rice, not fried.** If the restaurant serves brown rice, ask for it.
- **Use the 2:1 ratio.** Two times as much rice as main dish.
- **Avoid menu items described as crispy, golden brown, or sweet-and-sour.** They're all deep-fried.
- **Choose dishes rich in vegetables** and order at least one vegetarian entrée.
- **Ask for the sauce on the side.** Chinese restaurant chefs often stir-fry the main ingredients, then mix them together and ladle on the sauce. Get the sauce on the side and you'll use less.
- **Eat with chopsticks.** You'll get less of the high-calorie, high-sodium sauce that way.

Deadly Secrets of the Restaurant Trade

How do restaurants make their food taste so good? Here is the unhealthy truth:

Butter. In the soup. In the sauce. On the meat. On the vegetables. Butter is the easiest, quickest way to make things taste rich and wonderful.

Oil. Another way to make foods taste richer is to use lots of oil (remember, oil is a fat). This is why fried foods taste good: They are sponges for the oil they are cooked in.

Animal fat. Want to make anything taste better? Add bacon or other forms of pork fat—to vegetables, soups, and mashed potatoes.

Salt. Cook at home, you shake a little salt in while you go. At a restaurant, you *pour* it in to extract maximum flavor.

Sweeteners. Ever have vegetables that tasted sweeter than a dessert? That's because the cook added lots of sugar.

---

22 Stealth Healthy Italian dining means you:

▶ **Split and share.** One order of pasta is usually enough for two people, especially if you also have a salad.

▶ **Dine on pasta rather than pizza.** Pizza dough is dense with calories— about 1,250 per pound (without the cheese, sausage, and pepperoni). When you're dining Italian, a much better choice is pasta. A linguini puttanesca (olives, mushrooms, tomato sauce, and fresh basil), arrabbiata (spicy tomato sauce), or vongole (clams with marinara sauce) takes you down to 600 or 700 calories per pound, says Novick. You can further decrease the calorie density of a meal by ordering a side of fresh veggies or spinach and mixing it in with your pasta dish. Thus you eat more fiber, less fat.

▶ **Pick tomato-based sauces**—marinara, Bolognese, red clam, or puttanesca. Avoid cream-based sauces: Alfredo and primavera are two of the worst.

A Bloomin' Health Bomb

Do we even have to tell you to skip the Bloomin' Onion, cheese fries, cheese quesadillas, and fried mozzarella sticks that begin many chain restaurant menus? Take the popular fried onion. When researchers at the Center for Science in the Public Interest looked at the nutritional content, they found the typical appetizer portion contains 1,690 calories and 116 grams of fat—44 of them saturated. And that's *without* the dipping sauce. You say you're going to share? Well, CSPI found even half gives you about a day's fat and saturated fat along with more than half a day's sodium.

Bottom line: Skip the fried appetizers and order a salad or a fat-free broth-based soup instead.

▶ **Skip the garlic bread or breadsticks, often slathered in butter.** Instead, ask for a dish of olive oil and plain bread, and dip.

▶ **Go with fagioli**—Italian for "beans."

▶ **Skip the side of pasta.** If you've ordered veal piccata, you don't need the heaping dish of pasta that often comes with it. Get a vegetable instead.

▶ **Go all-you-can-eat on salad and soup—***not* **pasta.**

▶ **Steer clear of the following words on the menu:** Alfredo, carbonara, saltimbocca, parmigiana, lasagna, manicotti, stuffed. All mean heavy amounts of cream and cheese. Another dangerous word: frito (fried). Instead, look for "griglia," which means grill.

▶ **Order the appetizer-size portion of pasta.** With a salad, it will be enough.

▶ **Order antipasto** with extra chickpeas, olives, kidney beans, lettuce, tomatoes, and other vegetables, and fewer cheeses and meats.

▶ **Order one entrée and two sides of pasta.** Then split the entrée between you and a friend and eat it mixed with the pasta. You've just reduced your overall calories and the caloric density of the meal.

23 Stealth Healthy Mexican dining means you:

▶ **Keep your hands away from the fried tortilla chips.** Instead, ask for a short stack of soft tortillas to scoop up the healthy salsa and get a couple of vegetable servings under your belt even before the main meal arrives.

▶ **Ask for your salads on a plate,** not in a fried bowl.

▶ **Pick beans** to fill your burritos instead of beef or cheese.

▶ **Choose fajitas.** Not only can you load up on the vegetables, but you can pick and choose how much cheese, to add.

- **Ask for black beans or pinto beans, not refried.**
- **Nix the sour cream.**
- **Go for soft tacos, not hard tacos.** Hard taco shells are fried; soft taco shells are baked.
- **Avoid dishes with the following words in their names:** chimichanga (fried burrito), relleno (deep-fried pepper), chalupa (deep-fried tortilla), charra or charro beans (refried), con queso (with cheese), crispy.
- **Substitute a side salad for the rice on platters.** Spanish-rice recipes usually call for the raw rice to be fried in oil before it gets steamed (often using high-sodium chicken broth).

24 Stealth Healthy Indian dining means you:

- **Skip the appetizers (most are fried).**
- **Avoid the chapati, nan, kulcha, or roti breads.** They've all been fried or soaked in fat. A better bet: pappadam, made from lentils. It's usually baked, but check first.
- **Order side dishes with vegetables, beans, or peas, such as dal or chutney.**
- **Look for the healthy dishes:** chicken masala, shrimp bhuna, fish vindaloo, and tandoori (baked). Avoid dishes made with ghee (clarified butter) or malai (a thick cream).
- **Ask what kind of oil is used in cooking.** Most often, it's coconut— nearly all saturated fat. If that's what they use, ask if they can switch to canola oil for you.
- **Avoid dishes made with coconut, which is another hidden source of fat and calories.**
- **Choose a vegetable dish for your main course.**

Fast Food

23 WAYS TO MAKE THE RIGHT CHOICE

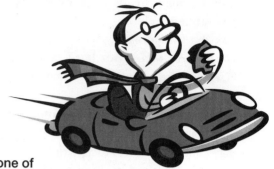

If you're like most Americans, you frequent one of the country's more than 72,000 fast-food restaurants at least once a week. After all, industry data show that fast-food accounts for 86 percent of meals taken home from restaurants. Stick to double cheeseburgers, supersize your fries and sodas, and add a few high-fat breakfast items a couple times a month, and you could see your waistline and cholesterol levels grow like weeds in a summer garden.

But something has been happening to fast-food restaurants. As Americans have become fatter and more concerned about what they eat, the McDonald's and Burger Kings of the world have taken notice. They've added salads that actually fill you up (sales of salads in fast-food restaurants were up 12 percent between 2002 and 2003), reduced serving sizes, and added more healthful options to their menus. Here's how to take advantage of it.

1 **Go for the salad, minus the fried toppings.** Although most fast-food restaurants offer decent-sized salads these days, if you top them with fried chicken, fried noodles, and the entire contents of the dressing packet, you will wind up with as much artery-clogging saturated fat and calories as if you'd had the double-cheese and fries. Instead, choose broiled or roasted chicken as your protein source, skip the croutons, and ask for the low-fat dressing—then only use half.

2 **Skip the cheese.** Craving a hamburger? That's okay—just get a plain hamburger without the cheese. For instance, at McDonald's, that saves you 50 calories, 40 of them from fat, and 2 grams of saturated fat.

3 **Ask for extra onions, lettuce, and tomato.** Whatever sandwich you choose, it'll be healthier, crunchier, and more filling if you add these classics. And it ticks off one more serving of vegetables from your day's quota.

4 **Order unsweetened iced tea or bottled water.** A king-size Sprite at Burger King is 420 calories. This one change might save you the same number of calories as the meal you're about to eat!

5 **Choose 1% or skim milk as your drink.** At just 100 calories (less for skim), it provides much of your daily dose of bone-building calcium, as opposed to soft drinks, which can suck the calcium from your bones.

6 Always say no to the special sauce. Many are just dressed-up mayonnaise, and thus overflowing with fat and calories. The best topping for your chicken, fish, or burgers? Mustard (no calories, lots of flavor). Second best? Ketchup (no fat, but a fair amount of sweetener). Other good choices: olive oil and vinegar (in moderation), hot sauces, red pepper spreads. Worst choices: butter or mayonnaise.

7 Use hot sauce, not ketchup, on your french fries. Hot sauce is low in calories, has a big, adventurous flavor, and contains nutrients that are particularly good for your body. Plus, it gets you drinking lots of water, which reduces your appetite.

8 Do not supersize. Ever. Even McDonald's has finally wised up to the evil of its ways, and is phasing out some of its supersized items.

9 In fact, order a kid's meal. A small hamburger, a small fries, and an orange juice is surprisingly filling for most adults, and much fewer calories than the adult version. Plus, you get a free toy!

10 Get a sub sandwich. A six-inch sub (or hoagie, wedge, grinder, or whatever it's called in your area) with roast beef or turkey and lots of vegetables is an outstanding fast-food choice. Choose a whole grain bread, and as we said, skip the mayo—a little bit of vinegar and olive oil is acceptable, or choose mustard. As with the burger stores, skip the value meal—chips and soda are no match for an apple or salad and a low-fat milk or orange juice.

11 Don't be fooled by low-carb claims. Although many fast-food outlets have added low-carb offerings to their menus, it doesn't mean the selections are any healthier for you. For instance, the Carl's Jr. Breakfast Bowl has only 5 grams of carbs, but, composed of two scrambled eggs, a sausage patty, and a slice of Swiss cheese, it packs a whopping 900 calories and 73 grams of fat, nearly half of them saturated.

12 Use a fast-food item as part of a meal. In other words, rather than buying the entire meal through the drive-through window and eating it in your car, buy a sandwich or salad, bring it home, then add to it with some raw veggies dipped in low-fat ranch dressing, a cup of yogurt, or some other healthy side dish that still doesn't involve cooking.

13 Get some kind of vegetable and/or fruit with every fast-food meal. Salads are an obvious choice, and as mentioned, you could also ask for extra tomatoes and lettuce on sandwiches, tacos, and burritos. Other ways: Order a

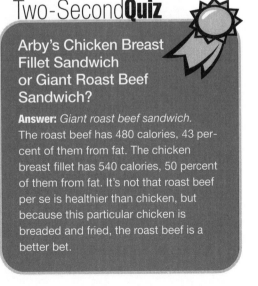

Two-Second Quiz

Arby's Chicken Breast Fillet Sandwich or Giant Roast Beef Sandwich?

Answer: *Giant roast beef sandwich.* The roast beef has 480 calories, 43 percent of them from fat. The chicken breast fillet has 540 calories, 50 percent of them from fat. It's not that roast beef per se is healthier than chicken, but because this particular chicken is breaded and fried, the roast beef is a better bet.

veggie burger (available at Burger King), add broccoli to your baked potato, and pick a fruit and yogurt parfait from McDonald's.

14 Get skinless chicken. This is particularly important when you're hitting KFC, home of the finger-lickin' good fried chicken. Ditch the skin—and much of the batter—and you'll save 240 calories and 16 grams of fat on a typical serving.

15 Order a taco salad without the shell or sour cream, and ask for only half the cheese. You still get the spicy meat and save about 300 calories and 10 grams of fat.

16 Look for ways to sneak in fiber. That means the baked potato (with skin) and chili (without cheese) from Wendy's, bean burritos and tacos from Taco Bell instead of meat (a Bean Burrito packs 12 grams of fiber—nearly half your daily needs met!), and baked beans and corn on the cob (without butter) as side dishes (or even main dishes) at KFC.

17 Look for the word "Jr." You'll get a smaller portion. Ironically, what's considered a junior portion today used to be considered a regular size 20 years ago.

18 Avoid value meals. An oversized sandwich (fat), lots of french fries (fat), and a large soda (sugar) add up to major calories and minimal nutrition. Burger King's Value Meals are some of the least healthful among fast-food chains, says Michael F. Jacobson, Ph.D., executive director of the Center for Science in the Public Interest and coauthor of the book *Restaurant Confidential.* One of the lowest-calorie value meals, he notes, is the Whopper Jr., medium fries, and medium Coca-Cola Classic, with a whopping 1,000 calories. McDonald's value meals average about 1,200 calories. In comparison, the typical woman needs to eat just 1,800 calories in a whole day.

19 Look for the words "grilled," "baked," or "broiled." If they're cooked that way, they're not fried—and you'll automatically be reaping some savings in terms of fat and calories.

20 Have an apple, banana, nonfat yogurt, or some other healthy snack an hour before you hit the fast-food

Healthy **Investments**

A Case of Granola Bars

We prefer the crunchy type—more substantial and pleasing to eat. We buy them in cases of 36 packets (each packet has two bars, totaling about 140 high-nutrition calories) for the cost of a large combo meal at a fast-food joint. We keep them in the car as a preventive measure against impulse visits to the drive-through window. Next time your stomach growls when driving down restaurant-filled Main Street, have a granola bar instead. Then have a healthy meal at home.

line. That way you're not showing up starving. If you're too hungry, one whiff of the enticing fast-food smells will send all your good intentions of a salad right out the drive-through window.

21 **Eat breakfast at home and save fast food for lunch or dinner.** At least you'll know you're getting one wholesome meal. Plus, since it's hard to eat high-fiber cereal in your car, you're more likely to order a high-fat option, like a sausage biscuit.

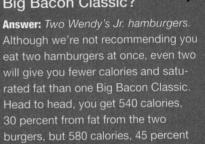

22 **Make a supermarket your fast-food restaurant.** Run in, grab a piece or two of fruit, a cup of yogurt, an energy bar, a salad at the salad bar, a turkey sandwich at the deli counter, and you're out through the express lane with breakfast, lunch, and snacks in 10 minutes.

Two-Second**Quiz**

Two Wendy's Jr. Hamburgers or One Big Bacon Classic?

Answer: *Two Wendy's Jr. hamburgers.* Although we're not recommending you eat two hamburgers at once, even two will give you fewer calories and saturated fat than one Big Bacon Classic. Head to head, you get 540 calories, 30 percent from fat from the two burgers, but 580 calories, 45 percent from fat, from the Big Bacon Classic.

23 **Avoid processed or cured meats.** We're talking hot dogs, salami, bologna, and ham. These heavily processed meats are filled with fat, salt, chemical additives, and in some cases, sugar. At a deli or a sub shop, go for turkey breast, chicken breast, or roast beef instead.

Take-Out Food

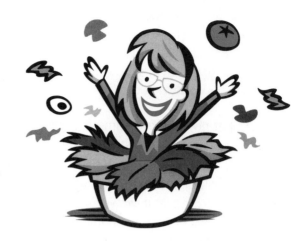

16 WAYS TO MAKE IT AS HEALTHY AS HOME COOKING

These days, many of us stop at the supermarket on our way home, not for the raw ingredients of supper but for already-prepared "home cooked" meals that just need to be slipped into the microwave for a few minutes. They're called "prepared meals," and more and more supermarkets are turning over large swaths of floor space to them.

In fact, a 2004 survey by the Food Marketing Institute found that 27 percent of respondents said they got most of their take-out from supermarkets, compared with 35 percent from fast-food restaurants and 18 percent from full-service eateries. That's nearly twice as many who got grocery take-out in 2002. Meanwhile, industry researchers at the NPD Group, a food industry consulting company, say dinners from a take-out counter or a grocery freezer will likely overtake meals from scratch within the next five years.

While most grocery stores offer the basics—fried and rotisserie chickens, deli salads, and so on—if you're lucky enough to live near an upscale grocery like Wegmans or Publix, you know take-out goes far beyond greasy chicken. These chains offer hot buffet lines, sushi, salad bars, and even Thai noodle bars. Not to mention pizza, chicken wings, hoagies, and other delectables. In fact, if you're willing to spend the money, you may never need to cook at home again.

As with everything in life, however, how you choose helps determine your health. Here's how to choose wisely, be it at a grocery store or your neighborhood hoagie shop, pizzeria, or Chinese take-out restaurant.

1 **If you buy take-out food to save time, only buy those things you don't have time to make.** "The less you buy pre-made, the more control you have over what you're eating," says Joan Salge Blake, R.D., clinical assistant professor of nutrition at Boston University's Sargent College. So pick up that rotisserie chicken, but also go to the produce department for a potato to microwave and some baby carrots instead of buying the twice-baked potatoes and candied carrots in the take-out case.

2 **Always think vegetables.** How are you going to get veggies into the meal? If you don't want to cook, then fill a salad bar container with raw veggies,

says Blake, but stay away from too many marinated veggies. And, of course, those pre-washed mixed greens in the produce aisle make salad preparation about as complicated as finding a bowl!

3 **Hit the seafood section.** Many upscale grocers will steam or broil your fish selection for free or for just a small charge. That way, you're getting the unadulterated fish without the hassle of cooking it. Try some steamed shrimp, clams, or lobster. The price alone will keep your portions healthy!

4 **Get two meals at a time.** Again, you're trying to save time. So that whole roasted chicken you got for tonight can double as a chicken Caesar salad tomorrow night. If you're making a bowl of couscous to go with your take-out dinner tonight, double the amount and pick up some extra veggies and feta cheese at the salad bar for a Mediterranean salad the following night. Or perhaps for lunch tomorrow.

5 **Grab a can of low-sodium beans before you pay for your food.** Then add the beans to the salad bar salad you just purchased. You will save a ton of money (because beans are so heavy) while still adding valuable fiber and other nutrients to the salad.

6 **Have an indoor picnic for dinner.** For a fresh take on healthy eating, buy a loaf of wheaty bread, a pint of strawberries, a favorite low-fat cheese, some thinly sliced roast beef or turkey, a small tub of olives, pre-cooked shrimp, cherry tomatoes, pre-sliced green or red peppers, and bite-size carrots. When you get home, throw it all on the table and—after properly cleaning the produce—declare dinner served. This type of "grazing" dinner is fun, easy and a pleasant surprise. Make it a bimonthly ritual.

7 **Skip the buffets.** Those by-the-pound Chinese, noodle, and chicken wing buffets at large grocery stores can be a health nightmare. First, the containers are large, so you tend to buy too much. Second, many of the foods are fried, and many more are packed with oil, salt, and sugar to boost the flavor.

8 **Order by the serving size, not the pound.** When ordering prepared foods from behind the counter, ask the server to give you enough for as many people as will be eating, for example, "I need enough to serve three people, and I'm serving a salad and brown rice along with it." If the server is no help, then go by the palm of your hand. You want a serving size of meat or protein about the size of your hand. The rest of the meal you can round out with vegetables and whole grains.

Two-Second**Quiz**

Soup or Salad?

Answer: *Salad.*
We know: Some soups are far healthier than some salads. But in general, you're better off with a salad of mixed greens and raw vegetables, coupled with a light, healthy dressing. You'll get more fiber and thus more filling for your calories, not to mention the healthy dose of disease-fighting antioxidants found in raw vegetables. Many soups are very healthy, but the cooking process can diminish some of the ingredients' nutritional value.

9 Order grocery-store hoagies and subs with turkey or chicken, lots of vegetable fillings like tomato, lettuce, peppers, and cucumber, with the spread on the side. Ask for whole grain bread.

10 Go for sushi. Low in fat, high in healthy omega-3 fatty acids, sushi is one of your best bets when running into your local grocer for dinner. Can't stand the thought of raw fish? Most groceries stock a selection of cooked fish sushi or even veggie-only sushi.

11 Order twice as much of the prepared vegetables as you do of the main entrée.

12 If you can see mayonnaise pooling around the chicken, tuna, seafood, or pasta salads, skip them. Mayonnaise is a combination of eggs and oil—primarily fat.

13 Start a conversation with your server. Among the talking points: How was that fish prepared? How much salt does the chef use? Can I see the recipe for the meat loaf?

14 Pick up a rotisserie chicken... Add a salad-in-a-bag, a box of instant brown rice, and some sliced tomatoes and you've got a healthy, easy, barely-have-to-cook meal.

15 ...But remove the skin. Much of the internal fat from a rotisserie chicken drips out in the cooking, but the skin still holds lots of the stuff.

16 Choose prepared soups made with veggies in place of meat, like black bean soup, lentil soup, or minestrone. Little fat is added to these soups. However, avoid creamy or cheesy soups like broccoli-and-cheese or cream of asparagus. If you're not sure, ask about the composition of the soup stock. The best is vegetable broth, followed by chicken broth, then beef, and finally cream.

Stealth Healthy Pizza

Americans order 3 *billion* pizzas a year, mainly from the more than 60,000 pizza restaurants found in every burg with a ZIP code. There's no reason to cut pizza out of your life—it offers a quick, easy, tasty way to get loads of vegetables, fruit, fiber, and even fish without much artery-clogging saturated fat. But pizza, like any other take-out/order-in food, has its own pitfalls. When the Center for Science in the Public Interest evaluated pizza slices from the top chains, it discovered fat levels approaching—and sometimes surpassing—a fast-food cheeseburger. The main culprit: way too much cheese. Add to that fatty meat like sausage and pepperoni, and you are in the unhealthiest reaches of the food world. Here's how to make pizza a healthy delight:

- Order half cheese or no cheese.

- Ask for extra veggies.

- Steer clear of stuffed crust pizzas. You don't need the extra cheese.

- Avoid anything called Meat Lover's, All the Meat, or Super Supreme. In fact, order your toppings individually.

- Best toppings: After veggies and fruit (ever tried pineapple-topped pizza?), chicken, ham, clams, shrimp, and anchovies offer the greatest nutritional punch with the lowest saturated fat.

Coffee and Doughnut Shops

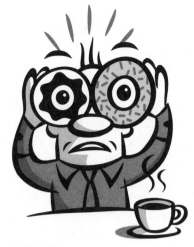

11 WAYS TO GET OUT HEALTHY

What would the world be like without Starbucks and Dunkin' Donuts? Well, somewhat thinner, perhaps. These chains, which specialize in sweet coffee and tea drinks to wash down their hard-to-resist pastries, have become a staple in American cities and suburbs, with 4,500 Starbucks and 4,000 Dunkin' Donuts alone. That's not counting all the smaller chains and mom-and-pop coffee shops. Yet beyond the caffeine and wireless hot spots, they're a major, albeit often hidden, source of fat and calories.

As Michael F. Jacobson, Ph.D., executive director of the Center for Science in the Public Interest and coauthor of the book *Restaurant Confidential*, notes, a Starbucks venti-size White Chocolate Mocha made with whole milk and whipped cream has more calories and saturated fat than a McDonald's Quarter Pounder With Cheese. Yowza!

1 **Order a glazed yeast doughnut.** We know most people want a doughnut when they walk into a doughnut shop. So have one. But make it a glazed yeast doughnut, that is, plain except for a sugar coating if you're at Dunkin' Donuts (180 calories and 8 grams fat) or a traditional cake doughnut at Krispy Kreme (200 calories and 11 grams fat). In comparison, that Vanilla Kreme Filled at Dunkin' Donuts has 270 calories and 13 grams fat.

2 **Classify doughnuts as treats, not breakfast.** A doughnut or other pastry as an occasional treat is fine, but as a breakfast it's disastrous. Not only will the simple carbohydrates and high sugar load leave you drooping and hungry an hour later, but you get little to no nutritional benefit for the fat and calories you're ingesting. If you must eat on the run at your friendly coffee shop, order a whole wheat bagel.

3 **Classify specialty coffee drinks as dessert, not coffee.** Fancy-flavored, whipped-cream, hard-to-pronounce coffee drinks can be worse for you than a big slice of cake. For example, a medium Java Chip Frappuccino with whipped cream at Starbucks has 510 calories, 22 grams fat, and 59 grams sugar. Of the 27 types of cakes Starbucks lists on its Web site, 21 have fewer calories per serving than the drink! If you must have a fancy coffee drink, treat it like a banana split or a big slice of

cake—a rare indulgence, to be had by itself and not as a mere beverage.

4 Choose biscotti. These twice-baked Italian delicacies are perfect for dunking, and at Starbucks carry just 110 calories and 5 grams fat. Compare that to the Caramel Pecan Sticky Roll, with 730 calories and 40 grams fat.

5 Order plain coffee and add the extras yourself. Not only are many of the specialty coffee drinks loaded with fat and calories, but some items are made from mixes, many of which contain large amounts of trans fats. The solution: Get a black coffee and add in healthy amounts of skim milk, sugar, or sugar substitute, and if you wish, unique flavorings like ground chocolate or cinnamon.

6 If you must order specialty beverages, order ones made with milk, like cappuccino or latte. And ask that they be made with low-fat or skim milk. You'll get a goodly amount of calcium along with the warmth and caffeine but without the saturated fat.

7 Forget the whipped topping. You'll instantly save 100 calories and 10 grams fat.

8 Share a muffin between you and two other people. With Dunkin' Donuts muffins weighing in at a hefty 5 ounces, each packs 500-600 calories, along with 15-24 grams of fat, notes Dr. Jacobson. As with a doughnut, think "treat" rather than breakfast when you get a muffin at a store. Muffins—even bran

Two-Second Quiz

Starbucks Café Au Lait or Caffe Latte?

Answer: *Café Au Lait.*
Café Au Lait is equal parts brewed coffee and steamed milk. A Caffe Latte is one or two shots of espresso with steamed milk and foam filling the rest of the cup. The Au Lait is just 140 calories, 70 from fat (assuming whole milk). The latte, because it uses so much more milk, is 260 calories, 120 from fat. To us, the Au Lait has a bolder, more coffee-rich flavor!

muffins—tend to be more about good taste than good nutrition.

9 Substitute skim milk when adding your own "creamer." You'll save upward of 50 calories, depending on the size of your drink. Chances are, you won't notice the difference between the skim dairy and the half-and-half.

10 Go for a flavored bagel. If you're ordering blueberry, cinnamon raisin, or some other tasty flavor, you won't need the extra cream cheese, butter, or other spreads, Dr. Jacobson notes. Skip the salt bagel, though. It has more than a day's worth of sodium, he says. Better still, go for whole wheat, multigrain, or oat bran bagels—you can eat your bagel and have some good nutrition too!

11 Pick the low-fat option. Many bakeries (even Dunkin' Donuts) do offer low-fat options of their tasty treats. This is still a long way from health food, but it's a Stealth Healthy step closer.

Picnics

17 WAYS TO GO BEYOND FRIED CHICKEN AND POTATO SALAD

Eating outside under the sun, with the crash of waves on the beach or the wind through the trees as your musical accompaniment, makes any meal taste better. That's why we've included this chapter on picnics. If the word "picnic" is synonymous in your mind with fried chicken, potato salad topped with bacon, and overstuffed hoagies, this is for you. Here are 17 Stealth Health ways to ensure that dining *al fresco* doesn't translate to dining *al fatso*.

1 Try these easy-to-transport entrées:

▸ Turkey or chicken breast sandwiches with low-fat cheese, sandwich pickles, tomatoes, and spinach leaves.

▸ Hummus stuffed into whole wheat pita bread with bean sprouts, diced tomatoes, and sliced grapes.

▸ A green salad topped with grilled chicken. Pack the dressing separately.

▸ Whole wheat wraps with smoked salmon, capers, tomato, avocado, hummus, spinach, and shredded carrots.

▸ Cumin, black bean, and corn salad. Rinse and drain a can of black beans and a can of sweet corn. Mix with a drizzle of olive oil, 1 tablespoon balsamic vinegar, and a pinch of cumin.

▸ Ricotta, spinach, and Parmesan whole wheat wrap. Place 2 cups loosely packed raw spinach leaves in food processor and grind. Mix in ½ cup fat-free ricotta and 1 tablespoon Parmesan cheese, and wrap in a whole wheat burrito.

▸ Mediterranean tomato salad in whole wheat pita. Dice fresh tomato and cucumber, mix with a thinly sliced red onion and black olives, drizzle with a little olive oil, red wine vinegar, salt, and pepper and stuff into a pita pocket.

2 Pack angel food cake for dessert. Bring sliced strawberries and nonfat whipped topping along for your own version of strawberry shortcake. Freeze the whipped topping the night before; it will thaw by the time you're ready to serve and still be cold enough to be safe. Or even easier, pick up a can of it.

3 Stuff celery with nonfat cream cheese, peanut butter, or goat cheese for appetizers. Baked corn chips with fat-free salsa or fat-free bean dip also works great as a meal opener.

4 Substitute this for fried chicken. Brush boneless, skinless chicken thighs with olive oil and sprinkle with rosemary, salt, and pepper. Bake or grill until juices run clear, about 45 minutes. Chill overnight and bring along on your picnic. For another option that's just as finger-lickin' messy as the real thing, mix the juice of 1 lemon with 1 tablespoon Dijon mustard, ¼ cup honey, a pinch of curry powder, and a pinch of salt. Roll skinless chicken drumsticks in the mixture to coat well and bake until done, 45-60 minutes.

5 Freeze turkey burgers the night before.
By the time you're ready to grill, they should be thawed and ready to go. Other good burger options: salmon burgers, lentil burgers, veggie burgers, and ground chicken burgers.

6 Instead of mayonnaise-dripping coleslaw,
buy a package of coleslaw mix and drizzle on fat-free Italian dressing once you're ready to eat.

7 Replace mayonnaise in summer salads
with nonfat yogurt, sour cream, or a mustard vinaigrette.

8 Pack baby veggies for dipping.
Another good use for baby vegetables (tiny corn, squashes, cauliflower, etc.) is to pickle them the day before by soaking them in a jar of vinegar.

9 Instead of sweetened sodas or fruit juices,
bring seltzer mixed with all-natural fruit juice; unsweetened, flavored iced tea; or bottles of water. Freeze the bottled water the night before, to use as cold packs to keep food cold. When you're ready to eat, you'll have an icy bottle of water ready to drink.

10 Instead of hot dogs,
take along turkey kielbasa or apple chicken sausages for grilling.

11 Make a Thanksgiving-in-the-summer salad.
This recipe comes from Joan Salge Blake, R.D., clinical assistant professor of nutrition at Boston University's Sargent College. Mix leftover chicken or turkey with dried cranberries, 2 tablespoons light mayonnaise, and 1 teaspoon cinnamon and stuff into a whole wheat pizza pita.

12 Go Mediterranean.
Microwave two boxes of whole wheat couscous (boil the water in a Pyrex measuring cup, add the couscous, cover with a plate, and let steam) and add fresh or roasted vegetables, a can of chickpeas, a sprinkling of feta cheese and sliced black olives, and a drizzle of olive oil. "Now you've got a gorgeous Mediterranean salad that goes great on a picnic," says Blake.

13 Pack frozen mango cubes.
They provide a sweet accompaniment to any picnic. Or mix several bags of frozen fruits in a container. By the time you're ready to eat, you'll have a sorbet-like treat.

Two-Second Quiz

Charcoal or Propane?

Answer: *Propane.*
Of course, grilling aficionados will debate this point for hours. But from a safety standpoint, there are more reported deaths and injuries due to carbon monoxide poisoning from charcoal grills than there are burns due to propane-grill fires. From a cooking standpoint, propane cooks more evenly, so you have fewer issues of raw on one end, well-done on the other. Plus, the smoke from charcoal is unhealthy for you, whether breathed in while cooking or eaten via the grilled food.

14 Make your own salsa. Drain a 15-ounce can of diced tomatoes with green chiles and add a handful of fresh cilantro leaves and a pinch or two of cumin and salt to taste. Put through the food processor or mini chopper and voilà! Salsa. Serve with baked tortilla chips or add to black beans for a cold salad just perfect for picnicking, says Lisa C. Andrews, R.D., a nutritionist at the VA Medical Center in Cincinnati.

15 Make your pasta salad a meal. Before the picnic, Andrews recommends grilling skinless chicken breasts, cutting them into strips, and adding them to pasta salad. Toss in some fresh broccoli, peppers, and tomatoes with low-fat dressing and you've got a main course.

16 Try a sweet potato salad. In a great variation on the original that's chock-full of valuable antioxidants

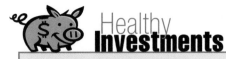

Healthy Investments

An Oversized Cooler and Plenty of Ice Packs

Stuffing a cooler to the brim prevents air from circulating, leading to unsafe temperatures.

and beta-carotene, Andrews suggests peeling and boiling a few sweet potatoes, then letting them cool. Cut into chunks and toss with enough orange juice to cover, a pinch of cinnamon, and your favorite dried fruit (Andrews prefers cranberries). Serve cold.

 17 Bring a whole watermelon, cantaloupe, or honeydew and slice it open on the spot. Nature's packing works beautifully to keep fresh fruit cool and fresh.

Healthy Food Storage

To keep unwanted guests like *Salmonella* and *E. coli* from your picnic, follow this basic advice:

- Keep hot foods hot and cold foods cold. Anything perishable should be kept at room temperature for no more than two hours.

- Bring along antibacterial wipes or hand-washing liquid to clean your hands before laying out (and eating) the food.

- Bring two coolers: one for food and one for drinks. Since you'll probably open

the drinks cooler more often than the food cooler, this prevents warm air from reaching your perishables.

- Avoid bringing anything made with fresh eggs, which can become a breeding ground for bacteria.

- Avoid bringing meats, fish, potatoes, and pasta mixed with mayo. These foods can reduce the acidity of the mayonnaise (which keeps bacteria at bay) encouraging the growth of bacteria. Instead, bring your salad ingredients in sepa-

rate containers and mix when you're ready to serve.

- Keep your cooler in the air-conditioned car.

- Thaw meat before grilling so it cooks evenly. Cook to an internal temperature of 160°F. Poultry should cook to 180°F.

- Keep raw meats, fish, and poultry (and the containers on which they sat) separate from cooked foods.

- Wash the outer surface of fruits, including melons, well before cutting.

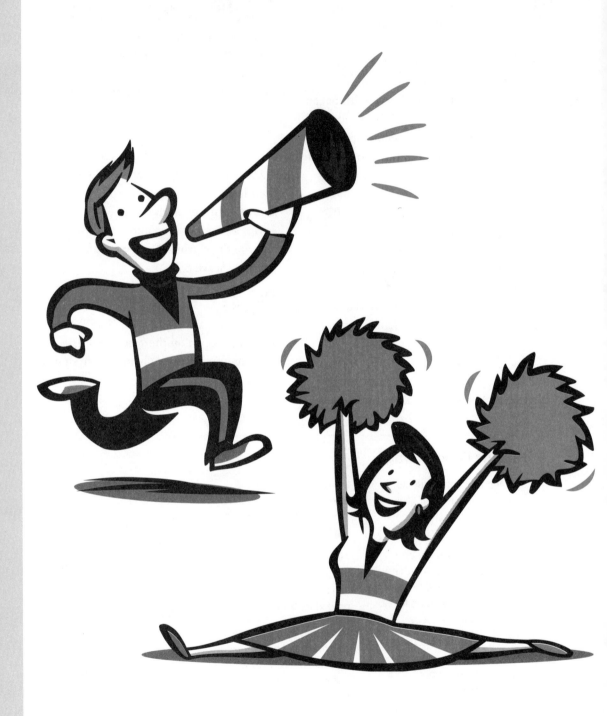

PART FOUR

Stealth Healthy

EXERCISE

After food, there's no better way to improve your health than by getting up and moving. Here's how to sneak extra movement into your days without hassle or sweat.

Stretching
14 Ways to Sneak In
Some Limbering

Walking
30 Ideas for Doing More
and Better

Weekends
23 Ideas for More
Active Days Off

Vacations
13 Tips for Actively
Indulgent Travel

Family Fun
47 Ways to Use the Ultimate
Exercise Machines—Children

Arm Strength
20 Ways to Exercise With—
or Without—Weights

Abs and Back Strength
19 Ways to Feel Less
Crunched During Your Routine

Leg Strength
19 Ways to Firm Your Hips,
Thighs, and Buttocks

**Neck and Shoulder
Strength**
12 Simple Strategies That
Decrease Pain and Stiffness

Self-Massage
17 Ways to Reduce
Tension in Seconds

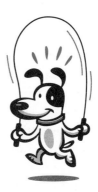

Stretching

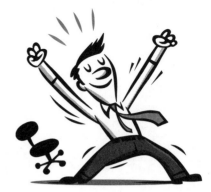

14 WAYS TO SNEAK IN SOME LIMBERING

The human body was engineered for standing and moving. Sitting all day long—as so many office workers and TV watchers do—is unnatural, and takes its toll on our well-being. Chronic sitting can shorten the muscles in the front of your thighs, tighten your back muscles and shoulders, and generally wreak havoc on your posture and body alignment. To survive the daily marathon known as the office job without eventually suffering from some form of chronic pain or injury, you must stretch regularly.

Of course, stretching is good for more than just that. Of the many injustices of aging, one of the most complained about is stiffness and joint pain. Stretching regularly helps keep you lithe, active, and injury resistant, no matter what your age.

A regular stretching routine not only improves how you feel and how you move, but may also improve your sleep. A study published in the journal *Sleep* found that people who began a stretching program were less likely to use sleep medication or experience trouble falling asleep than before they began stretching.

The following 14 tips will show you how to sneak in life-affirming stretches throughout your day.

1 **Stretch during your shower routine.** The perfect time of day to sneak in a little stretching is right after—or during—a warm shower in the morning. "Your muscles are warm and it is a great way to energize your day," says Jenny Hadfield, a Chicago-based fitness coach and author of *Marathoning for Mortals.* Hadfield suggests the following shower and just-after-the-shower stretching routine:

- While in the shower, raise your arms above your head, clasp your hands, and reach upward to stretch your shoulders and back.
- With the water spray hitting the back of your neck, slowly turn your head to the right until your chin is over your shoulder. Pause, then slowly turn your head all the way to the left. Repeat five times in each direction.
- Dry off with one foot on the toilet, lean forward, and stretch your hamstring.
- While drying your hair, hold a calf stretch by extending one leg 2-3 feet behind the other.

2 **Stretch with each bite of breakfast.** Do this sitting down. As you eat, roll your ankles in clockwise and counterclockwise circles. Then draw large, imaginary letters with your big toes, spelling your first, middle, and last name with each foot.

3 Every morning, roll out of bed and do these stretches.

Can you get away with just three stretches for the entire body? Yes, if your main goal is overall body health, says Phil Wharton, a musculoskeletal therapist and co-founder of the Wharton Performance Center in New York City. Wharton suggests the following gentle mini-stretching routine first thing in the morning just after getting out of bed. This stretching routine is safe to perform even when your muscles are cold.

▼ HAMSTRING STRETCH

The hamstrings along the backs of your thighs work hard during the day supporting your body weight as you walk. This stretch helps lengthen the hamstrings first thing in the morning, so you'll walk with more power and ease all day.

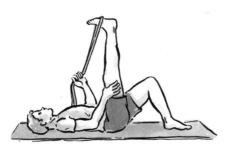

Lie on your back with your knees bent and feet on the floor. Lift your right knee in toward your chest and thread a rope, necktie, or towel around the arch of your right foot. Hold the ends of the rope, tie, or towel with your left hand. Extend your leg toward the ceiling. Place your right palm against your right thigh and press into it as you use the rope to increase the stretch. Hold for two seconds, release, and repeat 10 times. Switch legs and repeat.

▼ TRUNK EXTENSOR STRETCH

If you're going to be sitting at a desk all day long, you want your back to be ready for the challenge. This stretch helps. Repeat this stretch periodically during the day to release tension in your lower back.

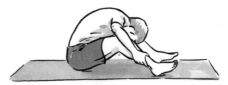

Sit on the floor with your knees bent and feet flat on the floor. Lift your toes until only your heels touch the floor. Sit tall with your back straight and spine long and extended. Place your hands on your shins. Tuck your chin into your chest, bend forward from the hips, and pull your torso as far down as you can. Hold two seconds, release, and repeat 10 times.

▼ PELVIC TILT

This stretch helps increase blood flow to your midsection, relaxes your back muscles, and helps realign your sacrum, one of the large, flat bones that forms your pelvis.

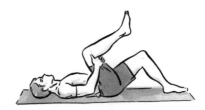

Lie on your back with your knees bent and feet flat on the floor. Lift your right thigh toward your chest, grasping the back of your thigh with both hands. Bring your knee as close to your chest as you can. Hold two seconds, release, and repeat 10 times. Switch legs and repeat.

4 Better yet, do a more thorough three-minute stretching routine every morning. We like this routine for two reasons: First, it is made up of extremely simple, natural moves; second, it is particularly good for those people who have stiff joints or mild arthritis. It gently warms your muscles and moves your shoulders, knees, elbows, wrists, and neck through a full range of motion, stimulating the release of synovial fluid, a thick secretion that lubricates and cushions your joints. Complete the following stretches from a standing position, starting with whatever range of motion you feel comfortable with and gradually increasing it as your joints warm up. Complete 10-12 slow repetitions of each stretch, moving clockwise and counter-clockwise, pausing for a moment at the full extension on each stretch.

Neck roll. Bring your chin to your chest and then move your chin in a half-circle, bringing your left ear over your left shoulder and then your right ear over your right shoulder.

Shoulder shrug. Lift your shoulders to your ears and then slowly drop them.

Shoulder circle. Slowly roll your shoulders in circles.

Arm circle. Extend your arms straight out to your sides, so they are parallel to the ground. Slowly whirl them in circles as if they were propellers on an airplane.

Hip circle. With your knees slightly bent and your feet placed slightly wider than your hips, circle your hips in one direction and then the other, as if you were balancing a hula hoop.

5 Stretch after every walk, run, bike ride, aerobic class, or any other cardiovascular activity. Your muscles are their most flexible and pliable after your workout, making your stretching more effective. After any activity designed to increase your heart rate, spend about 5-10 minutes cooling down and bringing your heart rate back to normal. Then complete the same stretches that are outlined in Tip 3.

6 Stretch during TV time. Sprawl out on the floor and go through your stretching routine, doing the stretches from Tip 1 or Tip 2. If you feel good, do them a second and third time. It's best to do this later in the day, when your muscles are warmed up from your daily activities. If you don't want to stretch the entire time you are watching the tube, make a point of stretching during the commercials.

7 Dance your way to flexibility once a week in a dance class. A Swedish study published in the *Journal of Strength Conditioning Research* tested 20 cross-country skiers for flexibility. Half the skiers took a dance class, and the other half served as a control group. Within three months, the skiers who took the weekly dance class improved the flexibility of their spines, and consequently, also increased their agility and ski speed on a slalom and hurdle test.

8 Stretch your legs as you wait in line. Stuck standing on line at the bank or grocery store? Stand on your toes, as high as you can, for as long as you can. Then, with feet back on the ground, lift the toes on your right foot as high as they can go without lifting your heel, and hold for 20 seconds. Then do your left foot. These simple moves are also good for boring parties, lengthy museum visits, and any other time you are on your feet for a long time.

9 Near the end of your workday, do another two-minute stretch routine. Because your muscles are relatively warm and pliable from walking around all day at work, now is the perfect time to do the following static stretches. Some research also suggests that flexibility peaks during the afternoon between 2:30 p.m. and 4 p.m., due to the body's natural circadian rhythms. Thus, although you'll achieve some benefit no matter what time of day you stretch, an afternoon stretching routine may help you gain more flexibility faster.

▼ SEATED HAMSTRING STRETCH

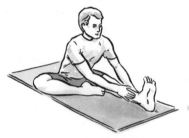

Sit on the floor with your left leg extended. Place your right foot against your left thigh. Lengthen your spine and bend forward from the hips. Hold 20 seconds. Repeat with right leg extended.

▼ LATERAL SIDE STRETCH

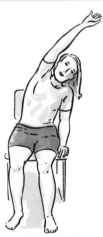

Sit on the edge of your office chair with your feet on the floor. Place your left palm against the seat of the chair. Reach your right arm overhead. Extend upward through your spine and then bend sideways to the left. Hold 20 seconds, release, and repeat on the other side.

▼ HIP OPENER

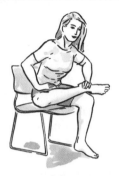

Sit on the edge of a chair with your feet on the floor. Lift your right leg and place your right foot on your left thigh. Lean forward from the hips. Hold 20 seconds, release, and repeat with left leg.

▼ CHEST STRETCH

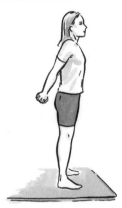

Stand with your feet under your hips. Clasp your hands behind your back. Roll your shoulders up, back, and then down, feeling your chest open. To increase the stretch, lift your arms. Hold 20 seconds and release.

Good Stretching Technique

Follow these tips to increase the effectiveness of your stretching routine:

Feel the muscle you are targeting. As you slowly proceed through the movement, you should feel a stretching sensation in your muscle as it lengthens and relaxes. If you feel a sharp pain in a joint, such as your knee or elbow, you have either gone too far or are using improper technique. If you feel nothing at all, you either have not gone far enough or are using improper technique.

Relax. It sounds simple, but many people tense up as they stretch. They clench their jaws or hunch their shoulders toward their ears. Stop doing this! Notice whether you are clenching with any other muscles in your body and gently allow those muscles to release as you exhale.

Breathe into it. Deep breathing helps relax your muscles, enabling you to stretch farther. If you breathe slowly and deeply as you stretch, you'll increase blood flow throughout your body, making your stretching more effective. Always exhale as you move into the stretch. As you hold, inhale by expanding the abdomen, rib cage, *and* chest, then exhale as you visualize your breath flowing through the tension you feel in your muscle.

Hold a stretch on the tighter side of your body twice as long as on the more flexible side. Prevent muscle imbalances by training the major muscle groups equally. If you are tighter on one side of your body (you'll know because each stretch on that side of your body will feel a lot harder and you won't be able to go as deeply into the stretch), stretch that muscle for twice as long or repeat a stretch on that side to even things out.

Stretch each and every day. When it comes to flexibility, what you don't use, you lose—and quickly. Studies have shown that clearly. The lesson: It is much better to stretch a little every day than to do a large stretching routine once or twice a week.

Use proper body alignment. It's easy to cheat when you stretch, but then you fail to get the stretch you need. The most typical "cheating" is rounding your back. In 95 percent of all stretches, you want to keep your spine long

10 **Release your neck whenever you're on hold.** Get a speakerphone or a headset. The next time someone puts you on hold, do some neck rolls or get down on the floor and start doing your stretching routine.

11 **Stretch every time you get out of the car.** Even just short periods of driving can do a number on your back if you don't periodically stretch it out. When you get out of the car, gently reach to the sky as far as you can without lifting your heels. Hold the position for 20 seconds, gently pushing higher as your body adjusts to the stretch. Then bend forward and place your hands on your knees. Exhale as you round your back and tuck your chin. Then flatten your back, inhaling as you go. Hold each position for a count of two, repeating in both directions 10 times.

12 **Rest your legs up a wall before bed every night.** Sit with one hip as close to the wall as you can get it. Then lie on your back and extend your legs up the wall, so your buttocks, backs of your thighs, and heels touch the wall. You'll feel a mild stretch in your legs as gravity encourages fluids to drain out of your legs and back up to your heart. Hold this position for five minutes.

and flat. Before bending forward into any stretch, first inhale and extend upward, creating as much space as you can between each vertebra in your spine. When you bend forward into a stretch, bend from the hips, not the waist. As you bend forward, your pubic bone should move forward while your tailbone moves back and up.

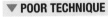
▼ GOOD TECHNIQUE

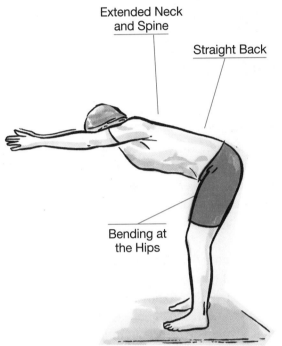

Extended Neck and Spine

Straight Back

Bending at the Hips

▼ POOR TECHNIQUE

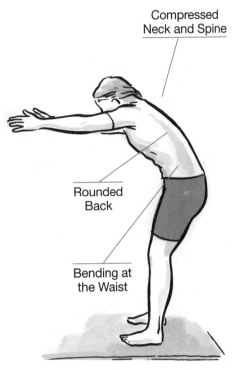

Compressed Neck and Spine

Rounded Back

Bending at the Waist

13 **Hang.** That is, grab a pull-up bar and just hang from it—no pulling or swinging—for a minute or two. It is surprisingly refreshing and can do considerable good for your spine, as well as your arm, shoulder, and chest muscles. A great place to do this is on the monkey bars at a children's playground. However, if you haven't exercised for a while, ask your doctor first about this one, since you are asking your hands and shoulders to hold your entire body weight.

14 **Do finger stretches** regularly to keep your hands limber and strong. Do one hand at a time for best effect.

Finger stretch. Place a hand on a tabletop or thigh, with palm facing down. Spread your fingers as far as you can and hold for 20 to 30 seconds.

Thumb touch. Place your hand, palm up, on a table with your fingers open and relaxed. Smoothly touch the tips of your thumb and index finger. Hold for a second, then return to the starting position. In a similar manner, touch the tip of your thumb to each of your other fingertips.

Spider walk. Place your hand palm-down on a tabletop. Using your fingers, pull your palm across the table as far as you can reach.

Walking

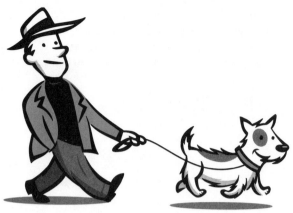

30 IDEAS FOR DOING MORE AND BETTER

I t's so simple and convenient it couldn't possibly count as exercise, right? Wrong. Study after study shows that regular moderate walking can help you lose weight and reduce your risk of heart disease. If you don't believe us, then trust the research. In a study published in *Diabetes Research in Clinical Practice,* Japanese researchers tested obese men before and after they joined a one-year modest walking plan. All they did was up the number of steps they took during their daily activities, such as walking from the car to the grocery store. The result: Their blood pressure and cholesterol levels improved and the amount of body fat around their abdomen—the dangerous kind of fat that leads to higher rates of heart disease and diabetes—significantly decreased.

That's good news, because walking has now become the most popular fitness activity in the United States. Convenient, simple, and gentle on the joints, walking is perhaps the easiest form of exercise to maintain. According to surveys, four out of five women who start a walking program continue to walk, while half of women who attempt other types of aerobic exercise, such as swimming, drop out during the first few months.

Here are some ways both to sneak more walking into your life, and to get the most out of every step you take.

1 Learn the basics. Before you take your next step outdoors, you need to know how much walking to do, and how often. Here are the facts:

▶ For it to be exercise, walk at a pace that has you breathing heavily, but still able to talk.

▶ Your goal, first and foremost, is to walk five days a week, 30 minutes a walk. Do that, and you are getting the base-level amount of exercise that research says should maintain your health and vigor.

▶ Don't assume you can reach that goal quickly. Walking hard for 30 minutes is, well, hard! Walk for as long as you are comfortable the first week, even if it's just to your mailbox and back. Each subsequent week, increase that amount by no more than 10 percent.

▶ Start every walk with five minutes of easy-paced walking, about the same pace at which you'd do your grocery shopping, to get your body warmed up. Then, cool down at the end of each walk with another five minutes of easy-paced walking. This allows your heart rate to *gradually* speed up and slow down.

▶ When you reach the target of 30 minutes a day, five days a week, set a new target. Either you should grow your walking habit by increasing your time, or you might be ready for new forms of exercise, such as strength-building exercises twice a week.

2 Pick a charity—it could be breast cancer, the American Red Cross, the United Way—and pledge to contribute $1 for every mile you walk.

You'll take pride in the fact that you are walking for something beyond yourself, which will motivate you to go longer and faster. After every walk, mark the amount you owe on a chart, and when you reach $100, send a check. Whoever thought exercise could be tax deductible?

3 Walk with a friend. If she's expecting you, you're more likely to get out of bed on cold winter mornings or skip the cafeteria for a lunchtime walk. If one of you backs out for any reason, put $5 in a kitty. Hopefully this will never happen, but if you manage to build up any substantial sum, donate it to charity.

4 Walk for entertainment one day a week. Instead of walking around your neighborhood, walk through the zoo, an art museum, or an upscale shopping mall. First circle the perimeter of your location at your usual brisk pace. Then wander through again more slowly to take in the sights.

5 Use a pedometer. These nifty gadgets measure how far you've walked in steps and miles. They provide motivation by spurring you to meet a particular goal and showing you if you've met it. And research shows that they work. In one study of 510 people completed at Gundersen Lutheran Medical Center in La Crosse, Wisconsin, people who wore a pedometer automatically increased the amount of steps they took in a day. Often, pedometers hook onto your belt and are small and easy to use.

6 Shoot for 10,000 steps a day. Don't let that amount scare you. Most people walk about 5,500 to 7,500 steps during an average day as they amble to and from meetings, to the water cooler, to the mailbox. In fact, researchers who study these types of things consider 5,000 steps a day a "sedentary lifestyle." According to researchers at Arizona State University in Mesa, you can cover 7,499 steps a day without participating in formal sports or exercise. If you garner 10,000 steps a day, you're considered "active," while 12,500 steps a day garners you the title "highly active." Using your pedometer, find your baseline of how many steps you normally take in a day. Then increase that amount by at least 200 steps a day until you reach 10,000 to 12,500 daily steps.

Two-Second Quiz

Walk or Run?

Answer: *Walk.*
Although runners and other high-energy athletes pooh-pooh walking, saying that it doesn't burn enough calories to result in real weight loss, research has shown time and time again that a regular walking program, mile for mile, packs about the same punch when it comes to your waistline. And as is clearly documented, people are far more likely to stay with a walking regimen than a running regimen.

7 Take the entire family on your daily walks. Not only will you be modeling good fitness habits for your children, but you'll also be able to supervise them while you walk rather than getting a sitter. If your children walk too slowly, ask them to ride their bikes or roller-skate alongside you. To keep everyone entertained, play your usual repertoire of long car trip games such as "I Spy." You can also try a scavenger walk, where you start out with a list of items to find during your walk and check off the list as you spot them.

8 Once a week, complete your errands on foot. If you live within a mile of town, or even a convenience store, start from your house. If you live out in the middle of nowhere, drive to within a mile of your destination, park, and walk the rest of the way there and back. You'll be surprised how much you can accomplish on foot, and even better, how many people you'll meet along the way.

9 Improve your walking posture. Proper posture will reduce discomfort as you walk and help you burn more fat and calories. So when you go on your next walk, readjust yourself to the following standards:

- Stand tall with your spine elongated and breastbone lifted. This allows room for your lungs to fully expand.
- Keep your head straight with your eyes focused forward and shoulders relaxed. Avoid slumping your shoulders forward or hunching them toward your ears.
- Roll your feet from heel to toe.
- As you speed up, take smaller, more frequent steps. This protects your knees and gives your butt a good workout.
- Allow your arms to swing freely.

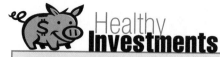

Healthy Investments

Walking Shoes

Why? A good pair of walking shoes will help you travel farther and faster with more comfort. Go to a respected athletic-shoe store so a skilled salesperson can size your feet and find the best shoe for your foot shape and size. Tell the salesperson what type of terrain you'll be walking on and how many miles on average you plan to walk a week.

If you have an old pair of sneakers, bring them to the store with you. The salesperson can look at the wear pattern on your shoes to determine your foot type. For example, if the inner heel is more worn than the outer heel, your foot probably turns in excessively as you walk. In this case, you'll want some extra arch support and a shoe designed for "motion control."

Try on your shoes and walk around the store. Make sure the shoe hugs your heel; your heel should not slide up and down as you walk. The shoe should also have a firm arch support and the forefoot of the shoe should bend with the natural bend in your foot. Most important, the shoes should feel comfortable when you walk. A good walking shoe lasts about 350 miles. If you walk 10 miles a week, that's about eight months.

- Firm your tummy and flatten your back as you walk to prevent low back pain.

10 Breathe deeply as you walk to a count of 1-2-3. Many people unintentionally hold their breath when they exercise and then suddenly feel breathless and tired. Oxygen is invigorating, and muscles need oxygen to create the energy for movement. So as you inhale, bring the air to the deepest part of your lungs by expanding your ribs outward and your tummy forward and inhale for a count of three. Then exhale fully either through your nose or mouth, also to the count of three.

11 Periodically pick up the pace. Boredom can quickly bring a walk to a premature end. Keep your mind and your body engaged by periodically picking up the pace or challenging yourself by trudging up a hill. Every 10 to 15 minutes, complete a 2- to 3-minute surge. During your surge, try to catch a real or imaginary walker ahead of you.

12 Explore on your walks. You can walk anywhere at any time, from your neighborhood to your local mall to your downtown main street to a local trail. You can even walk laps around your office building! Rather than walking the same old tired route day in and day out, use your walks as a way to experience and explore the great outdoors. Varying your route and terrain will do more than keep you mentally engaged. It will also help you to target different leg muscles, improving the effectiveness of every outing. One day you might walk through a section of your neighborhood that allows you to marvel at your neighbors' gardens or home improvement projects. Another day you might head to the local park. Still another day you might walk downtown.

13 Take your dog with you (or get a dog). Once your dog gets used to your walks, he or she will look forward to them and give you a gentle nudge (or annoying whine) on the days you try to get out of it. There's nothing more effective than a set of puppy dog eyes to extract your butt from the couch and get it out the door. In addition to walking the neighborhood, consider signing up for a dog agility class. During the class, you and your dog will circumvent a course with seesaws, hurdles, tunnels, and other obstacles. (Your dog tackles the obstacles. You run or walk

alongside and yell the appropriate command.) Both you and your dog will get a great workout and you'll end up with a better-behaved and calmer dog as a result. Don't have a dog? Offer to walk a neighbor's dog twice a week. That commitment thing will keep you motivated.

14 Pump up the volume. In a study published in the journal *Chest,* people with severe respiratory disease who listened to music while walking covered four more miles during the eight-week study than a similar group that did not listen to music while walking. Researchers speculate that listening to music made the participants feel less hindered by shortness of breath and distracted them from possible boredom and fatigue. You don't have to have lung disease to benefit from music during your walks. Bring along a headset and play your favorite tunes.

15 Sign up for a stroller walk. If you're a new mom, you don't need us to tell you how hard it is to fit in time for fitness—not to mention time for other basics like taking a shower. The good news is you can take your infant on your walk. A growing number of hospitals and fitness centers, including the YMCA, offer group stroller walks for new moms. Entire franchises, such as StrollerFit and Stroller Strides, have popped up in communities around the country. These franchises promote 50-minute to one-hour workouts that combine walking, stretching, and strength training with elastic tubing for stretches and resistance work.

16 When you feel like blowing off your walk, promise yourself you'll do just 10 minutes. "Head out the door for a short walk. Chances are, once you've warmed up, you'll exercise for longer than you anticipated," says Liz Applegate, Ph.D., nutrition and fitness expert at the University of California at Davis and author of *Bounce Your Body Beautiful*. "Even if you don't walk longer, 10 minutes is better than no minutes at all."

17 **Five times a day, climb up and down a flight of stairs for two minutes.** You'll garner the same heart-rate-enhancing results in those 10 minutes as you would get from 36 minutes of walking on a level surface.

18 **Roll out of bed, get dressed, put on your shoes, and go.** It's easy to get caught up in your day-to-day activities and tell yourself that you don't have time for a walk. If you exercise first thing in the morning, however, you have no excuse. Research shows that people who plan to exercise in the morning are more likely to fit in their workouts than people who plan to exercise later in the day. Exercising in the morning may offer a side benefit: You'll sleep better at night. When researchers at the Fred Hutchinson Cancer Research Center in Seattle, Washington, compared morning and evening exercise, people who exercised at least 225 minutes per week in the morning had an easier time falling asleep at night than those who completed the same amount of exercise in the evening.

19 **Or, walk in the evening.** That sleep study aside, we still like after-dinner walks. They get you away from the television, they keep you from eating too much at dinner, it's when your neighbors are outside, and it's just a lovely time of day. Don't let unlovely weather stop you either—that's what jackets, boots, and umbrellas were invented for. There's something childlike and fun about a walk in the rain or snow.

20 **Learn your m.p.h.** That's miles per hour, of course, just like a car. Knowing it isn't that useful, but we're a nation of statistics lovers, and if monitoring your speed helps keep you motivated, then more power to you. A leisurely pace is 2 miles per hour, a healthy, brisk pace is 3.5 miles per hour, and going over 4 miles per hour is downright fast. A pedometer will measure this for you, but if you don't have one, you can simply count your steps during various 15-second periods. For a normal grown-up stride, if you walk 15 steps in 15 seconds, you're walking at a leisurely pace of 2 miles per hour, At 23 steps, you're walking a moderate pace of 3 miles per hour, and at 30 steps, you're walking about 4 miles per hour.

21 **Walk in the prettiest area in your town (or the next town over).** It just might encourage you to walk more often. When researchers from the University of Wollongong in New South Wales, Australia, surveyed walkers about their walking habits, they found that men who perceived their neighborhoods to be "aesthetic" were more consistent about walking around their neighborhoods. Other research finds that neighborhoods with well-maintained sidewalks and safe and well-lit walking areas encourage walking over neighborhoods that don't have those features. In fact, people who live in so-called walkable neighborhoods walk an average of 70 more minutes each week than people who live in neighborhoods lacking such characteristics, according to a study completed at Cincinnati Children's Hospital Medical Center.

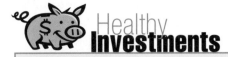

Healthy Investments

Walking Poles

Why? These lightweight walking poles sold at most sporting goods stores can help you feel more steady and safe when walking on trails. The poles encourage you to bend your elbows and use your arms as you walk, which will prevent swelling in your hands. The movement also provides a great upper and lower body workout, which burns more calories as well as strengthens your muscles. Finally, the poles take stress off your knees.

22 **If you're over 60, walk on soft surfaces.** As you age, the fat padding in your feet deteriorates. The absence of this natural shock absorber can make walking on sidewalks and other hard surfaces feel like foot torture. Flat grass and dirt paths will provide more cushioning for your feet than roads or sidewalks.

23 **Train for an event.** It's a great motivator. Check your local sporting goods stores for calendars or flyers on walks being held in your area. Generally, these fun runs and walks raise money for a good cause. For example, the Leukemia and Lymphoma Society offers a Team in Training program that will get you in marathon walking shape. Yes, that's right, lots of people walk an entire 26.2 miles in one shot. The society assigns you a coach and walking plan, and you raise money through donations.

24 **Apply some lube.** If you're a long-distance walker or somewhat overweight, chafing clothes can make you want to call it quits. You can solve the problem by wearing skin-hugging clothing and lubing up your sensitive areas with Vaseline. The Vaseline acts like a barrier to protect your skin.

25 **Split it up.** When you're too busy to go for your usual 30- to 60-minute walk, split it up and get out there for 5 or 10 minutes at a time. That may be as simple as taking a 5-minute walk break around the building after completing a big project at work. Such short walking breaks will refresh your mind, so you can return to work with more vigor. In fact, research shows that most of us can only focus at top capacity for 30 minutes at a time. After that, concentration begins to drop off. Your intermittent walk breaks may actually make you more productive!

26 **Shop at the mall instead of online.** Walking around the mall can burn about 200 calories an hour, much more than what you will burn sitting on your tush as you surf the Net for great deals. You can increase the effectiveness of your walk and shop time by doing a lap around the mall between store visits.

27 **Walk and talk.** Use a cordless phone and walk around the house as you chat with friends or conduct your business. This is a great way to make use of those long times spent on hold with the IRS, phone company, or Internet service provider. Not only will you get some heart-healthy exercise, but the exercise will help you maintain your mental cool. Use your pedometer to count your steps and you'll get the added bonus of feeling like you accomplished something rather than just wasting time.

28 **Walk faster earlier in your walk.** If you want to increase the amount of fat you burn during your walk, add some bursts of faster walking toward the *beginning* of your walk. Many walkers wait until the end of the walk to speed up, treating their faster walking as a finishing kick. Yet a study published in the *European Journal of Applied Physiology* found that exercisers burned more fat and felt less fatigued when they inserted their faster segments toward the beginning of a workout. It works because you speed up your heart rate early and keep it elevated for the rest of your walk.

29 **Feel each muscle you use in your walk.** Concentrate on different muscle areas: calves, hamstrings, glutes, and quadriceps. Feel the movement in each area as you walk. The motivation you'll get from realizing the bang you're getting for your walking buck (all those muscles!) will keep you walking longer.

30 **Take light weights (3 to 5 pounds) on your walks.** Periodically work in arm exercises as you walk. This does more than increase the benefit of the workout. Carrying weights also builds muscle, and each pound of muscle burns about 30-50 more calories a day. Build a couple of pounds of muscle in your arms alone and you'll burn an extra 100 calories a day—even while you're just channel surfing. Not into weights? Try isometric exercises of the arms, chest, and abdominal muscles. For instance, as you walk, go through the motion of throwing a punch in slow motion. As you extend your arm, tense the muscles along it and do the same as you retract it. You should feel tension in your triceps, biceps, deltoids, and pectoral muscles. Then repeat with your arms going straight up and down, or out to the side, rather than straight ahead. You can also tense your chest muscles by bringing your hands together in front of your body and contracting across the chest and shoulders. Do this rhythmically to match your gait. Also try doing curls with no weights. Simply curl your arms alternately, in rhythm with your gait. Each time you curl your forearms, tense your biceps.

Weekends

23 IDEAS FOR MORE ACTIVE DAYS OFF

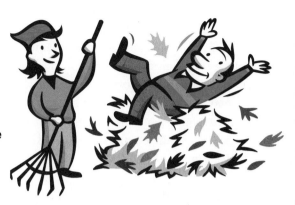

If you believe the car commercials you see every day on television, the majority of us spend our weekends blazing through the hills, on the way to a day of bicycling, rock climbing, beach frolicking, picnicking, and generally being active.

A look at the parking lot of the local mall come Saturday afternoon shows the reality. Our weekends have become a time of errands, shopping, and finishing up the work we didn't get to during the week. For too many of us, our spirit of adventure is being fulfilled by finding a great bargain at a store. And for parents, our thrill seeking is being fulfilled through our kids—we shuttle them to and from their sports matches, and cheer from the sidelines.

It's time to reclaim our weekends—or at least, a good-sized chunk of them. There is no better time for exercise and stress relief than a sunny Saturday afternoon outdoors. Here, then, are ways to sneak in some life-affirming weekend activity.

1 To determine the scope of your weekend hassles, keep a log of your activities this coming weekend. Jot them down in your day planner. Then, come Sunday night, take stock of the weekend that passed you by. Where did you spend your time? How can you cut back on those activities to make time for fun and fitness? You'll likely find that working, shopping, cleaning, cooking, and shuttling are dominating your weekend. Once you document what's chewing up your time, it gets easier to come up with a fix.

2 Shift weekend duties to weekday evening duties. There's no need to wait until the weekend to go to the supermarket, clean the house, or cut the lawn. Make Tuesday and Thursday evenings your "weekend duty" evenings and get the housework out of the way rather than sitting in front of the TV. This way, come the weekend, you'll have free days to do as you wish!

3 Designate each Thursday evening as the weekend planning time. Start by getting the weather report. Next, detail the "must do" stuff, such as attending church or taking your kid to a birthday party. Then, get creative and be bold by filling in the open space with great, refreshing activities. Work the phone—make reservations, call friends or family for invitations. Too many of us enter the weekend without solid plans,

and end up watching TV and baking cookies we don't really need.

4 **If you must work, get it out of the way early.** A good way to reclaim your weekend from your work is to get up an hour earlier than normal, set the alarm for two to three hours, work in a very focused manner, and then when the alarm rings, turn off the computer. The rest of the weekend is yours!

5 **Save enough money to hire a cleaning service.** That way, you won't spend your weekends cleaning. Want to know how to fund it? Easy. Just cut out the little extras that cost you big bucks. For example, borrow videos from the library instead of renting them. Brew your own coffee instead of hitting Starbucks. Pack your lunch, color your own hair, cook your own gourmet dinner instead of heading to a restaurant. The sacrifices will be worth it when you walk into your home and see and smell the cleanliness. *Now* you have time to enjoy your weekend!

6 **Get out of bed at the same time as during the week.** We often have great intentions to be active on the weekend—that is, until we sleep in until noon. When you lose half the day to the covers, it's hard to find time for fun and exercise. Make it a habit to get out of bed the same time on weekends as during the week. In addition to freeing up more time for your weekend fitness forays, you'll also regulate your body clock better. Once your body gets used to a regular wake and sleep schedule, you'll fall asleep faster, feel more refreshed when you wake, and avoid that Monday morning "hungover" feeling.

7 **Go for a walk first thing in the morning.** Head out the door before the Sunday newspaper, rolls, and coffee. Walking first thing in the morning ensures you fit in your workout. Once you return, you'll feel invigorated and be more likely to move more during the rest of the day.

8 **Make nature part of your weekend worship routine.** For many of us, the great outdoors has a way of sparking our love of life and God. So don't limit the family ritual to a trip to the church or synagogue; add in a weekly family walk through the park or woods or desert, either before or after services. It will lift your heart, as well as exercise it!

9 **Always commit one day to fun.** Never, ever let errands and work spread to both Saturday and Sunday. Whether you live alone or with a family, pick one of those days and go to a water park, take a hike in the mountains, or spend the day playing softball, badminton, or other games in the backyard. You and your companions will soon look forward to this day, devoted not to formal exercise but to fun activities you can do together.

Healthy Investments

Wiffle Balls

If you play golf or baseball, you typically need lots of space—and hours of time—to pursue your game. Plastic balls let you play in a small space, and at any time you want. With plastic golf balls you can whack away in your backyard with the full range of clubs, without risking damage and using up lots of space. And with a Wiffle baseball, anyone can play—even without baseball gloves.

10 Match your time watching sports with playing sports.

Too many men—and women!—have become addicted to watching sports on television. So we issue you this challenge: For every hour you watch sports on TV, commit to 30 minutes of doing a sport or some other exercise. Gradually increase the ratio to one-to-one; that is, an hour watching, an hour doing. For all the joys of major league sports, nothing compares to hitting a home run, scoring a goal, making a birdie, finishing the race, or winning the tennis match yourself.

11 Spiff up the yard—manually.

Many types of yard work, from leaf raking to garden digging to mowing, build upper body strength and burn excess calories. In fact, one major study found that gardening was the best physical activity for preventing osteoporosis. And don't make it too convenient for yourself. Physically rake the leaves rather than using a leaf blower. Use a push mower rather than a self-propelled one. The more you use your own body, the more calories you'll burn. As an added bonus, you can feel good knowing that the less you use gas-powered equipment, the less pollution you've released into the air.

12 If you cycle, go for a long ride.

During the week you probably can't ride much, but weekends allow you the luxury of riding for half the day or more, if you're so inclined. Scout out a local route or put the bike in the car and drive to a great riding location. Bring along plenty of food and stash it in your bike jersey. Take some cash as well. You never know when you'll ride past a bagel or coffee shop and want to take a pit stop.

Two-Second**Quiz**

Movie Theater or Rental?

Answer: *Movie theater.*
Assuming cost is not an issue, going to a movie theater provides more fun, activity, and social interaction than sitting in front of your television at home—all of which are good for your health. Plus, you don't have a refrigerator to raid during the slow parts.

13 Join a club.

Many outdoors organizations, such as the Audubon Society and Sierra Club, sponsor group hikes and other outings on the weekends. You need only show up with food and water, and your guide will take you on a half-day to full-day excursion. In fact, there are surprisingly large numbers of walking, biking, bird-watching, or running clubs in most areas that have regular weekend events. Fitness centers and regional parks are a great place to start your search for the right one for you.

14 Make a list of weekend fitness activities and choose one activity from the list every weekend.

The more varied your weekend fitness routine, the more likely you'll stay active on the weekends. On your list, you might write hiking, canoeing, walking, cycling, bird-watching and other activities.

15 Keep a fitness kit in your car.

Stock your car with a volleyball, soccer ball, baseball and mitts, basketball, or other favorite fitness items. Make sure to include a pair of sneakers. You never know when you'll find yourself away from home with a little downtime. If your fitness kit is stocked and ready, you'll have everything you need for fun.

16 Train for a race. Whether you walk, run, cycle, or do some other sport, signing up for a race will give you the incentive to train on the weekends. Suddenly fitness becomes the top priority in your life. Plus, this is what serious athletes do—complete their longer workout sessions on the weekends, when they have time away from work.

17 Take calisthenics breaks. If you find yourself working at the office (or in your home office) over the weekend, take a 10-minute break every hour and do jumping jacks, lunges, push-ups, and crunches. Over the course of the day, you'll have exercised for more than 60 minutes—and finished that big project on time.

18 Combine physically active work with pure indulgence. For instance, split some wood or gather kindling in the woods as the physical activity part of your day, then sit in front of the fire with someone special for the pure indulgence part. Or clean up the yard by day, and have a barbecue that evening. Or take a long hike, and have a wonderful picnic basket waiting for you in the car.

19 If your kids play sports, coach or assist their team. Instead of spending the weekend with your butt glued to the driver's seat of your car as you shuttle your kids from one activity to another, join them. Sign up to coach their Little League, soccer, or swim team. Or help manage things along the sidelines. It'll get you out of the car and you'll exercise all parts of your body—and soul.

20 Take the family to the mall and powerwalk as your spouse and kids get their shopping done. Just because everyone else wants to shop all day doesn't mean you have to forgo exercise. Bring your cell phones and watches. When you get to the mall, split up, agreeing to meet in a certain spot at a certain time. You walk loops through the mall as your spouse and kids do their shopping.

21 Keep a Frisbee in your car in case of emergency. No matter where you find yourself, you can always play a game of Frisbee golf—assuming you have a Frisbee with you. You don't need a fancy Frisbee golf course to play. Just designate your own targets. Pick out 18 trees, telephone poles, and other targets. Whoever hits all the targets in the least amount of throws wins.

22 Be one of the kids. Don't just push them out the door and spend the afternoon inside reading or cleaning. Join them. Find a tall tree and climb it with them. Play a friendly game of hoops in the driveway. Spend the day skating or cycling or playing tag. After all, even if our bodies are aging, we all have a some childishness inside us, still aching to get out. See page 168, "Family Fun," for more ways to stay fit with your family.

23 Take the family camping. There's nothing quite like the great outdoors to put your body in a calorie-burning state, or to create happily memorable times for your kids. After you've pitched your tent, built your campfire, and secured your site, you can look into other activities such as swimming, canoeing, and hiking. Yes, it is worth all the hassle.

Vacations

13 TIPS FOR ACTIVELY INDULGENT TRAVEL

When many of us take a vacation from work and home, more than anything, we seek to relax. We spend long, lazy days on a beach chair or in a hammock and socialize the night away with rum drinks, fancy martinis, and indulgent desserts. Too often, we return home heavier and flabbier than we've been since, well, our last vacation.

It doesn't have to be this way.

Active vacations are often the most relaxing of all. Wait! Don't toss the book out the window! It's all in defining what an active vacation is. We don't expect you to take up jogging, backpacking, or hang gliding. Rather, we ask the sedentary vacationers among you to spend two to four hours a day *doing things*. Walking the city streets. Exploring a nature preserve. Going to a zoo. Biking along the ocean. Taking a leisurely rowboat ride. These kinds of activities aren't just good for your physical health. They improve your mental health, even your spiritual health. And they make vacations memorable and worthwhile. And after all, isn't that what you want from your vacation? Here are some fresh ideas to make your vacations as pleasurable as they are active and healthy. On page 389, you'll also find ways to sneak health and exercise while traveling by airplane or on business trips.

1 **Make morning time your activity time.** Most likely the weather will be friendlier, your energy level higher, and your agenda emptier than later in the day.

2 **Reacquaint yourself with sunrises and sunsets.** A walk at dawn or dusk is rejuvenation defined. Try to make this a daily ritual of life away from home, and you will guarantee yourself both physical and spiritual replenishment.

3 **Get into the water as much as you can.** Don't allow yourself to spend all your time sitting in front of the water. Whether it is the ocean, a swimming pool, or a tree-lined lake, make sure you get into the water for swimming or games or even walking. Heck, merely *standing* in waist-high water is a good workout, thanks to the action of the water. And you'll feel so much more alive!

4 **Get *on* the water as much as you can.** Paddleboats are a blast. Canoeing is a joy. Rowboats are romantic. Powerboats exhilarating. Sailboats serene. Kayaks pure adventure. Inner tubes can erase 50 years from your attitude in a matter of minutes. Even standing at the rail of a

steamboat is exciting. Boats make you feel young, and whether you are propelling them or not, they all burn calories and engage your muscles more than being on dry land.

5 **Choose a cruise for your trip.** It's amazing how active you can be being stuck on a boat in the middle of the Atlantic. Most cruise ships offer numerous options for seaworthy exercise. Most ships house pools, golf simulators, rock walls, basketball hoops, fitness centers, jogging and walking areas, and instructor-led fitness classes—and that's just what's on board. During your sea and land excursions you can burn calories as you snorkel, swim, hike, scuba dive, and horseback ride.

6 **Get out of the car every two hours.** Many of us spend a large chunk of our vacations on the road, either getting to and from our destinations, or using the car for sightseeing. But no matter how beautiful the scenery is, great, memorable vacations don't happen in a car seat. Don't wait for exhaustion or nature's

Two-Second Quiz

Bowling, Billiards, Badminton, Croquet, or Darts?

Answer: *Badminton.*
In terms of exertion, badminton considerably beats the competition at 266 calories burned per hour, since it requires jumping, swinging, and lots of leg movement. Second is bowling (177 calories per hour). Billiards, croquet, and darts all burn about the same amount of calories per hour (148). By comparison, a moderately paced walk burns 207 calories per hour.

call to get you to pull over. Frequently get out and stretch, walk, picnic, shop, visit, and have fun. It's important for your health and energy, and it makes traveling a lot more active and interesting.

7 **Play active games.** When most people think of outdoor games, they think of team sports like baseball, football, or volleyball, all of which can be both intimidating and excessively strenuous for grown-ups who stopped playing such things a long time back. So forget about the standard games. All types of fun outdoor games are available today. Start with the old-fashioned ones—badminton, shuffleboard, horseshoes, Wiffle ball, or bocce. Try some new ones too—they make great balls out of Nerf these days, and if you haven't bought a squirt gun in a while, be prepared for today's amazing supersoakers. Plus all types of new paddle games are available that are easy and fun. Your goal: Play an outdoor game every day while on vacation.

8 **Create a silly tournament.** Particularly if there are kids on the vacation, it can be a hoot to create your own mini-Olympics. For example, if you use the swimming pool every day, have a daily competition, such as holding your breath underwater, or swimming between people's legs, or having a big splash contest. Or maybe a weeklong badminton competition. "Silly" is the operative word—don't make it serious competition, but just a chance to have active fun in which everyone participates.

9 **Play miniature golf.** You burn more calories sitting than lying, standing than sitting, and walking than standing. Although miniature golf won't incinerate fat, it will burn more calories than lying in a hammock. Plus, your kids will have a great time. You probably will too.

10 Beware the food obsession. Let's be honest: For many of us, vacations are about eating splurges. It's fresh seafood by the ocean, amazing restaurants in great cities, unlimited breakfast buffets at the hotel, that ice cream/candy/cake/jambalaya that you remember as a child and come back for every few years. This is the stuff of great vacations, and don't deny yourself these pleasures. Our suggestion: Limit yourself to one food splurge a day. If you do more, the uniqueness and specialness of the splurges fade away. And you'll spend too much time sitting in restaurants—and then sitting some more, recuperating from the overindulgence.

11 Explore on foot. Yes, you can use the concierge, the travel guides, the map, or the bus tours to get acquainted with a new location. But only by getting out and walking can you truly get the feel of a village, city, resort, or wilderness. We recommend that you plan to spend the first several hours at your vacation destination walking the area. If you are in a city, pick a few restaurants to try while you are walking and make your reservations in person. Be sure to locate the parks, museums, and shopping areas.

12 Fly a stunt kite. If there's a good wind blowing at your destination, purchase a stunt kite and take it to the

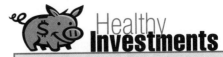

Healthy Investments

An Upgraded Hotel Room

Why? Many hotels, including the Omni chain, now offer special fitness guest rooms complete with treadmill or other exercise machine, dumbbells, rubber tubing, floor mat, radio headset, energy bars, and other handy fitness items. The Omni "Get Fit Guest Room" costs $14.99 more a night than other guest rooms, a drop in the bucket when your health is concerned.

beach or other large open area. These kites can be easily assembled and then taken apart, making them perfect for traveling. You'll give your upper body a great workout as you struggle to control the kite. You may also have to run or walk to keep the kite in the air—or chase it down once it plummets to the earth.

13 Schedule an activity-based vacation. Ready to commit to even more action? Wrap your entire vacation around an activity, such as sailing, skiing, hiking, biking, or exploring. No expertise is necessary—just a willingness to take on a new challenge. Travel agents can hook you up with any number of vacation packages targeted from novice to expert, adolescent to senior, single or whole family. If you have children, look for packages that include excavating dinosaur bones and other anthropological expeditions, or that teach them a new sport. A ski vacation with lessons for different ages and ability levels works beautifully.

Family Fun

47 WAYS TO USE THE ULTIMATE EXERCISE MACHINES—CHILDREN

If you happen to have children living at home, this chapter is for you. It's also for grandparents, and for all you uncles and aunts who love to spend time with your nieces and nephews, and all of you babysitters, day care workers, friendly neighbors, and school and church volunteers. In short, it's for any adult who spends time with children.

The message of this chapter is twofold: First, that you have a wonderful opportunity to get some very fun, high-quality exercise by playing with kids; second, that you have a responsibility to teach the kids in your life about the joys and importance of exercise.

You know why *you* need to be active. You may not know to what extent obesity and sedentary living is crippling our youth. More than 60 percent of children do not exercise on a regular basis. Overall, the Centers for Disease Control finds that just 8 percent of elementary schools, 6 percent of middle schools, and 5 percent of high schools offer daily physical education classes. Small wonder, then, that the CDC also finds that at least 15 percent of U.S. children and teens are now overweight, more than triple the number in 1970. These fast-rising numbers have serious implications:

- Children are now subject to an epidemic of type 2 diabetes, a disease that once occurred exclusively at or beyond middle age in adults.

- The obesity epidemic holds more harm for today's children than exposure to tobacco, drugs, and alcohol combined.

- Today's kids have a shorter life expectancy than their parents, the first time this has ever occurred in this country.

So engaging your kids in a health-promoting lifestyle should be a priority for every loving parent. But if you want trim and healthy kids, you have to get trim and healthy yourself. Studies show that family environment is one of the strongest predictors of childhood obesity. In one study, children of sedentary parents (a.k.a. couch potatoes) were more likely to gain weight and become overweight than children of active parents.

Some of the movement suggestions in this chapter seem too easy to be considered exercise. But remember: You and your child burn more calories standing than sitting, walking than standing. The more you move, the more you burn. It doesn't matter how wacky your antics, if you are moving and having fun, you're burning calories and getting in shape. It's that simple.

1 **Go on a treasure hunt.** Here's a great way to keep the family fit and teach your kids about trust, teamwork, and problem solving at the same time. Take them to a local park and set an expedition course on a map, circling various "checkpoints." Take turns navigating to each point on the map and leading the team to each destination. "Start out with an easy course in an open park and then progress to a trail system," suggests Jenny Hadfield, a Chicago-based fitness coach and author of *Marathoning for Mortals.* "Stay together and explore terrain features, study map clues, and look for the secret treasure." Sound too complicated? Then merely go hunting for bugs, animals, or flowers. You can't entertain a young kid much better than finding a colorful salamander under a log or rock.

2 **Plan 10-minute spurts of activity** followed by 5-minute rest periods. Don't force your adult exercise program on your children. That's a recipe for disaster. Studies published in the journal *Medicine & Science in Sports & Exercise* show

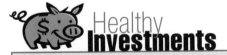

Healthy Investments

A Mini-Trampoline

Your children will probably turn up their noses at most adult types of fitness equipment such as a treadmill or hand weights. A mini-trampoline, however, is another story. You can set one up in your living room and line it with pillows. When you feel tempted to babysit your child with the TV, suggest she jump on the trampoline for 15 minutes. She will burn about 100 calories rather than the mere 10 calories burned during 15 minutes of watching television. Buy a trampoline designed for indoor use that contains handles for safety.

that forcing children to participate in structured exercise turns them off to exercise later in life. Instead, take advantage of their natural tendency to participate in intermittent and sporadic play and exercise bouts. A game of tag is a perfect example. Children's bodies are designed to sprint and rest, sprint and rest. Because they are easily distracted and incapable of long periods of focused activity, they will resist long exercise sessions that don't include rest periods.

3 **Train for school fitness tests as a family.** In 2004, 75 percent of the 1.3 million students in California who took an annual fitness test failed at least six basic categories, including running, lifting, and stretching. Only 49 percent of the state's ninth graders could run a mile in under 12.5 minutes. Learn which fitness tests your child is required to pass in physical education class and train for them as a family. Set goals, such as running a quarter-mile and then a half and then a full mile in a certain amount of time—and reward each family member for meeting each goal.

4 **Hold a sports party.** Rather than the typical pin-the-tail-on-the-donkey birthday party, hold your child's birthday party in an active location, such as a roller-skating or ice-skating rink, laser tag center, wall-climbing gym, or indoor playground center. You don't have to limit this to parties. A growing number of indoor playgrounds offer such structured games weekly. Or you can have your own "no particular reason" party. Kids won't think of what they're doing as exercise—but it is.

5 **Play follow the leader with one or more children.** Line up single file and weave your way through the house or backyard. Every few steps, hop, skip, do

the grapevine or some other movement that your followers must imitate. Once the kids get the hang of the game, let them take turns as leader. Their naturally creative minds will come up with all sorts of fun movements for the followers to imitate. You'll be out of breath before you know it.

6 **Purchase some family-friendly aerobics tapes for cold or rainy days.** Choose tapes that describe the workout as "low intensity" or "low impact" says Melinda S. Sothern, Ph.D., director of the Prevention of Childhood Obesity Lab at Louisiana State University in Baton Rouge and author of *Trim Kids.* These types of aerobic exercise are better for children's developing bodies. Good options include Elmocize, Workout with Mommy and Me, the Richard Simmons series, YogaKids, and Tae Bo Junior.

7 **Give your child a head start—and race around the house.** You can do the same with calisthenics. You do 10 crunches, and your child does 5. See who can complete them first.

8 **Spend an hour doing yard work together.** Raking leaves, pulling weeds, and spreading out mulch all help to build strength and endurance. Plus, when your kids help, it doesn't take as long or seem as much of a chore (depending on the age of the child, of course). There are numerous ways to make yard work more fun for kids. For instance, when you finish raking a pile of leaves, you get to jump in them.

9 **Wash the car together.** The scrubbing is good exercise, but everyone getting wet and soapy is just plain fun for kids.

10 **Give your kids a list of indoor chores—then join them.** Younger children often like to feel helpful and will enjoy helping you with household chores. Ask them to help you make the beds, fold the laundry and put it away, set the table, and put dishes in the dishwasher—all physical activities that can help get your heart rate up, stretch your body, and build your muscles.

11 **Join the President's Challenge as a family.** In this challenge, children and adults log daily physical activity levels and earn points for each activity. For details, go to www.presidentschallenge.org.

12 **Plan a garden together.** As you dig holes, plant seeds, and pull weeds, you'll build your child's and your upper body strength. As an added bonus, research shows children are more likely to eat the vegetables they help grow, which means your gardening forays will help your child follow a more nutritious diet.

13 Take a hike at least twice a month. Grab a backpack, plenty of water (everyone should drink 8 ounces every half-hour), and a light lunch and head to a local trail for a hiking expedition. Wear hiking boots for rocky terrain or sneakers for smoother trails, and pack sunscreen and insect repellent. To make this more fun for kids, make it about something else, such as looking for a particular animal or bird, climbing to see a lake or pond, or seeing how many rocks you can scamper over without touching the ground. Kids like hiking much better when they don't realize it's about hiking! Bring a picnic, of course; this is a great opportunity to share a delicious but healthful meal and cultivate good family eating habits.

14 Dance during commercial breaks. Make it a family rule that whenever you watch television, you have to stand up and dance around during the commercials. This goes for everyone! Whoever gets caught sitting on the couch during a commercial break must perform his or her least-liked household chore for one week.

15 Sign up for a race. Check your local paper for a list of 5K and 10K walk/run events in your area. Many of these events also raise money for charity, which can inspire your children to train for the event. "You'll not only contribute to your family's health, but also to research to help find cures for many diseases," says Dr. Sothern. Don't worry about finishing; the

motivation involved in training for it is enough on its own.

16 Play volleyball once a week in warm weather. Set up a net, get a ball, and invite other neighborhood children and their parents over for a game. You can get in even more fitness if you add these rules:

▶ When the opposing team scores a point, the receiving team must do 10 calisthenic moves, such as jumping jacks, push-ups, or crunches.
▶ Whoever is responsible for fumbling a shot must walk, dance, skip, or jog around the court.

17 Try a family-friendly game of flag football. Purchase table napkins in two colors. Divide your family into two teams and ask everyone to tuck one of the colored napkins into his waistband. When an opposing team member pulls a napkin from the ball carrier's waistband and places it on the ground, the play has ended. Allow only 20 seconds to prepare for kickoff and 10 seconds after a down. Switch positions every 15 minutes to keep the entire family active. Not only will you get in some family fitness time, but you'll also be teaching your children valuable lessons about practice, perseverance, cooperation, and teamwork.

18 Dance, dance, dance. Put on your favorite music and dance with your children. Teach your children dance moves from your generation and have them show you moves from theirs (or make up moves for you to try). Vigorous dancing burns just as many calories as brisk walking or playing basketball. And kids love it—particularly when the grown-ups pick them up and swing them around every now and then. And don't just leave dancing to chance, or when you happen to be in the mood—make sure to have one or two family dance sessions a week. Perhaps a Friday night dance can become family tradition. Let everyone choose some of the music, play it in turns, and shake that thang!

19 **Walk your children to and from school.** By walking with them, you not only get peace of mind that they're safe, but you also get to hear about their upcoming day on the way there, and how their day went on the way home.

20 **Make like an animal.** If you have young children ages 3–8, organize an animal race. Let everyone in the family pick an animal, such as a snake, monkey, or crab. Then race across the room as you imitate how that animal might move. For example, if you choose a monkey, you must race using your hands and feet, but not your knees or torso. If you are imitating a snake, you must slither across the room. Add some proper animal noises for real fun. You'll be out of breath before you know it.

21 **Walk around the world.** Place a map of the country, state, or world somewhere prominently in your home. Work with your children to arrive at a walking destination. Then, based on your daily family walks, plot your progress on the map using thumbtacks. There are about 2,000 steps in a mile, so you can plot your progress by using a pedometer. To add some incentive, promise to actually take a vacation to your walking destination once you complete the number of steps to get there.

Setting Limits on Television Time

One study of children ages 2-18 found kids spend an average of 5 hours and 29 minutes per day watching television, playing video games, and using various other types of electronic media. You can increase your kids' physical activity and decrease sedentary behavior with the following simple switches.

- Remove TVs and computers from children's bedrooms. According to Kaiser Family Foundation research, two-thirds of children ages 8 and older have a TV in their bedroom, half have a video game, and one-third a VCR. Almost half of children live in a house where the TV is on at all times, even when no one is watching it. According to research done at Johns Hopkins University, a child's weight increases with the number of hours he or she watches television.

- Place active toys such as jump ropes, mini-trampolines, Sit 'n Spin, and hula hoops within easy access in kids' bedrooms or playrooms.

- Require that your kids exercise during commercial breaks.

- Put a curfew on electronics. For instance, nothing that requires batteries or electricity may be used until 5 p.m. on school days.

- Set a tit-for-tat rule. For every 30 minutes of television watching or Internet surfing, your child must do 30 minutes of physical activity.

22 **Start a ball fight.** A large, air-filled stability ball can provide you and your children with plenty of fun, laughter, and a great workout, says Liz Applegate, Ph.D., author of *Bounce Your Body Beautiful*. Applegate suggests the following ball exercises.

- Stand facing your child with the ball between you. You should both grasp the ball about chest level. This may mean you need to get on your knees depending on the height of your child. Then fight over the ball, rotating it from side to side for 15-20 seconds at a time.
- Stand holding the ball at chest level with your arms extended. Ask your child to try to knock the ball out of your hands by tapping different parts of it from different directions. To really up the ante, try it with your eyes closed.

23 **Toss a ball or a Frisbee.** It seems more like relaxation than structured exercise, but you'll get your heart rate up every time you have to run for an errant ball or Frisbee. Plus, you'll both improve your hand-eye coordination.

24 **Act like a child.** Remember duck-duck-goose, hopscotch, and red-light-green-light-one-two-three? You probably thought of these games as just that, games. But they also require movement and count as exercise. Teach them to your kids and play along. As you laugh, you'll burn extra calories. Don't forget Simon says!

25 **Hold a night of active family games every week.** Organize a night of matchups of the three-legged race, wheelbarrow races, and others and challenge another family from the neighborhood to a friendly competition.

26 **Place small children on the floor at least once a day—and let them crawl, move, and toddle.** Children are inherently active when given the opportunity to move, says Dr. Sothern. Yet we often confine children and prevent the very exercise they need. For example, have you ever placed your baby in a swing or portable car seat to give yourself some free time? Ever settled your children in front of the VCR, DVD player, or television when you needed a break? Instead of automatically finding a stationary activity for your children when you need your own personal time-out, encourage more activity. For toddlers and crawlers, find a safe space on the floor where you can plop them and let them move. Have other children play in the sandbox, run through the backyard, or climb your backyard tree as you do your own thing nearby.

27 **Waltz with your baby.** If your baby is crying for attention, don't just stick a pacifier in her mouth or take her for a drive. Instead, take her in your arms and waltz around the room. The more exaggerated and smooth your movements, the better. The waltzing will give your baby new sights to focus on, soothing the crying. You'll burn extra calories and tone the muscles in your arms by holding her.

28 **Make your child a superhero, lifting and spinning him with your arms and/or legs.** Basically, you're using your infant or toddler as resistance to

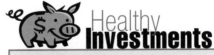

Healthy Investments

Water Bottles With Carrying Straps

Get one for every member of the family, strap them on, and head out for a two-mile hike/walk. Handy, and cost effective, since you bypass buying bottles of water to carry with you.

strengthen your muscles. Try doing biceps curls with your baby on your forearms. Lie on your back and press your baby or toddler away from your chest. As he giggles, you'll get stronger. For larger children, lie on your back and press them away with your feet and hands, getting an upper and lower body workout. Also try swinging them up and down in your forearms. Not only will you get a great workout, your kids will have to use the muscles that control their posture and everyone will bond and have fun.

29 Design your backyard for activity.

What you put in your backyard helps determine how fit your children become. If they see it, they will play. If they don't, they will watch TV. Older children enjoy climbing on ropes or ladders and playing in forts. Make sure you have a swing set, sprinkler attachment for your hose, sandbox, wagon for hauling toys and dolls, and outdoor sporting equipment for basketball, badminton, soccer, and other games.

30 Play active video games.

Although most video games only exercise the muscles in the fingers and eyes, a few can instill a pretty good workout. At the video arcade, challenge your child to a game of Dance Dance Revolution. In this game, you must step on floor squares in the order they light up, simulating dancing. Whack-a-Mole and Skee Ball offer other good options. At home, buy a Power Pad for your computer. You connect it to your or your child's body. As you move, it records your actions in the computer screen in abstract images. Another game available on Game Boy is called Boktai. It requires users to physically go outside to charge up their gun with actual sunlight.

Players find themselves running indoors and out to keep the gun charged and the game in play.

31 Create an obstacle course.

Set out hula hoops, pillows, and other devices that you can imagine as "rocks." Then tell your children that the hoops are rocks in a turbulent river. You all must jump from rock to rock to avoid falling in and getting swept away.

32 Master the hula hoop and other toys.

You and your children will bond, and you'll be the coolest parent on the block if you personally master the hula hoop, Lemon Twist, and other active toys along with your child.

33 Crawl with your baby.

Too often, once babies start to crawl, we confine them to a bouncy chair or some other device so we can work or even work out. Crawling helps develop upper body strength for both you and your baby, and it's a great aerobic activity. So get down on all fours and crawl around the room with your baby. To add to the challenge, take a large, air-filled ball (perhaps your stability ball) and push it with your nose as you crawl. Encourage your baby to do the same.

34 Take your kids for a wagon ride.

Place small children in a wagon and pull them around the neighborhood. As you pull the wagon, you can get an upper body workout by mimicking typical exercises you would do in a gym. For example, you can walk backward as you pull the wagon, bringing your hands toward your shoulders to simulate a biceps curl. You can walk sideways—doing the grapevine—as you lift and lower your arm out to the side. When you walk forward, bend and extend your elbows for triceps presses. You can also raise your bent elbows toward your shoulders to mimic upright rows. Plus, to make it a better workout for the kids, have them get out of the wagon and walk periodically.

35 **Play tug-of-war.** You'll develop upper body and lower body strength as you tug on the rope. To level out the playing field, place two children on one side of the rope and yourself on the other. Bend your knees and bring your legs into a lunge position to get a leg workout as you tug the rope.

36 **Learn a sport together, such as skiing.** Don't live near a slope? How about in-line skating or golf (no carts allowed).

37 **Forget lying by the pool—play.** If you have a pool in your backyard, or belong to a community pool, turn pool time into activity time. Chase your kids in the water, play pirates, water polo, or just swim and frolic. Hoist your kid onto your shoulders, have your spouse hoist another kid, and have a chicken fight. Whoever gets knocked into the water loses (but you all win given the extra energy required to play the game).

38 **Play Pinja.** A favorite game in the Katz household (with its five children) this is based on the Lion King movie, in which Nala plays with Simba and says "pinned ya" every time she manages to get him on his back. Pretend you and your kids are all characters from *The Lion King* and wrestle each other around the living room floor. The game is over when you are wiped out; the kids, however, could probably go all night.

39 **Put malls to use.** Older kids love to go to the mall. Tell them that you'll take them to the mall, but set up the following ground rules first: No junk food (most malls provide healthy options, or you can bring a snack pack), and you must cruise the entire mall. A good mall provides several miles of walking. To really get a sense of the benefits, all of you should wear a pedometer.

40 **Plan pedometer competitions.** Pick a week in which each member of the family wears a pedometer and you compete to see who can garner the greatest number of steps. The winner gets a prize.

41 **Set a good example with simple habits.** Take the stairs instead of the elevator, walk to the store if possible, park far from the entrance of a building. Your children will grow up figuring this is simply the way things are done, and will carry these good health habits into adulthood.

42 **Add fun to physically active obligations.** Put on music when sweeping, vacuuming, or doing the dishes. Create a game out of chores (who can find the most dust bunnies) and turn grocery shopping into a scavenger hunt.

43 **Play "chase my shadow."** The kids have to jump and run to catch your shadow.

44 **Hit a hotel or office building (during off-hours) and play the staircase game.** The family splits into two teams. One team takes the elevator, and the other takes the stairs. The goal is to see who gets to the set floor the fastest. Then you switch teams.

45 **Learn martial arts together.** Many local community colleges and fitness centers offer martial arts classes designed for adults and children, and many forms of martial arts, including karate, judo, and tai bo, provide aerobic, strength, and flexibility training. In these classes, your children will also learn self-control and discipline as well as boost their self-esteem, balance, and posture.

46 **Look into family fitness programs at your local health club.** A growing number of fitness clubs now offer these programs for families, ranging from aerobics to swimming to in-line skating. Don't, however, just sign everyone up and hope for the best. Sit down with your family and go over your options. You get the best results if you pick a family fitness option that is pre-approved by all.

47 **Organize a playgroup with other parents and children in your neighborhood.** As the toddlers actively play in the center of the yard, the adults exercise around the periphery, doing calisthenics, marching, walking, and jogging in place.

Arm Strength

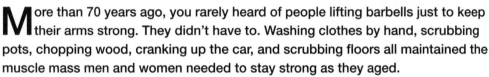

20 WAYS TO EXERCISE WITH—OR WITHOUT—WEIGHTS

More than 70 years ago, you rarely heard of people lifting barbells just to keep their arms strong. They didn't have to. Washing clothes by hand, scrubbing pots, chopping wood, cranking up the car, and scrubbing floors all maintained the muscle mass men and women needed to stay strong as they aged.

Today, of course, things have changed. Modern-day conveniences have made using your arms almost as unnecessary as using a typewriter. Thanks to laser-guided vacuum cleaners, electric car windows, sit-on mowers, electric bread makers, and automatic dishwashing machines, we rarely call upon the muscles in our arms to do much of anything. Over a lifetime, this can cause your muscles to shrink and wither away. You get weaker and weaker, daily tasks become harder and harder, and your body puts on weight and grows more susceptible to disease as you become more and more sedentary.

So don't think that strengthening your arms is an act of vanity. Well-exercised biceps (along the top front of your arms) and triceps (along the top back of your arms) not only contribute to overall health, but make lifting grandchildren, lugging groceries, moving furniture, and carrying laundry feel like a breeze. Even better, most arm-strengthening exercises also build up your wrists and hand grip, making it easier to open tight jars and hold on to heavy items.

The tips in this chapter will help you sneak some arm-strengthening moves into your daily and weekly routines the old-fashioned way. By reacquainting yourself with some arm-strengthening tasks from long ago, you'll not only build back your arm muscles, but you'll also reduce stress and, in many cases, enjoy life more fully. Plus, we've thrown in a few exercises using dumbbells in case you want to go to the next level.

1 **Each fall, plant bulbs on three consecutive weekends.** Make each planting session last at least an hour. Congratulations—that's your arm workout for the week. Digging in your garden will strengthen your hands, wrists, forearms, upper arms, and shoulders. Your hard work will pay off in the spring, when your daffodils and tulips sprout.

2 **Stop using weed killer on your garden.** Yes, this will encourage weeds to grow with wild abandon (even with mulch). That's good, because your job is to get down on your hands and knees once a week to rip weeds out of the ground. Leaning onto your hands as you weed will build arm, shoulder, and upper back strength, and yanking the weeds provides an extra dollop of arm-building strength. Just remember to alternate hands as you reach and pull so you work both arms equally.

3 Cut your own wood. If you use a fireplace, then chances are you are burning prepackaged logs bought at the grocery store or split wood delivered and stacked by that burly lawn-service guy. If you have the option, though, go out and chop your own wood. Starting in July and continuing through the first snow of winter, do 30 minutes of log splitting every weekend. Too much at once and it's bad for your back. But in small doses, cutting wood is amazingly good exercise. One medium-sized tree cut down makes for more than enough wood for one or two years of chopping.

4 Scrub the floors on your hands and knees once a week. Not only will you have cleaner floors than a mop provides, but you'll strengthen your arms at the same time.

5 Bake bread once a week. You'll strengthen your arms, shoulders, and hands as you simultaneously soothe away stress. There's nothing more soothing than the repetitive motion of kneading dough and nothing more pleasing than the smell of bread rising in the oven. Plus, home-baked bread—kneaded with your own two hands—tastes better than anything you can buy in the store or make in the bread maker.

6 Make your own pizza and pie dough instead of buying pre-made crusts. The forward and back action of using a rolling pin is a great arm and shoulder workout. Plus, your family will thank you for your effort later, as no commercial crust compares to homemade.

7 Trade in your electric mixer for a whisk and wooden spoon. You'll build arm strength as you use your own elbow grease to mix batter. Make sure to use both hands to work your arms evenly.

8 Make an omelet rather than fried eggs. Fill it with at least three different vegetables, such as spinach, mushrooms, and onions. You'll not only use your arms to whisk the eggs and chop the veggies, but you'll also improve your health by incorporating vegetables into your morning meal.

9 Use a cast-iron skillet for most of your cooking—and store it in the drawer under the oven. That way you must lift the heavy skillet onto the stove each time you need it—building more arm strength with every meal.

10 Use a large cleaver for your everyday chopping and cooking. Professional chefs love cleavers for their heft, weight, and super-sharp, slightly rounded edge. We love them because they are heavy and give your hand and arm a great workout while you cook.

11 Pour water out of a gallon jug. Although, as the popular joke goes, you probably won't build much arm strength lifting a 16-ounce beer can to your mouth, the weight of a gallon jug just may do the trick (a gallon of water weighs more than 8 pounds!). Plus, this is roughly how much water you need to drink in a typical day to stay hydrated. Curl your gallon jug five times—by bending your elbow and bringing your hand to your shoulder—before pouring.

12 **Hang your laundry outside instead of using the clothes dryer.** You'll save money on your electric bill and get in a mild arm workout at the same time. As you carry the laundry basket to the clothesline, curl it up and down, bringing your hands to your shoulders. You can also press it overhead, bending and then extending your elbows, to build some extra strength.

13 **Use a push mower rather than a sit-on variety.** Even better, opt for a non-powered mower. You'll save money on gas and do your part to help reduce air pollution. (Next to cars and power plants, lawn mowers are one of the biggest contributors to dirty air.)

 In**Perspective**

Strength

When someone in his twenties is described as "strong," chances are the subject is muscles. Call someone in his sixties "strong," and chances are the subject is character. Time to change the perception.

The benefits of strong muscles—particularly for people above 50, and particularly for women—are vast. In fact, in the hierarchy of Stealth Health pursuits, building stronger muscles is near the very top. Why? Here are just a few reasons:

- Strong muscles help you lose weight. And it's not just the exercise involved to become strong that matters. Muscle tissue burns as much as 15 times more calories per day than does fat tissue—even when at rest! Nothing stokes your metabolism better than muscle.

- Strong muscles are healthy for your heart. That's because they can perform better with less oxygen, meaning the heart doesn't have to pump hard when you are active. By extension, strong muscles are good for your blood pressure.

- Strong muscles protect your joints and your back. More muscle power means you put less strain on joints and connective tissue when lifting or exerting. And that's awfully important both for treating and preventing arthritis.

- Strong muscles improve your looks. Lean muscles are taut against your body, as opposed to flab, which hangs and sags.

- Strong muscles give you a mental boost. You feel more energized, and you feel prouder about yourself.

- Strong muscles require active living. You can't get strong muscles from a pill, a meal, or an herb. The mere fact that you have strong muscles means you are being active, and as we have been saying, nothing drags your health down like sedentary living.

- Strong muscles help fight free radicals. Research shows that when regular folks lift weights regularly, they have less damage to their body from free radicals than those who are sedentary.

The consensus is growing: Strong muscles are good for everyone. In fact, the American Heart Association now recommends that *all* adults strength train their major muscle groups at least twice a week. Time for you to get on board.

⭐ 14 **Do each of the following exercises** at least once a week. For even better effect, do each of them twice a week. An easy system: do one exercise each night during a three-minute commercial break on television (you get to rest on Sunday). Do three slow sets of 10 to 12 repetitions, with 20 seconds of breathing time between sets. This will require keeping a set of dumbbells next to the couch. Beginners should use 5-pound dumbbells, and more active adults should try 10- or 15-pound versions. These simple exercises are suggested by Wayne Westcott, Ph.D., research director at the South Shore YMCA in Quincy, Massachusetts, who has completed hundreds of studies on strength training and written numerous books on the topic.

▼ BENT-OVER ROW

You'll strengthen your biceps as well as your upper back muscles with this exercise.

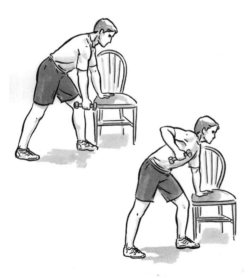

Stand with your left foot about two to three feet in front of your right foot. Bend forward from the hips and place your left

palm on the seat of a chair. Grasp a dumbbell in your right hand and extend your right arm toward the floor. Exhale as you bend your right elbow and lift the dumbbell toward the side of your chest. Inhale as you lower and repeat.

▼ CHAIR DIP

This exercise strengthens your triceps, the muscles along the back of your upper arms (the ones that flap about when you wave good-bye) and your chest muscles.

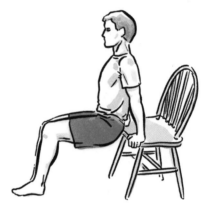

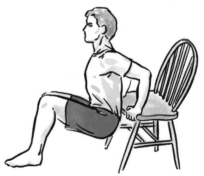

Sit on the edge of a sturdy chair. Place your palms on the seat of the chair, on either side of your buttocks, with your fingers facing forward. Place your feet flat on the floor with your knees bent. Press into your hands and lift your buttocks about an inch up and forward, until you can clear the seat of the chair. Inhale as you bend your elbows, lowering your buttocks toward the floor. Keeping your elbows close to your sides, exhale as you extend your arms and return to the starting position. Be careful you're not cheating by pushing yourself back up with your legs rather than your arms.

As you gain strength, you can increase the challenge by extending your legs and placing only your heels on the floor. To increase the challenge even more, elevate your legs by placing your heels on a separate chair in front of you.

▼ BICEPS CURL

This exercise strengthens your biceps, the muscles along the front of your upper arms.

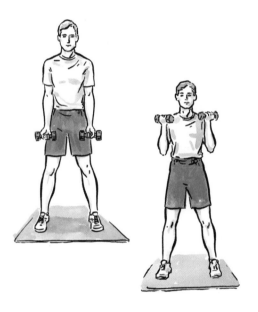

Grasp a dumbbell in each hand. Extend your arms at your sides with your palms facing forward. Exhale as you curl your hands toward your shoulders, keeping your elbows close to your sides. Inhale as you lower the weights. You can also do this exercise with elastic tubing, securing the middle of the tubing under your feet and curling the ends.

15 Eat a steak on the nights you work out.

What does red meat have to do with muscle strength? Apparently quite a bit, particularly if you are older. Researchers at the University of Wollongong in New South Wales, Australia, put 28 participants ages 60-plus on one of two diet and exercise programs. Both programs included weightlifting exercises and a diet composed of 20 percent protein. One diet, however, included 25 weekly ounces of red meat (the amount in 3 medium steaks), whereas the other included only 13 weekly ounces of red meat (the amount in 1½ medium steaks). After 12 weeks, participants who got the extra red meat increased their muscle strength more than those who ate less red meat. Researchers suspect the extra red meat supplies additional amino acids needed for muscle growth. If you plan to increase your consumption of red meat in order to increase your arm strength, choose lean cuts of meat, such as sirloin, rather than porterhouse. That helps protect your heart as you build your strength.

16 Spend 10 minutes every workday building resistance in your office.

Just because you're stuck at work putting out yet another fire doesn't mean you have a good excuse to skip your arm-strengthening routine. You have everything you need in your office to keep your arms in great shape. Here are some great office-based arm exercises:

▶ **Desk curl.** Place your palms against the underside of your desk with your elbows bent. Push up into the desk with your palms, as if you were trying to lift the desk off the floor. Hold for a count of five, release, and repeat until you feel the burn. This strengthens your biceps.

▶ **Desk push.** Place your palms against the top of your desk with your elbows bent. Press into the desktop with all your might. Hold for a count of five, release, and repeat until you feel the burn. This strengthens your triceps.

▶ **Desk push-up.** Stand about two feet away from your desk. Keep your feet in place and lean forward from the ankles, placing your palms on top of the desk. Your body should form a straight line from your ankles to your head. Bend your elbows as you lower your chest toward the desk. Straighten your elbows as you push away. Keep your elbows in close to your sides the entire time. This works your triceps.

17 **Play tug-of-war with a large-breed dog.** We're talking retrievers, Doberman pinschers, German shepherds, Weimaraners, and other dogs that weigh more than 40 pounds. Hold a rope with one hand and encourage your dog to pull it. Keep your elbow close to your side as you resist your dog's pull by bringing the rope toward your shoulder. Do this over and over on one side of your body until your dog gets the best of you, then switch arms. Once you've completely fatigued your biceps, move on to your triceps. Holding the rope with one arm, try to extend your arm behind your torso as your dog yanks it forward. By the time you fatigue the front and back of your arms, you'll have fatigued your dog as well, thus saving your couch or remote control from one bored dog's gnawing.

18 **Use your arms on your fitness walks.** Imagine you are holding ski poles in your hands and must pump them forward and back to keep moving. As you

bring each elbow back, squeeze your shoulder blades together.

19 **Curl your groceries.** When you arrive home from the grocery store, carry one bag in each hand. As you walk from the car to the kitchen, curl your groceries by lifting your hands toward your shoulders, keeping your elbows close to your sides. By the time you bring in all of the bags of groceries, you'll have completely fatigued your biceps—and you'll have burned some extra calories by making the extra trips to and from the car.

20 **Try these isometric exercises.** Isometric exercises are performed against something that doesn't move, like a wall. You don't actually move here, but by pushing against the immovable object, tension builds up in your muscles, increasing their strength.

Hold each position for 6–8 seconds, and repeat 5–10 times each. Here are some to try throughout the day:

▶ **Press your hands together as hard as you can 10 times for 5 seconds at a time.** Seems like a small thing, but this isometric exercise will really make a difference in your arm strength (and look) after a couple of weeks. Try this every time you go to the bathroom (even while sitting on the toilet!).

▶ **Stand with your legs apart about a foot from the wall and push against the wall as if you were trying to move it.** A great thing to do while you're waiting for water to boil, scrambled eggs to set, or pasta to cook.

▶ **Stand in the doorway with your legs straight and knees locked.** Press your hands upward against the top of the door frame, holding for several seconds, then relaxing. Repeat at least 10 times.

▶ **Extend both arms to the side of the doorway with your palms shoulder high, facing outward.** With both arms, press hard against the sides of the door frame. Hold for several seconds, relax, then repeat up to 10 times.

Two-Second Quiz

Heavy or Light Weights?

Answer: *Light weights.*
Lifting heavy weights for a few reps is good for you … if you want to hit massive home runs, bust your shirt seams when you scratch your head, or impress kids with your grunting capabilities. For the rest of us, lifting lighter weights through lots of repetition is probably the better way to go. This approach shapes and sculpts muscle without adding size. It also builds endurance, which for most of us is more important, not just for our muscles, but also for our heart and lungs. And in general, lighter weights pose less risk of injury and muscle strain. For this approach, pick weights that you can lift 15–20 times per set.

▶ **Extend both arms to the sides of the doorway, arms down, palms facing inward.** With the back of your hands, press hard against the sides of the frame. Hold several seconds, relax, then repeat up to 10 times.

Abs and Back Strength

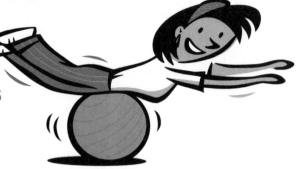

19 WAYS TO FEEL LESS CRUNCHED DURING YOUR ROUTINE

Your abs and back are the core of your body, the power center from which all movement originates. Strengthen this area and you'll move with more power and grace. You'll more easily hoist your kids or grandkids out of harm's way, spring up from the couch to answer a ringing phone, and, if you play sports, whack tennis balls with more oomph, swim the freestyle with gusto, drive golf balls farther, and generally complete every task you tackle with greater ease and energy.

Strong abdominal muscles also help support and move your spine, protecting your back from injury. Strengthen your abs and you'll be less likely to throw your back out reaching behind you to pick up a map from the floor of your car, or miss a step walking out the door. Finally, strengthen the lowest part of your core—your pelvic floor muscles—and you'll prevent incontinence and may even improve your sex life.

The best news is that you don't have to do the same old exercises to build core strength. So if you've avoided abdominal work because you hate crunches, do not fear. In this chapter, you'll not only learn how to make crunches more effective and less taxing, you'll also discover a whole new world of opportunities for abdominal and back strengthening beyond the basic crunch.

1 If you walk for fitness, squeeze your butt. As you walk, imagine you are holding a $50 bill between your butt cheeks. As you firm and lift your buttocks muscles to hold your imaginary bill, you'll strengthen your back muscles. You can also work your abs as you walk by imagining you have a zipper along the midline of your abdomen. Picture yourself zipping up a tight pair of jeans. As you pull the zipper up your abdomen, feel your torso lengthen and abdomen firm. Keep your abs zipped up and your butt clenched throughout your walks and you'll strengthen your core even as you burn fat.

2 While driving, tighten your tummy and pelvic floor muscles. Starting with your pubic area, begin to tighten from the bottom up. Once you squeeze your pelvic floor, suck your lower belly and then upper belly in toward your spine as you exhale. Hold for a count of 5, then release and repeat 10-20 times.

3 When you're nervous, tighten and release your abdominal muscles over and over again. You'll strengthen your abs and take your mind off your anxiety. This is a particularly good exercise for when you are nervous about an upcoming speech or presentation.

4 During commercial breaks on the nightly news, sit on the edge of your chair and lift your feet off the floor, bringing your knees into your chest. Lower and repeat 10-15 times.

5 Whenever you find yourself standing on line, lift one foot off the floor and try to hold your balance. You'll feel myriad muscles in your abdomen and back firing up to help steady your body. Make sure to alternate your feet.

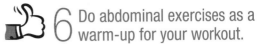

6 Do abdominal exercises as a warm-up for your workout. The typical workout starts out with 5 or 10 minutes of walking or marching to get your body warmed up and blood flowing. But let's face it, that's boring. Instead, do your abdominal work. Because your abdomen consists of large muscle groups, abdominal work is very warming for the body. Five to 10 minutes of abdominal exercises will warm you up as well as walking, and give you some good muscle building at the same time.

7 Strengthen your waist and back with a medicine ball twist. Stand back-to-back with a friend. Hold a medicine ball with both hands and rotate to your right to hand the ball off to your buddy. Your friend takes the ball, rotates

In Perspective

Achieving Flat Abs

So what does it take to have an abdomen that is so strong, so lean, that it reveals beautifully symmetric, perfectly arranged muscles? There are a few surprises in the answers.

Most of all, it takes being very, very lean. For most people, much of their fat lies in the abdomen, and much of that abdominal fat lies between the skin and abdominal muscles. That layer of fat covers up the shapeliness of the muscles. So models and athletes with "six-pack abs" must have very low body fat to reveal that musculature. Sit-ups

didn't get them that way — you cannot "spot reduce" fat from your belly using abs exercises. To melt the fat off your body, it requires a low-calorie diet and lots of aerobic exercise like biking, walking, or running.

Of course, it does take targeted exercise to create big, shapely abdominal muscles. A lot, in fact. While most of us think of abs as a simple band of muscles across the top of our belly, there are many separate abdominal muscles, with names like "obliques" and "transversus abdominis." People serious about their

abs know all these muscles, and target each one for exercise. A thorough abs workout for someone who is serious about his appearance could involve 10 different abdominal exercises.

Is all this necessary? Maybe for models, but not for you. What's important is that your ab muscles be conditioned well enough to support your back and allow you to twist and turn and lift without a challenge. If you are at a healthy weight but have a little belly fat covering your abdominal muscles, consider yourself well ahead of the game.

and hands it off to your left. Continue to receive and hand off the ball for one minute and then switch direction.

8 As you watch television, fly like Superman. This simple exercise will strengthen your lower back. Lie on the floor with your legs extended. Extend your

arms in front. Inhale as you lift your shoulders and feet, reaching your hands and feet away from each other. Hold 10-20 seconds. Lower and repeat 1-2 times.

9 Trade in your office chair for a stability ball. Found in most sporting goods stores, large air-filled stability balls

10 Use your stability ball to do abs and back exercises. Whether you are at work or at home, you can perform abdominal or back exercises on your new desk chair—uh, ball—that are nicely effective. When you perform abdominal-strengthening movements on a stability ball, you use more of your core muscles for every movement. Try the traditional crunch on the ball, shown on page 188, along with these additional ball moves, courtesy of Liz Applegate, Ph.D., a nutrition and fitness expert at the University of California at Davis and author of *Bounce Your Body Beautiful*.

▼ **KNEE FOLD-UP**

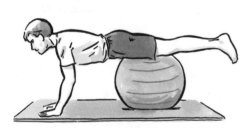

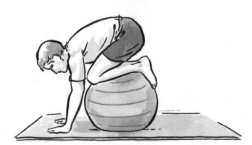

Start in a push-up position with your thighs or shins on the ball and your palms on the floor under your chest. Exhale as you bend your knees and bring your shins and ball in toward your chest. Inhale as you straighten your legs. Repeat 10-15 times.

▼ **ARM SWING**

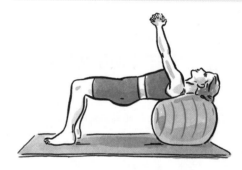

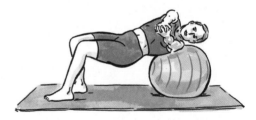

Lie with your upper back on the ball, your knees bent, and feet on the floor. Clasp your hands together and extend your arms toward the ceiling, so they are perpendicular with your torso. Exhale and roll your torso to the left, lifting your right shoulder

are all the rage in gym settings these days and are slowly making their way into office settings as well. If you sit on a stability ball rather than your desk chair, you'll work your abdomen as you type away at your keyboard. That's because your abs and back must continually firm as they support your torso to help you keep your balance on

off the ball. Return to the starting position and repeat to the right, alternating sides. Complete 10-15 rolls on each side.

▼ KNEELING LAYOUT

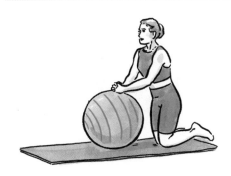

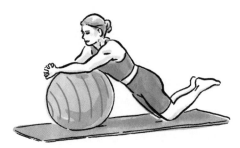

Kneel on the floor with the ball in front of you. Clasp your hands and press the bottoms of your hands and forearms into the ball. Lift your feet and shins and balance on your knees. Exhale as you press your hands into the ball and roll the ball forward. Your knees will stay in place, but your feet and shins will rise and your torso will lean forward. Rise and repeat 15 times.

that bouncy ball. As an added bonus, you'll wiggle around more, burning a few extra calories and keeping your mind fresh.

11 Set the alarm on your watch or computer to do hourly posture checks. Your abdominal muscles support your spine. Strengthening them will help improve your posture, and improving your posture will help strengthen your abdominal muscles. So do a posture check. Every hour, imagine you are zipping up a tight pair of jeans. Extend your spine, bringing the top of your head toward the ceiling. As you do so, your lower belly should pull up and in toward your spine and your lower back should flatten slightly as your tailbone reaches toward the floor.

12 Take a Pilates class once a week. This exercise method was developed by Joseph Pilates in the early 1920s. It places a heavy emphasis on the abdominals and core as it simultaneously strengthens the arms and legs. Although many books and videos teach the Pilates method, you'll have best results by taking a few classes from a certified instructor. Once you learn the basic technique, you can then practice at home with a video.

13 For a simple, effective back stretch, lie flat on your back. Lift one knee to your chest, then the other, keeping your lower back on the floor. Wrap your arms behind your knees, using them to support your legs and if necessary, pulling them so your buttocks rise off the floor. You should feel your back muscles stretching. Hold the position for 30 seconds, then release.

The Most Effective Abdominal Exercises

Researchers at San Diego State University have tested numerous abdominal exercises for their effectiveness, and surprisingly, the quintessential crunch ranked only 11 out of the 13 exercises tested. The following exercises ranked within the top five.

▼ BICYCLE

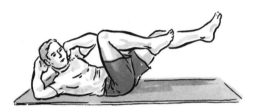

Lie on your back. Tuck your tailbone and press your lower back against the floor. Place your fingertips behind your head and your elbows out to the sides. Bend your knees and lift your feet off the floor, keeping a 45-degree bend in your knees. Begin to pedal your legs, bringing your opposite elbow to the opposite knee as you extend your free leg.

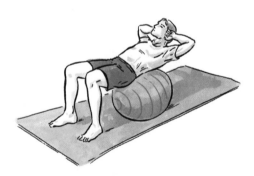

▼ BALL CRUNCH

A large, air-filled fitness ball will wiggle under your back, causing you to recruit more muscles as you crunch.

Sit on the ball with your feet on the floor. Walk your feet away from the ball as you recline onto it. The ball should rest against your lower back and the top of your buttocks. Your upper back and shoulders should not rest on the ball. With your fingertips behind your head, open your elbows to the sides. Tuck your tailbone and exhale as you lift your shoulders. Lower and repeat.

▼ CAPTAIN'S CHAIR

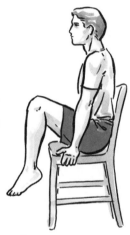

Most gyms have a device that allows you to place your forearms on padding and lift your feet off the ground. It's usually connected to a dip bar. If you have this equipment, grip the handholds and press your lower back against the back pad. Start with your legs extended and feet off the floor. Slowly lift your knees toward your chest, then return to the starting position and repeat. You can also do this exercise at home if you have a sturdy, armless chair. Sit up straight, and grab the chair's edges just in front of your hips. While supporting yourself with your hands, slowly draw your knees up toward your chest, keeping your lower back against the chair. Hold, then slowly lower and repeat.

▼ EXTENDED LEG CRUNCH

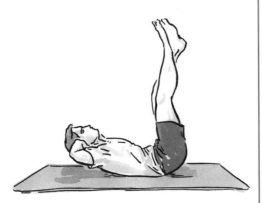

Lie on your back. Extend your legs toward the ceiling and cross one ankle over the other. Keep a slight bend in your knees. Place your fingertips behind your head with your elbows open to the sides. Tuck your tailbone. Slowly lift your shoulders off the floor as you exhale. Lower and repeat.

▼ REVERSE CRUNCH

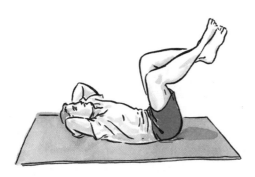

Lie on your back. Bend your knees and lift your feet off the floor, forming a 90-degree angle between your thighs and calves. Place your fingertips behind your head with your elbows open to the sides. Cross your ankles. Press your lower back into the floor, tuck your tailbone, and reach your shins toward the ceiling. Lower and repeat.

14 **Three times a week, when you get home from work, reach an arm and a leg away from each other.** You can strengthen your abs and back at the same time with an exercise called the reciprocal reach (also sometimes called opposite limb extension). Get on all fours with your hands under your shoulders and knees under your hips. Extend your left leg behind, placing the ball of your left foot against the floor. Tuck your tailbone and try to keep it tucked throughout the exercise. Lift your left foot off the floor as you lift your right arm, reaching your right hand and left foot away from each other. Keep your hips level. Hold for 10-20 seconds, release, and repeat on the other side. Work up to 2-3 sets.

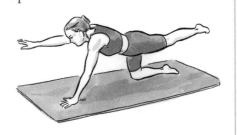

15 **Try a purse or briefcase side bend.** This is another exercise that's great for your obliques and can be done anywhere, anytime. Stand upright with your briefcase or purse in your right hand, palm facing in, your feet about shoulder-width apart. Slowly bend to your right, allowing the item to drop directly down your right leg until you feel a stretch along your left side. Keep your body facing forward the whole time. Once you've gone as low as possible, slowly return to upright, repeat for a set of 10-20 repetitions, then switch hands and repeat on the other side.

16 Use a 6- to 8-inch ball as an abdominal strengthening

companion. Children's balls called Gerti balls or small, light fitness balls make great workout aids. To start, use one in the kitchen while cooking. Place the ball between your thighs, just above your knees. As you stir your food at the stove or chop vegetables, squeeze your inner thighs to hold the ball in place. This action fires up your pelvic floor and lower abdominal muscles.

You can also use the small ball to increase the effectiveness of traditional abdominal exercises. Here are a few exercises to try with the ball:

▼ THE MOUNTAIN

This exercise stretches your calves, helps your posture, and by adding in the exercise ball, works your lower abdominals as well.

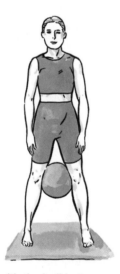

Stand tall with the ball between your thighs. Lift your arches and squeeze the ball. Hold 10-20 seconds. Release the ball, walk around, then repeat 1-2 times.

▼ THE PLANK

This simple exercise challenges several body areas, including the shoulders, backs, and abs. The exercise ball brings even more pelvic muscles into the mix.

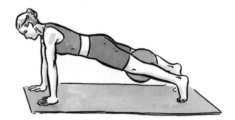

With the small ball between your knees or thighs, come into a push-up position with your hands under your chest. Reach back through your heels and forward through the top of your head. Tuck in your tailbone. Hold 10-20 seconds. Repeat 1-2 times.

▼ THE BRIDGE

This exercise works your lower abdominal area, lower back, and buttocks.

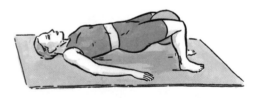

Lie on your back with your knees bent, feet on the floor and ball between your thighs. Rest your arms at your sides with your palms down. Tuck your tailbone and lift your hips and lower back off the floor. Only lift as high as you can keep your tailbone tucked. Hold 10-20 seconds. Lower and repeat 1-2 times.

17 For upper-back strength, do shrugs—with weights. Hold a light dumbbell in each hand, allowing your arms to hang down naturally at your sides, palms facing in. Your legs should be about shoulder width apart. Slowly shrug your shoulders straight up toward your ears. Pause, then lower them back to starting position. Repeat until your muscles feel fatigued. Don't rotate your shoulders—that will strain them. Instead, concentrate on going straight up and down.

18 Do the twist, using a broomstick or long cardboard tube to keep yourself properly aligned. This exercise is easy yet effective at building the oblique muscles that line the sides of your abdomen. Stand upright with your feet about shoulder width apart. Hold a broomstick across your shoulders and behind your neck so it is resting on the top of your back. Your hands should be near the ends of the broomstick or tube. Keeping your hips as still as possible, twist to your left as far as you can go, moving your head with your torso (otherwise, you might strain your neck). Then come back to the starting position, pause, then twist in the opposite direction. Repeat at a slow, steady pace until you tire. Don't jerk your body—move smoothly! This is a particularly good exercise for golfers, since a golf swing involves lots of twisting.

19 Once in the morning and once at night, pretend you're a scared cat. Get on the floor on your hands and knees. Exhale as you curl your spine toward the ceiling, tucking your tailbone and bringing your chin to your chest. As you do so, bring your navel up and in toward your spine. Inhale as you flatten your back. Continue to curl and flatten your spine as you breathe, doing 10 repetitions. This stretch will help work the kinks out of your spine before bed and first thing in the morning, helping you to sleep better and feel better during the day. It will also strengthen your abdomen.

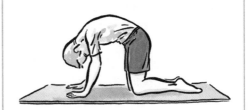

Leg Strength

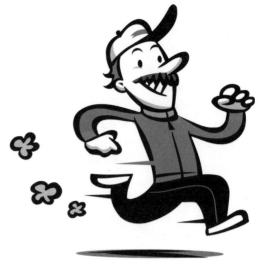

19 WAYS TO FIRM YOUR HIPS, THIGHS, AND BUTTOCKS

Your legs are perhaps the easiest muscles in your body to keep in shape. After all, they support the weight of your body and you use them every time you walk. Just being on the go can help you tone and fine-tune them, and they, in turn, will help you burn calories and keep the rest of you toned. Add some leg-strengthening exercises, and you'll garner even more benefits without a lot of extra effort.

A set of stronger legs will help you accomplish more every day. You'll climb stairs with less effort, walk uphill without feeling winded, and be able to bend your knees and squat down to pick up heavy objects, protecting your lower back from strain. To strengthen your legs and avoid injury, you must work all of the muscles in your legs equally. Include exercises that zero in on the inner thighs, outer thighs, back of the thighs, front of the thighs, and buttocks. The following tips will seamlessly incorporate leg work into your day so you can keep your legs strong no matter where you find yourself.

1 Whenever you find yourself stopped at a traffic light, tighten your thighs and butt, over and over again. You will firm your leg muscles, boost blood flow (thus preventing that pins-and-needles sensation that tends to attack your rear end when you've parked it in a car seat for too long), and keep yourself entertained.

2 Before you get out of bed in the morning, do the clam. Lie on your back, bring your feet together, and open your knees out to the sides. Then, as you exhale, lift your knees, bringing them together. Lower and repeat 10-15 times to strengthen your inner thighs.

3 Do leg lifts as you cook dinner. Flex your foot and lift your leg out to the side, lower, and repeat 10-15 times. Then switch legs. You'll finish your leg workout before dinnertime.

4 If you walk for fitness, switch to a softer surface. Your legs get a better workout when you walk on trails or sand rather than pavement. And, softer surfaces transfer less impact to your joints, preventing strain to your knees and back.

5 Get up, place your palms against your desk, and do a series of donkey kicks when you find yourself falling asleep at your keyboard.

Bend one knee, flex that foot, and kick your leg back, as if you were a donkey kicking someone behind you. Alternate legs for 15 total kicks. Then return to work refreshed and with a stronger backside.

6 **Instead of straining and reaching to get something off a high shelf, step up on a stable chair or step stool.** You'll strengthen your legs *and* protect your back.

7 **Next time you find yourself at a wedding or other function with a dance floor, do the twist.** Or, do it in your living room tonight. Bend your knees and squat down as far as you comfortably can as you shimmy from side to side. You'll burn calories, have a few laughs, and strengthen your legs—all at the same time.

8 **Jump into the pool once or twice a week.** Literally. Sports coaches have typically told their runners, soccer players, and other athletes to increase their leg strength through plyometrics, which are a series of skipping, jumping, and bounding exercises usually done on land. Because of the force of gravity and the impact of the body as it hits the ground, these exercises result in quite a bit of post-exercise muscle soreness, which is why we're not recommending you do them. (So go ahead and breathe a sigh of relief.)

That said, researchers at Ohio State University have developed a way to get the leg-strength benefit from plyometrics without the post-exercise soreness: Complete the exercises in a swimming pool. Researchers split 32 women into two groups. One performed plyometrics on land for 8 weeks; the other did the same routine in the water. After 8 weeks, both groups increased their leg strength, but the group that did their exercises on land experienced much more muscle soreness.

So the next time you find yourself entertaining your grandchildren at the local pool, try the following routine from the shallow end and see if they can keep up with you:

▶ **Hop.** With your legs together, hop the width of the pool from one side to the other and back. Rest up to one minute, then repeat twice.

▶ **Exaggerated running.** Run the width of the pool slowly with an exaggerated motion, lifting your knees into your chest and pushing off with your rear foot just enough to lift your entire body off the bottom of the pool. Once you have reached the other side, turn around and run back. Rest up to a minute, then repeat twice.

▶ **Hop on one foot.** Hop in place on one foot for 30 seconds, trying to get as much

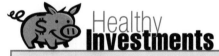

Healthy Investments

Ankle Weights

One set of ankle weights allows you to do just about any leg exercise at home and you'll never have to set foot in the gym again to maintain shapely legs. In addition to the traditional leg lifts, you can use ankle weights to do other popular leg exercises such as hamstring curls and leg extensions, often done on a machine at the gym. Look for ankle weights that allow you to add weight as you get stronger, and with Velcro straps rather than shoelaces for easy access and removal. Many of these weights contain small pockets into which you can insert or remove weighted bags. Try on the weights at the store to make sure they feel comfortable.

air as possible. Then switch legs. Rest up to one minute, then repeat twice.

9 **Mount the stairs two or three at a time.** Similar to a traditional step-up exercise done at the gym, this strengthens the gluteal muscles in your buttocks and revs up your heart rate, boosting your cardiovascular fitness.

10 **Do the "lunge walk" on the way to the mailbox.** Your neighbors might laugh if they see you, but you'll have the last laugh when, in just minutes each day, you sculpt a sexy set of legs. During each step forward to the mailbox, bend your knees and sink down until both legs form 90-degree angles. Then press into your front heel to rise. Lift your back leg and knee all the way into your chest before planting it in front of you for the next lunge. This will take a little practice, but if you do this "lunge walk" for 20 or more steps a day, your legs will be far stronger and shapelier.

11 **Add a hill to your walking route.** As you trudge up the hill, you'll feel the muscles in the backs of your legs working hard to push off with every step.

12 **Practice hot seats while you watch television.** Television time doesn't have to be couch potato time. Pledge to yourself that you won't sit down on your favorite recliner until you've done 15 hot seats. Then, during each commercial, get out of your chair and do 15-20 hot seats. To do a hot seat, stand with your feet slightly wider than your hips. Sit back into a squat, just until your tush touches the seat of the chair. As soon as you feel the seat of the chair under your buttocks, spring up to a standing position, as if the seat were "hot" and you wanted to get away from it as fast as you could.

13 **Whenever you stand in line, balance on one foot.** As soon as you lift one foot off the ground, the muscles in the foot, ankle, calf, thigh, and buttocks of the opposite leg firm as they work harder to keep you upright. If you're worried about what other people might think, you can balance on one foot without anyone noticing. Just lift one foot about an inch off the ground and tuck it behind the heel of the other foot. Each time you step forward in the line, switch legs. If you are one of the lucky few who rarely, if ever, stand in line, try standing on one foot when completing household tasks such as cooking dinner or folding laundry.

14 **Leapfrog with your grandkids.** Everyone will get in a good leg and cardiovascular workout—and lots of laughs. Everyone squats down as low as he can go, imitating a frog sitting on a lily pad. To leap over the person in front of you, place your hands on his back and then spring forward and up. Keep your legs and feet wide, in case you need to take two hops to clear your obstacle. Land with your knees soft and slightly bent to protect them from the impact.

15 **Do a squat every time you pick something up** off the floor. When most of us bend over to pick something up, we do exactly that, bend over from the waist, rounding the back. Over time, this can put stress on the lower back, especially if you're lifting something heavy. But a squat forces you to use your legs, building leg strength. The best way to squat: With your feet hip distance apart or wider, bend your knees and stick your butt

The Squat: King of the Leg Exercises

Can you do only one leg exercise and still see results? Yes, if that exercise is a squat. You can strengthen all of the muscles in your legs and butt with either full squats or quarter-squats, says Jose Antonio, Ph.D., director of Exercise and Sports Nutrition Research at the Institute of Human Performance in Boca Raton, Florida, and president of the International Society of Sports Nutrition.

▼ FULL SQUAT

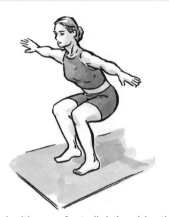

Stand with your feet slightly wider than hip distance apart. Tuck your tailbone, flatten your back, and firm your abdominal muscles. Inhale and slowly bend your knees as you sit back, as if you were going to sit back into a chair. Your upper body will lean slightly forward, but don't allow your lower back to arch or your spine to round. Bend your knees until your thighs are parallel with the floor. Then exhale as you press up through your heels and extend your legs in a fast, explosive motion. Repeat 10-15 times. Do this two or three times a week.

If you lack the leg strength to do a full squat or—more important—you feel pain in your knees or back, try one of two variations.
Variation 1. *Hold on to a doorknob with both hands as you squat. This removes* some of your body weight from your legs and helps keep your torso upright.
Variation 2. *Squat with your back against a wall and a small, 8-inch-diameter ball between your thighs. The ball keeps your thighs and knees in proper alignment, and the wall provides more support for your back.*

▼ QUARTER-SQUAT

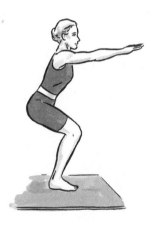

For this exercise, you'll do the same motion and use the same technique as the full squat, but you won't bend your knees quite so far. Rather than lowering your thighs to parallel, only bend your knees a quarter of the distance of the full squat before rising to the starting position. Repeat 10-15 times, two or three times a week.

out as you squat down. Then bend forward and pick up your object. Bring your torso upright and then rise by pressing up through your heels. Even if you just squat to pick up a pencil, it will help build more leg strength.

16 Practice kickboxing moves for 5 minutes every morning before putting on your pants or skirt. There's nothing like seeing your bare thighs in the mirror to motivate you to do your kicks. Kick in all directions, mixing in front kicks, side kicks, back kicks, and roundhouse kicks. No matter what kick you do, never fully extend your knee. This protects your knee joint.

▼ FRONT KICK

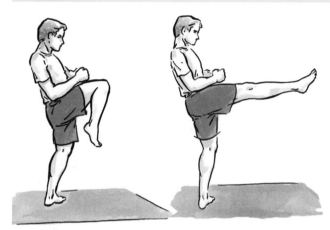

Pretend an opponent is standing in front of you and you wish to kick him in the groin (or her in the stomach). Lift one knee into your chest and then forcefully extend your leg, smacking the top of your foot into your imaginary target. Recoil your leg quickly and follow up with the other leg in quick succession.

▼ ROUNDHOUSE KICK

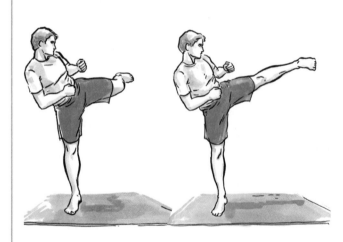

Pretend your opponent is standing in front of you and slightly to your left. Place your hands in a boxer's stance for balance. Bring your left knee diagonally into your chest. Snap your leg forward as you extend your foot and shin into your opponent's imaginary abdomen. Recoil quickly and follow up with 10-20 more kicks before switching sides.

17 Challenge your kids, grandkids, partner, or office mate to a toe-walking contest every other day. Rise onto the balls of your feet and walk across the room. Whoever lowers his or her heels to the floor first, loses. You'll have plenty of laughs as you strengthen your arches, ankles, and calves.

18 Exercise your calf muscles while you brush your teeth. Place your feet flat on the floor, then rise up onto the balls of your feet, hold for two seconds, and sink down. Repeat 20, 30, 50, or more times. You can do this not only while brushing your teeth, but any time you are waiting.

▼ SIDE KICK

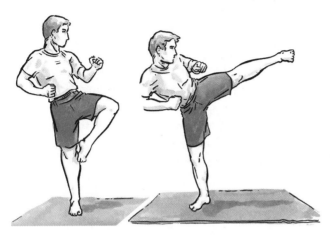

Pretend an opponent is standing to your left side. Place your hands in a boxer's stance for balance. Bring your left knee diagonally into your chest. Then thrust it sideways to the left, into your opponent's imaginary abdomen. Keep your foot either parallel to the floor or your heel slightly higher than your toes. If your toes are higher than your heel, you'll feel a twinge in your knee. Do 10-20 on one side, then switch sides.

▼ BACK KICK

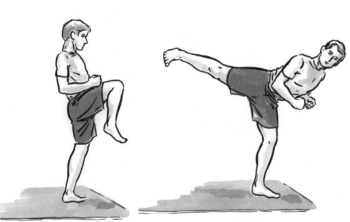

Pretend your opponent is standing behind you. Place your hands in a boxer's stance and turn your head and shoulders to look at your "attacker." Bring one leg in toward your chest and then thrust it behind you, trying to thrust your foot into your attacker's imaginary abdomen. Alternate with your other leg in rapid succession.

☆ 19 **Push against immovable objects.** We're talking isometric exercises, of course—the best way to exercise without moving! Your goal is to put your foot or upper thigh against a surface that won't move or break, and to press against it hard (but not so hard as to strain your muscles or joints). Hold each position for 6-8 seconds, relax for a few seconds, then repeat 5-10 times on each side. Sitting down, you can press your feet against the floor. Or, if you have your legs under a sturdy desk, try to lift it with your thighs. Standing up, you can face away from a wall, bend one knee so your foot moves behind you, place it against a wall, and push.

Four Other Great Leg Exercises

While squats strengthen all of the muscles in your legs, you should do other leg exercises to balance your muscles. So include the following leg-strengthening movements with your squats, completing the entire routine two to three times a week.

▼ LUNGE

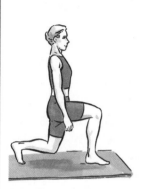

Stand with your feet under your hips. Take a large step forward with your right foot. Bend both knees up to 90 degrees until your right thigh is parallel with the floor. Exhale as you straighten your legs and step back to the starting position. Repeat with the left leg. Continue alternating stepping forward with your right and left leg for a total of 10-15 repetitions on each leg.

▼ LEG LIFT

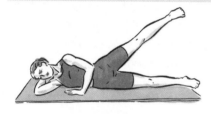

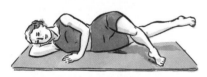

Lie on your right side with your legs extended. Lift your left leg toward the ceiling, keeping your foot flexed and the edge of your foot level (don't lead with your toes). Lower and repeat 15 times. Then bend your left knee and place your left foot on the floor in front of your torso.

Flex your right foot and lift your right leg, feeling the effort in your right inner thigh. Lower and repeat 15 times. Then switch sides. Once 15 repetitions begin to feel easy, strap an ankle weight on each ankle for extra resistance.

▼ HAMSTRING CURL

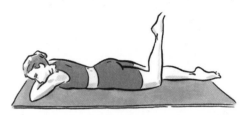

Lie on your tummy with your legs extended. Bend your left knee, lifting your left foot toward your buttocks. Lower and repeat 10-15 times. Then switch sides. Once 15 repetitions begin to feel easy, strap an ankle weight on each ankle for extra resistance.

▼ QUADRICEPS EXTENSION

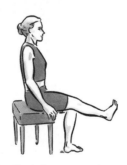

Sit in a chair with your knees bent and feet on the floor. Lift and extend your right leg, until your calf is parallel with the floor. Lower and repeat 15 times. Switch legs. Once 15 repetitions begin to feel easy, strap an ankle weight on each ankle for extra resistance.

Neck and Shoulder Strength

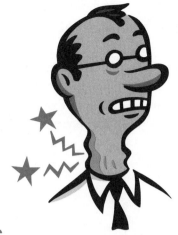

12 SIMPLE STRATEGIES THAT DECREASE PAIN AND STIFFNESS

You might wonder why the strength of your neck and shoulders matters. After all, you're not training for a football team or pulling a plow. Yet neck and shoulder strength are very important to overall well-being. Neck pain, be it caused by bad sleep, bad posture, a sudden twist, or too much stress, is among the most common everyday complaints. Research shows that neck-strengthening exercises may be more important than stretching when it comes to preventing neck pain. In one study published in the *Journal of the American Medical Association,* a year-long neck-strengthening program reduced neck pain and increased range of motion in 180 women who had, until that time, suffered from neck pain for more than six months. The program included neck, shoulder, and upper back exercises three times a week.

The same goes for shoulder strength. Strengthening your shoulders not only prevents shoulder stiffness and pain, it may also protect your elbow joints. That's because weak shoulders increase the stress placed on your elbows and wrists. Here are some simple ways to build neck and shoulder strength throughout the day:

1 **Whenever you feel exasperated at work, press your forehead into your palms.** Many of us tense up our neck muscles when under stress, which can lead to pain and stiffness over time. You can reduce tension and strengthen your neck at the same time with this simple exercise. The best part: No one in the office will know you're exercising; they'll think you're just frustrated.

▶ Sitting at your desk, lean forward and place your elbows on your desk. With your head centered over your shoulders, press your forehead into your palms, using your palms to resist the pressure of your head. Hold this position for 3-5 seconds, release, and repeat three to five times. Now sit up straight and place your palms on the back of your head with your elbows out to the sides. Press your head back into your palms as you use your palms to resist the pressure of your head. Hold for 3-5 seconds, release, then repeat three to five times.

2 Exercise your rotator cuff once a week.

Your rotator cuff is actually a group of muscles and tendons that hold your shoulder joint in place. Most people neglect to strengthen this area of the body because these deep muscles don't play much of a role in shaping sexy shoulder contours, and quite frankly, no one tells you about these muscles until after you've already injured them. Yet strengthening them will go a long way toward preventing shoulder problems later in life. You can do the following exercises at home.

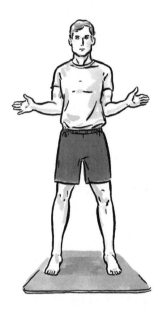

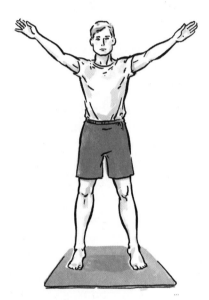

Stand with your elbows pressed into your waist, your upper arms snuggled next to your ribs, your elbows bent at 90 degrees, and your palms facing each other. Without allowing your upper arms and elbows to lose touch with your sides, increase the distance between your palms as you open your hands slowly out to your sides. If you do it correctly, you should feel some tension between your shoulder blades. Hold for a count of five, bring your palms back together, and repeat 10 times.

Stand with your feet under your hips and your arms at your sides. Raise your arms out to the sides and put them 45 degrees forward of your torso as high as you can with your pinkies facing up. Keep your shoulders relaxed away from your ears as you raise your arms. Lower and repeat 10-20 times. As the exercise becomes easier, attach ankle weights to your wrists to increase the challenge.

3 Boost yourself up twice a day.

Here's another great exercise for the office. Place your palms on the edge of your chair and press down into your hands, lifting your hips and buttocks an inch or two into the air. Hold for 5 seconds, lower, and repeat five times for a great shoulder muscle strengthener.

4 Rent a rowboat and take your spouse for a romantic excursion on a lake or pond. As you row out onto the water, you'll strengthen the weakest section of your shoulders, behind your shoulder blades. When these muscles are weak, your shoulders slump forward. Rowing impractical? Then simulate the motion for a few minutes, moving slowly and carefully. Or use a rowing machine at home or at the gym.

5 When you don't know the answer to a question, use body language and literally shrug your shoulders. The action of lifting your shoulders up to your ears will strengthen your neck and shoulder muscles. And when you are alone, do three sets of 10 shoulder shrugs for a fuller workout.

6 As you watch television at night, retract your shoulder blades. Sit on the edge of your chair and lengthen your spine, as if you were trying to grow taller. Place your hands in your lap. Bring your shoulders as far back as you can, pinching your shoulder blades together. Hold for the length of an entire commercial. Relax and then repeat one more time during the course of the evening.

7 When you get home from work, fill a tube sock three-fourths of the way with white rice, 2 cinnamon sticks, and 1 tablespoon cloves. Seal the end tightly with a rubber band. Heat for 2 minutes in the microwave and drape around your neck for a surprisingly pleasing aromatherapeutic remedy for sore shoulders and neck. No need to empty the sock—you can use it over and over, until the spices lose their fragrance.

8 Whenever you spend more than 45 minutes in the driver's seat or in front of the computer, practice the "turtle" exercise. Often during driving and when staring at a computer screen, we tend to jut our heads forward, as if sticking our nose out is going to get us to our

Do **Three** Things

The repetitive movements involved in working at a computer all day—making micro-movement after micro-movement with your mouse, typing at your keyboard, and staring at your computer screen for hours on end—can, over time, stiffen the muscles in your arms, shoulders, and neck, causing pain. Although a number of treatments have been used over the years to prevent and reverse "computer neck," ranging from chiropractic manipulation to massage, only three tactics have been proven by research to reduce neck pain, according to Charles Edwards II, M.D., a surgeon and research coordinator at the Maryland Spine Center at Mercy Medical Center in Baltimore.

1. **Exercise aerobically for at least 30 minutes three to four times a week.** Regular aerobic exercise increases blood flow to your muscles, helping them heal faster. It also reduces stress and may help you sleep better. A brisk walk works just fine.

2. **Lose weight.** Excess pounds not only encourage you to sit with poor posture, they also impede blood circulation, slowly the healing process. You can lose one pound a week by eliminating 250 daily calories from your diet and walking for 20 additional minutes a day.

3. **Quit smoking.** Research shows that regular smoking can cause all types of pain, including neck and back pain. The nicotine in tobacco is toxic to all body tissues and may damage the blood vessels in your neck and shoulders, preventing blood from getting to your spine.

destination faster or help us finish that project quicker. Because the head weighs about 10 pounds, this puts quite a bit of stress on the back of the neck. Before you know it, you've got a headache. You can both strengthen the muscles in the back of your neck and train yourself to sit with proper posture with the following exercise. As you drive or type, pretend you are a turtle retracting your head into your shell. Keeping your chin level, bring your head back, flattening the curve in the back of your neck. Hold for a count of five, release, and repeat 10 times.

9 Every hour, drop your chin to your chest, then roll your neck to the left, back, to the right, and down again in a circular motion. Repeat five times, then switch direction, starting with a roll to the right.

10 Start each workday with a chair exercise. Sit on the edge of a chair with your knees bent and feet on the floor. Extend one arm overhead and the other toward the floor, with your palms facing in. Keeping your shoulders low on your back and away from your ears, reach

11 Every morning before you get dressed, stretch into a yoga down dog. This quintessential yoga posture stretches your calves, hamstrings, chest, and spine while it strengthens and stretches your shoulders. Kneel with your palms on the floor under your shoulders and knees under your hips. Spread your fingers as wide as you can with your middle fingers pointing forward. Tuck your toes under, coming onto the balls of your feet. Roll your shoulder blades away from each other, bringing the creases of your elbows toward each other. Lift your tailbone. Then exhale as you extend your legs and lift your hips toward the ceiling, forming an upside-down **V** shape with your body. Relax your head between your arms. Press into your palms to bring more body weight back into your legs. Continue to roll your shoulder blades away from each other and the inner creases of your elbows toward each other. Hold for 5–10 breaths. Lower and repeat.

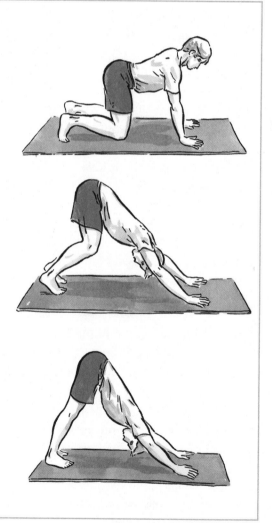

back through both arms, feeling a stretch through your top armpit and front of your

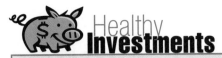

Rubber Tubing

Available at sporting goods stores under such brands as Thera-Band, rubber tubing can help you get in a more effective neck- and shoulder-strengthening session at home. You can easily store these stretchy, lightweight, elastic strips behind the couch or under the bed. Pull one out whenever you have a spare five minutes and do an exercise. For example, you can stand on the middle of your elastic tubing and hold an end in each hand. Then raise your arms out to the sides to strengthen your shoulders.

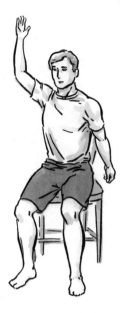

bottom shoulder. You'll also feel muscles in the backs of your shoulders and upper back firming as they work to keep your arms in place. Hold 2 seconds, then switch positions, so the top arm is now facing toward the floor and the bottom arm is facing the ceiling, and repeat. Continue to hold 2 seconds and then switch positions 20 times. Then do the same movement 20 times, but turn your hands so your

palms face behind your torso. Finally, repeat the exercise again, but turn your hands so your palms face forward. Each new palm position strengthens and stretches a slightly different area of your shoulders.

 12 **Make sure you're sleeping on the right pillow.** The best pillow for you depends on your own preferences, but generally stomach sleepers should go for soft, side sleepers for medium, and back sleepers for firm.

REMINDER

 Fast Results
These are bits of advice that deliver benefits particularly quickly—in some cases, immediately!

 Easy Gains
These are tips that give the biggest value for the least amount of effort.

 Super Effective
These are tips proven to be particularly effective through scientific research or widespread usage by experts.

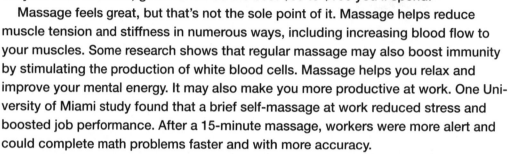

Self-Massage

17 WAYS TO REDUCE TENSION IN SECONDS

Have you ever had a professional massage? If yes, then you *know*. If you haven't, well, words can't describe what a terrific experience it is. On your next vacation, get one. It'll be the best $50 to $100 you'll spend.

Massage feels great, but that's not the sole point of it. Massage helps reduce muscle tension and stiffness in numerous ways, including increasing blood flow to your muscles. Some research shows that regular massage may also boost immunity by stimulating the production of white blood cells. Massage helps you relax and improve your mental energy. It may also make you more productive at work. One University of Miami study found that a brief self-massage at work reduced stress and boosted job performance. After a 15-minute massage, workers were more alert and could complete math problems faster and with more accuracy.

Fortunately, you have your very own massage therapist with you at all times—your hands! "Most people practice the art of self-massage without thinking about it, whether they are rubbing their forehead because of a headache, scrubbing themselves with a loofah sponge in the shower, or rubbing their feet after a long day," says Anna Walsemann, a yoga and Oriental healing instructor at New Age Health Spa in Neversink, New York. "These are all simple and natural self-massage techniques."

You don't have to take a class to give yourself a proper rubdown. In this chapter, you'll get the advice you need to reduce tension from head to foot—within seconds.

1 **Every morning and evening, hammer out the kinks.** Using your fists, gently thump the outside of your body, starting with your legs and arms, working from top to bottom. Then move inward to your torso and thump from bottom to top. "Pummeling your muscles and bones will help strengthen the body, stimulate blood circulation, and relax nerve endings," says Walsemann. When done in the morning, this self-massage technique will waken and prepare your body—and mind—for the day ahead. When done before bed, it calms down the mind and beats out the stress and tension of the day. One warning: If you're taking any kind of blood thinner, such as Coumadin (warfarin), avoid this one; you could wind up with bruising.

2 **Rub your belly after every meal.** Most of us do this instinctively, especially after overeating. Place one or both palms on your abdomen and rub it in clockwise circles. This is the same direction food naturally moves through your intestine, so your circular massage will help to stimulate digestion.

3 Rub yourself down before and after exercise. Massaging your body before your stretching, cardio, or strength training increases blood flow to the muscles. Massaging your muscles after exercise may help encourage waste removal and speed muscle recovery. Before exercise, use a pummeling motion with your fists to bring blood flow to your leg and arm muscles. After exercise, rub along your muscles with your palm or fist, moving in the direction of your heart.

4 Give your hands a massage every day—whenever you put on lotion. Start with the bottoms of your palms by clasping your fingers and rubbing the heels of your palms together in a circular motion. Then, with your hands still clasped, take one thumb and massage the area just below your other thumb in circular motions, moving outward to the center of the palm. Repeat with the other hand. Then release your fingers and use your thumbs and index fingers to knead your palms, wrists, and the webbing between your fingers. With one hand,

gently pull each finger of the other hand. Finish by using your thumb and index finger to pinch the webbing between your other thumb and index finger.

5 Roll on a tennis ball whenever you feel tight. If your foot feels tense, stand with one hand on a wall for support and place the arch of one foot on top of the ball. Gradually add more body weight over the foot, allowing the ball to press into your arch. Begin to slowly move your foot, allowing the ball to massage your heel, forefoot, and toes. Note: If the tennis ball seems too big for your foot, try a golf ball instead.

You can also lie on the ball to get at that hard-to-reach spot between the shoulder blades or to soothe tension in your low back. For tight hips, sit on the ball, wiggling your booty around and holding it in any spot that feels particularly good.

6 Fill the bottom of a shoe box with golf balls and stick it under your desk at work. Whenever you need to take a trip to podiatric paradise, take off a shoe and rub your foot over the golf balls.

7 Whenever you take off a pair of high heels, sit on the floor and give your calves some attention. Elevating your heels all day long can eventually shorten your calf muscles. To release them, sit with your knees bent and feet on the floor. Grasp one ankle, placing your thumb just above your Achilles tendon. Press your thumb into the bottom of your calf muscle, hold for 5 seconds, and release. Move an inch up your calf and repeat the pressure. Continue pressing and releasing until you get to your knee, then switch legs.

Two-Second Quiz

Hard or Soft Massage?

Answer: *Hard.*
The point of massage isn't to stimulate the skin; it's to relieve the muscles lying deep below the skin. While we're not saying to massage to the point of pain, you need to use enough effort to work the muscles thoroughly. And that takes more force than many home massagers assert. If your hands and arms aren't getting strained or tired giving a massage, you're probably not pressing hard enough.

8 Fill a tube-style athletic sock three-fourths full with uncooked rice, tie off the end tightly with a rubber band, and stick it in the microwave for 2 minutes. Remove the sock and rub it up and down your legs and arms for a gentle, soothing hot massage. Leave the sock filled with the rice; you can use it over and over. As noted on page 201, in "Neck and Shoulder Strength," you can add spices to the rice if you wish to have a pleasant scent while massaging.

9 Use your hands to *heel* your neck. Once an hour, take a break from staring at your computer and clasp your fingers behind your neck, pressing the heels of your palms into your neck on either side of your spinal column. Massage the heels of your hands up and down in slow, deliberate motions. Then place the fingers of your right hand on your trapezius muscle along the left side of your neck just below the base of your skull. Press into that muscle, tilt your head to the left, and rub downward until you reach your shoulder. Repeat three times, then switch sides.

Finish by stretching your head back so the top of your office chair presses into your neck just below your skull. This also stretches out the front of your neck, which tends to get tight during deskwork. Hold for 20 seconds.

10 Open your sinuses with some finger pressure. If you have clogged sinuses due to a cold or allergies, rub them with your index fingers. Start just above your brow line. Place your finger pads just above your nose, press down and rub outward, tracing your brow line as you go. Repeat two or three times. Then place the pads of your fingers below

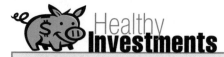

Healthy Investments

The Stick

Sold at most sporting goods stores and online sports stores, this plastic wand costs roughly $30 and contains rotating spindles. You can use it to rub just about any area of your body and store it under your couch at home or desk at work. Hold it in both hands and rub up the back of your calf or thigh or down the front of your thigh. Ask a friend or spouse to roll the stick up and down your back and over the tops of your shoulders.

your eyes and to the sides of the bridge of your nose, rubbing outward and moving downward with each stroke. Now use your thumbs to massage your cheekbones, making small circles starting at the center of your face and moving out toward your ears. Finally, place your thumbs on your temples and massage them in small circles.

11 When your eyes feel tired from staring at your computer screen all day long, give them some heat. Rub your hands together vigorously until you feel the skin on your palms begin to warm up. Then cup one hand over each eye, feeling the heat from your hands relax your eyes.

12 When your feet are sore after a long day of standing, take off your shoes and socks, wash your feet, and give them a rubdown. Sitting on a comfortable couch or chair, thread the fingers of one hand through the toes of one foot, spreading out your toes and placing the palm of your hand against the bottom of your foot. Use your palm to gently rotate the joints of your forefoot forward and back for one minute. Then remove your fingers from your toes, hold your ankle with one hand, and gently rotate the entire foot with the other hand, starting with small circles and progressing to larger circles as your ankle warms up. Switch directions, and then repeat with the other foot.

13 **Give yourself a bear hug to relax away shoulder tension.** Cross your arms over your chest and grab a shoulder with either hand. Squeeze each shoulder and release three times. Then move your hands down your arms, squeezing and releasing until you get to your wrists.

14 **Rub lavender oil onto your feet before bed.** Lavender-scented oils are available at most health food stores. The smell of lavender and the gentle massaging motions you make as you work the oil into your feet will help you to unwind. An added bonus: The nightly oil treatment softens and hydrates any rough, dry spots on your feet. Once you're done with your massage, put on a pair of socks to prevent the oil from rubbing off onto your sheets.

15 **After tennis, cycling, rock climbing, and other arm-tiring sports, give your arms a pinch.** Place your right arm across your chest with your elbow bent. Reach across your chest with your left arm and pinch your right arm's triceps, near the shoulder, with the thumb and index finger of your left hand. Hold for a few seconds, release, then pinch again an inch lower on the arm. Continue pinching and releasing until you've made your way to your elbow. Then pinch your right arm's biceps near your armpit and work your way in the same way down to the elbow. Then switch arms. This will release the tension in your muscles and help improve blood circulation.

16 **When you have a headache, stand up, bend forward from the hips, and place your forehead on a padded chair.** The chair will gently place pressure on your head as you relax in the forward bend. Hold about 30 seconds. When you rise, sit down and spread your fingers through your hair, making a fist. Gently pull the hair away from your head. Hold 2-3 seconds, then release. This stretches the fascia along your scalp, releasing tension. Continue to grab different clumps of hair all over your head, working from the top front of your head, progressing to the sides, and then to the back of your head. Once you have grabbed and released your entire scalp, return to work, feeling refreshed.

17 **Keep a tennis ball on your desk and squeeze it regularly.** The squeezing motion helps rejuvenate tired fingers and hands, and strengthens your hands for other self-massage techniques.

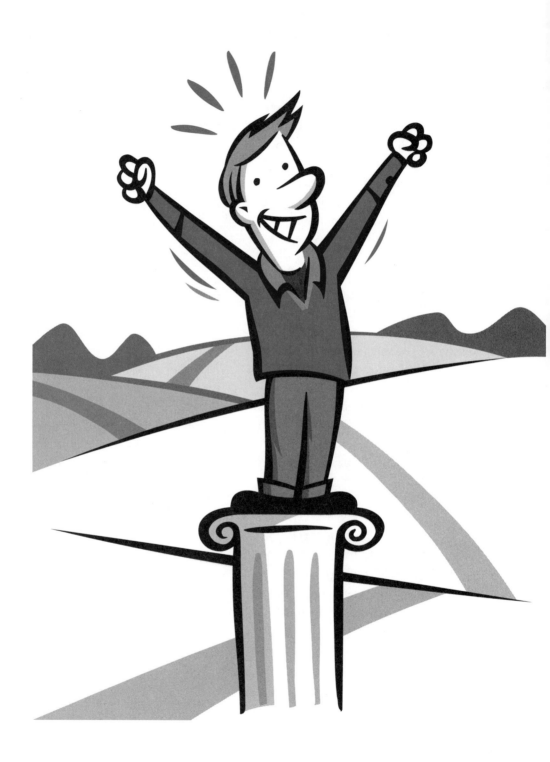

PART FIVE

Targeted Health

GOALS

As we travel through life, each of us encounters unique health challenges and concerns. To help you make your journey as disease- and hassle-free as possible, we've put together proven health tips for 18 common health goals, from losing weight to preventing cancer.

Burning More Calories
14 Ways to Boost Your Metabolism and Kick-Start Your Weight Loss

Losing Weight
58 Best Tips for Easy Slimming

Greater Energy
26 Ways to Find Your Get Up and Go After It Has Gotten Up and Gone

Monitor Your Health
16 Ways to Do It Without a Doctor

Preventing Colds and Flus
23 Ways to Stay Healthy Year-Round

Reduce Your Risk of Heart Disease and Stroke
30 Simple Solutions

Lower Your Cholesterol
18 Ways to Get The Numbers Down

Lowering Blood Pressure
20 Ways to Go Beyond Low-Sodium

Stabilizing Your Blood Sugar
20 Tips for Stable, Steady Glucose Levels

Preventing Cancer
31 Ways to Inoculate Yourself Against the Big C

Greater Lung Power
18 Ways to Breathe Easier

Greater Mobility
18 Ways to Keep Joints Limber and Arthritis at Bay

Stronger Bones
28 Ways to Help Prevent Osteoporosis

Stronger Libido, Better Sex
31 Ways to Get There

Combating Allergies
20 Ways to Stop Being Sneezy

Improving Your Vision
24 Ways to See Clearly Forever

Improving Your Hearing
18 Ways to Hear a Pin Drop

Sharpen Your Sense of Smell and Taste
20 Sensible Strategies

Burning More Calories

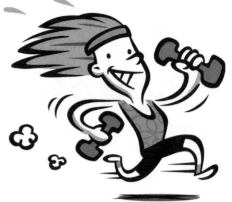

13 WAYS TO BOOST YOUR METABOLISM AND KICK-START YOUR WEIGHT LOSS

One frustrating thing about trying to lose weight is the snail's pace at which the pounds seem to drop. Then there's the harsh reality that the more weight you lose, the harder your body fights to hold on to the calories it gets and the fewer calories it burns. That's usually about the time you hit the infamous weight-loss plateau—and start losing steam. But what if you could turbo-charge your weight-loss efforts without a lot of sacrifice?

That's where this chapter comes in. We've come up with easy ways to boost your metabolism, or the rate at which you burn calories. We've also thrown in ideas for cranking up the calorie burn of your workout—without making it longer. Taken together, these tips should be more than enough to shift your weight loss out of neutral and move it full speed ahead again.

Still, it's important that you maintain a realistic expectation of what's considered "healthy" weight loss. About a pound or two a week is ideal; much more than that is unlikely to last long-term.

1 **Sip green tea three times a day.** A study from the University of Geneva in Switzerland found that in addition to caffeine, green tea contains catechin polyphenols, plant chemicals that may boost metabolism.

2 **Use interval training to rev up your workout.** Walk for the same amount of time at the same intensity day in and day out and your body gets as bored with your workout as you do. Throw it a curveball with interval training, which involves varying the intensity of your workout throughout your exercise session.

Every five minutes into your walk, jog for one minute. Every five minutes into your bike ride, shift into a higher gear and pedal hard for a minute. If you swim, turn on the speed every other lap. You'll burn more calories in the same amount of time.

3 **Fidget.** People who drum their fingers or bounce their knees burn at least 500 calories a day! That adds up to losing a pound a week.

4 **Keep a small squeeze ball with you** and work out your hands frequently during the day. It's one of the few exercises

you can do anytime. You'll build up the muscles in your hands—and muscle, whether in your hands or legs, burns a lot of calories.

5 **Don't starve yourself.** Cutting too many calories can backfire in more ways than one. Try to subsist on morsels and your metabolism will slow so much that you'll not only stop losing weight, but you'll be lucky if you can peel yourself off the couch.

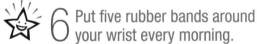

6 **Put five rubber bands around your wrist every morning.** That's how many 16-ounce bottles of water you should drink during the day to rev your metabolism, helping burn more calories. At least, that's what German researchers found when they had 14 participants drink about 17 ounces of water. The volunteers' metabolic rate—or how quickly they burned calories—jumped a third within 10 minutes of drinking the water and remained high for another 30 or 40 minutes. The researchers estimated that over a year, increasing your water consumption by 1.5 liters a day (about 50 ounces) would burn an extra 17,400 calories, or about five pounds' worth. Since much of the increased metabolic rate is due to the body's efforts to heat the water, make sure the water you're drinking is icy.

7 **Exercise outside.** Maybe it's the fresh air, maybe it's the sunshine, but something about exercising in the open makes you walk or run faster than doing the same exercise in the gym.

8 **Turn up the heat with hot peppers.** Some studies show that very spicy foods can temporarily increase your metabolism. Gourmet groceries often stock a dozen different kinds of peppers. Buy one a week and practice adding some to various meals. Spice up your scrambled eggs with minced jalapeño, add a little fire to your beef stew with half a diced banana

In**Perspective**

The Weight-Loss Plateau

There's nothing more frustrating than hitting a weight-loss plateau, particularly when you're still doing everything right—eating right, exercising, passing up the ice cream and doughnuts. So what gives?

First, you should know that it's not your fault. Weight-loss plateaus are perfectly normal and easily explained. Your basal metabolism, or the energy your body consumes just to survive, accounts for about 70 percent of all calories you burn—and it depends on how much you weigh. The less you weigh, the lower your basal metabolic rate (BMR). Lose enough weight, and boom! Your metabolism slows and you hit the weight-loss plateau. The only way to lose more weight is to decrease the amount of calories you take in, increase the amount of calories you burn through physical activity, or both.

You can boost your basal metabolism, but only indirectly, by building muscle. Muscle tissue requires more energy than fat does, even when you're at rest. In fact, every pound of muscle you add burns another 30-50 calories a day.

Best bets for building muscle? Walking will help a bit, but resistance training (such as lifting weights, doing push-ups, or using exercise bands) will help more.

pepper, or pull together a spicy jambalaya (using turkey sausage and lots of veggies).

9 Eat five small meals throughout the day instead of three large meals. You might think you should eat less often if you want to lose weight, but that's just not the case. By eating every few hours, you keep your metabolism fired up and ensure it doesn't slow between meals in order to hang on to calories. A "meal" can be as small as a cup of soup.

10 Sip a couple of cups of coffee throughout the day. Studies find that the caffeine in coffee increases the rate at which your body burns calories. This does not mean, however, that you can order one of those fancy calorie-packed frappuccinos! And skip the java if it makes you toss and turn at night.

11 Don't get discouraged because you've been yo-yo dieting. Somehow the myth got started that if you've spent your life losing and gaining the same 10 or 20 pounds, your metabolism gets out of whack and winds up slower than an airport security line. Don't believe it. When researchers reviewed 43 studies on the topic, they found no difference in the metabolic rates of yo-yo dieters versus those of everyone else.

12 Walk with intent—and intensity. Burn more calories in the same amount of time with these strategies:

▶ **Swing your arms when you walk.** You'll burn 5-10 percent more calories.
▶ **Wear a weighted vest.** Another great

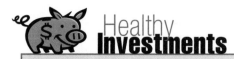

Healthy Investments

A Curves Membership

We've tried whenever possible to stay away from name brands in this book, but the case for joining Curves, the national chain of women-only health clubs, is compelling. Eight studies from a team of health and fitness experts at Baylor University found that sedentary and overweight women who followed the Curves program were able to significantly raise their metabolic rate, in some cases by as much as 400 calories a day. The best part: You get both aerobic and resistance training in one 30-minute workout.

way to crank up the calorie burn. Leave the hand and ankle weights at home, though. They throw you off balance and could result in injury.

▶ **Walk on grass, sand, or a gravel trail instead of the road.** It takes more muscle power to glide smoothly over these uneven surfaces (especially sand) than over asphalt.
▶ **Use walking poles.** A University of Wisconsin study found you get a much more intense workout than without the poles.
▶ **Walk along the shoreline of a beach, lake, or pond with your ankles in the water.** The resistance will cause you to burn more calories and give your muscles an added workout.

13 Bump up the protein in your diet. There is some evidence that by taking protein to the upper end of the recommended range (roughly 20 percent of your overall calories), the amount of energy you expend while resting remains the same even as you're losing weight (normally, it falls).

Losing Weight

58 BEST TIPS FOR EASY SLIMMING

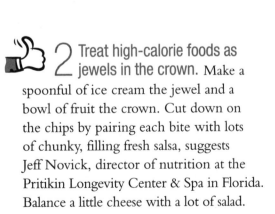

One of the best things you can do for your overall health is drop a few pounds. Or maybe more than a few pounds. Being overweight significantly increases your risk of heart disease, diabetes, stroke, high blood pressure, cancer...the list seems almost endless. Plus, if you do get sick or need surgery, being overweight can make any treatments riskier.

You know the drill when it comes to losing weight—take in fewer calories, burn more calories. But you also know that most diets and quick weight-loss plans have about as much substance as a politician's campaign pledges. You're better off finding several simple things you can do on a daily basis—along with following the cardinal rules of eating more vegetables and less fat and getting more physical activity. Together, they should send the scale numbers in the right direction: down.

1 Once a week, indulge in a high-calorie-tasting, but low-calorie, treat. This should help keep you from feeling deprived and binging on higher-calorie foods. For instance:

- **Lobster.** Just 83 calories in 3 ounces.
- **Shrimp.** Just 60 calories in 12 large.
- **Smoked salmon.** Just 66 calories in two ounces. Sprinkle with capers for an even more elegant treat.
- **Whipped cream.** Just 8 calories in one tablespoon. Drop a dollop over a bowl of fresh fruit for dessert.

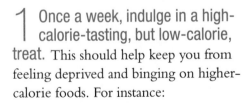 2 Treat high-calorie foods as jewels in the crown. Make a spoonful of ice cream the jewel and a bowl of fruit the crown. Cut down on the chips by pairing each bite with lots of chunky, filling fresh salsa, suggests Jeff Novick, director of nutrition at the Pritikin Longevity Center & Spa in Florida. Balance a little cheese with a lot of salad.

3 After breakfast, make water your primary drink. At breakfast, go ahead and drink orange juice. But throughout the rest of the day, focus on water instead

of juice or soda. The average American consumes an extra 245 calories a day from soft drinks. That's nearly 90,000 calories a year—or 25 pounds! And research shows that despite the calories, sugary drinks don't trigger a sense of fullness the way that food does.

4 **Carry a palm-size notebook everywhere you go for one week.** Write down every single morsel that enters your lips—even water. Studies have found that people who maintain food diaries wind up eating about 15 percent less food than those who don't.

5 **Buy a pedometer, clip it to your belt, and aim for an extra 1,000 steps a day.** On average, sedentary people take only 2,000 to 3,000 steps a day. Adding 2,000 steps will help you maintain your current weight and stop gaining weight; adding more than that will help you lose weight.

6 **Add 10 percent to the amount of daily calories you *think* you're eating, then adjust your eating habits** accordingly. If you think you're consuming 1,700 calories a day and don't understand why you're not losing weight, add another 170 calories to your guesstimate. Chances are, the new number is more accurate.

7 **Eat five or six small meals or snacks a day instead of three large meals.** A 1999 South African study found that when men ate parts of their morning meal at intervals over five hours, they consumed almost 30 percent fewer calories at lunch than when they ate a single breakfast. Other studies show that even if you eat the same number of calories distributed this way, your body releases less

insulin, which keeps blood sugar steady and helps control hunger.

8 **Walk for 45 minutes a day.** The reason we're suggesting 45 minutes instead of the typical 30 is that a Duke University study found that while 30 minutes of daily walking is enough to prevent weight gain in most relatively sedentary people, exercise *beyond* 30 minutes results in weight and fat loss. Burning an additional 300 calories a day with three miles of brisk walking (45 minutes should do it) could help you lose 30 pounds in a year without even changing how much you're eating. See "Walking," page 154, for Stealth Healthy ways to make doing this more fun.

9 **Find an online weight-loss buddy.** A University of Vermont study found that online weight-loss buddies help you keep the weight off. The researchers followed volunteers for 18 months. Those assigned to an Internet-based weight maintenance program sustained their weight loss better than those who met face-to-face in a support group.

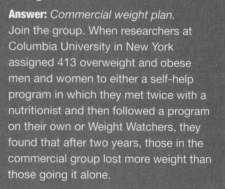

Two-Second**Quiz**

Commercial Weight Plan or Solo Weight Loss?

Answer: *Commercial weight plan.* Join the group. When researchers at Columbia University in New York assigned 413 overweight and obese men and women to either a self-help program in which they met twice with a nutritionist and then followed a program on their own or Weight Watchers, they found that after two years, those in the commercial group lost more weight than those going it alone.

10 Bring the color blue into your life more often. There's a good reason you won't see many fast-food restaurants decorated in blue: Believe it or not, the color blue functions as an appetite suppressant. So serve up dinner on blue plates, dress in blue while you eat, and cover your table with a blue tablecloth. Conversely, avoid red, yellow, and orange in your dining areas. Studies find they encourage eating.

11 Clean your closet of the "fat" clothes. Once you've reached your target weight, throw out or give away every piece of clothing that doesn't fit. The idea of having to buy a whole new wardrobe if you gain the weight back will serve as a strong incentive to maintain your new figure.

12 Downsize your dinner plates. Studies find that the less food put in front of you, the less food you'll eat. Conversely, the more food in front of you, the more you'll eat—regardless of how hungry you are. So instead of using regular dinner plates that range these days from 10-14 inches (making them look forlornly empty if they're not heaped with food), serve your main course on salad plates (about 7-9 inches wide). The same goes for liquids. Instead of 16-ounce glasses and oversized coffee mugs, return to the old days of 8-ounce glasses and 6-ounce coffee cups.

13 Serve your dinner restaurant style (food on the plates) rather than family style (food served in bowls and on platters on the table). When your plate is empty, you're finished; there's no reaching for seconds.

14 Hang a mirror opposite your seat at the table. One study found that eating in front of mirrors slashed the amount people ate by nearly one-third. Seems having to look yourself in the eye reflects back some of your own inner standards and goals, and reminds you of why you're trying to lose weight in the first place.

15 Put out a vegetable platter. A body of research out of Pennsylvania State University finds that eating water-rich foods such as zucchini, tomatoes, and cucumbers during meals reduces your overall calorie consumption. Other water-rich foods include soups and salads. You won't get the same benefits by just drinking your water, though. Because the body processes hunger and thirst through different mechanisms, it simply doesn't register a sense of fullness with water (or soda, tea, coffee, or juice).

16 Use vegetables to bulk up meals. You can eat twice as much pasta salad loaded with veggies like broccoli, carrots, and tomatoes for the same calories as a pasta salad sporting just mayonnaise. Same goes for stir-fries. And add veggies to make a fluffier, more satisfying omelet without having to up the number of eggs.

17 Eat one less cookie a day. Or consume one less can of regular soda, or one less glass of orange juice, or three fewer bites of a fast-food hamburger.

Doing any of these saves you about 100 calories a day, according to weight-loss researcher James O. Hill, Ph.D., of the University of Colorado. And that alone is enough to prevent you from gaining the 1.8 to 2 pounds most people pack on each year.

18 Avoid white foods. There is some scientific legitimacy to today's lower-carb diets: Large amounts of simple carbohydrates from white flour and added sugar can wreak havoc on your blood sugar and lead to weight gain. But you shouldn't toss out the baby with the bathwater. While avoiding sugar, white rice, and white flour, you should eat plenty of whole grain breads and brown rice. One Harvard study of 74,000 women found that those who ate more than two daily servings of whole grains were 49 percent less likely to be overweight than those who ate the white stuff.

19 Switch to ordinary coffee. Fancy coffee drinks from trendy coffee joints often pack several hundred calories, thanks to whole milk, whipped cream, sugar, and sugary syrups. A cup of regular coffee with skim milk has just a small fraction of those calories. And when brewed with good beans, it tastes just as great.

20 Use nonfat powdered milk in coffee. You get the nutritional benefits of skim milk, which is high in calcium and low in calories. And, because the water has been removed, powdered milk doesn't dilute the coffee the way skim milk does.

21 Eat cereal for breakfast five days a week. Studies find that people who eat cereal for breakfast every day are significantly less likely to

be obese and have diabetes than those who don't. They also consume more fiber and calcium—and less fat—than those who eat other breakfast foods. Of course, that doesn't mean reaching for the Cap'n Crunch. Instead, pour out a high-fiber, low-sugar cereal like Total or Grape Nuts.

22 Pare your portions. Whether you eat at home or in a restaurant, immediately remove one-third of the food on your plate. Arguably the worst food trend of the past few decades has been the explosion in portion sizes on America's dinner plates (and breakfast and lunch plates). We eat far, far more today than our bodies need. Studies find that if you serve people more food, they'll eat more food, regardless of their hunger level. The converse is also true: Serve yourself less and you'll eat less.

23 Eat 90 percent of your meals at home. You're more likely to eat more—and eat more high-fat, high-calorie foods—when you eat out than when you eat at home. Restaurants today serve such large portions that many have switched to larger plates and tables to accommodate them!

24 Avoid any prepared food that lists sugar, fructose, or corn syrup among the first four ingredients on the label. You should be able to find a lower-sugar version of the same type of food. If you can't, grab a piece of fruit instead! Look for sugar-free varieties of foods such as ketchup, mayonnaise, and salad dressing.

25 Eat slowly and calmly. Put your fork or spoon down between every bite. Sip water frequently. Intersperse your eating with stories for your dining partner of the amusing things that happened during your day. Your brain lags your stomach by about 20 minutes when it comes to satiety (fullness) signals. If you eat slowly enough, your brain will catch up to tell you that you are no longer in need of food.

26 Eat only when you hear your stomach growling. It's stunning how often we eat out of boredom, nervousness, habit, or frustration—so often, in fact, that many of us have actually forgotten what physical hunger feels like. Next time, wait until your stomach is growling before you reach for food. If you're hankering for a specific food, it's probably a craving, not hunger. If you'd eat anything you could get your hands on, chances are you're truly hungry.

27 Find ways other than eating to express love, tame stress, and relieve boredom. For instance, you might make your family a photo album of special events instead of a rich dessert, sign up for a stress-management course at the local hospital (or read the chapter on stress management that begins on page 290), or take up an active hobby, like bowling.

28 State the positive. You've heard of a self-fulfilling prophecy? Well, if you keep focusing on things you can't do, like resisting junk food or getting out the door for a daily walk, chances are you won't do them. Instead (whether you believe it or not) repeat positive thoughts to yourself. "I can lose weight." "I will get out for my walk today." "I know I can resist the pastry cart after dinner." Repeat these phrases like a mantra all day long. Before too long, they will become their own self-fulfilling prophecy.

29 Discover your dietary point of preference. If you work hard to control your weight, you may get pleasure from your appearance, but you may also feel sorry for yourself each time you forgo a favorite food. There is a balance to be struck between the immediate gratification of indulgent foods and the long-term pleasure of maintaining a

Two-Second **Quiz**

Hot or Dry Cereal?

Answer: *Hot cereal.*

Hot cooked cereal like oatmeal has one-fifth the calorie density of dried cereal, says Jeff Novick, director of nutrition at the Pritikin Longevity Center & Spa in Florida. Hot cereal has 300 calories per pound; dried cereals pack in 1,400 to 2,000 calories per pound. Plus, hot cereal is more filling. It keeps you fueled well into late morning, helping you avoid the 10 a.m. munchies.

desirable weight and good health. When you have that balance worked out, you have identified your own personal dietary pleasure "point of preference." This is where you want to stay.

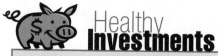

30 Use flavorings such as hot sauce, salsa, and Cajun seasonings instead of relying on butter and creamy or sugary sauces. Besides providing lots of flavor with no fat and few calories, many of these seasonings—the spicy ones—turn up your digestive fires, causing your body to temporarily burn more calories.

31 Eat fruit instead of drinking fruit juice. For the calories in one kid-size box of apple juice, you can enjoy an apple, orange, and a slice of watermelon. These whole foods will keep you satisfied much longer than that box of apple juice, so you'll eat less overall.

32 Spend 10 minutes a day walking up and down stairs. The Centers for Disease Control says that's all it takes to help you shed as much as 10 pounds a year (assuming you don't start eating more).

Healthy Investments

A Kitchen Timer

Set it for 30 minutes when you sit down to eat dinner, then eat slowly so your last bite coincides with the ding, allowing time for fullness signals to make it from your stomach to your brain. Once you're finished eating, set the timer for two hours. If you're really hungry when it dings, you may have dessert. Otherwise, pat yourself on the back.

33 Eat equal portions of vegetables and grains at dinner. A cup of cooked rice or pasta has about 200 calories, whereas a cup of cooked veggies doles out a mere 50 calories, on average, says Joan Salge Blake, R.D., clinical assistant professor of nutrition at Boston University's Sargent College. To avoid a grain calorie overload, eat a 1:1 ratio of grains to veggies. The high-fiber veggies will help satisfy your hunger before you overeat the grains.

34 Get up and walk around the office or your home for five minutes at least every two hours. Stuck at a desk all day? A brisk five-minute walk every two hours will parlay into an extra 20-minute walk by the end of the day. And getting a break will make you less likely to reach for snacks out of antsiness.

35 Wash something thoroughly once a week—a floor, a couple of windows, the shower stall, bathroom tile, or your car. A 150-pound person who dons rubber gloves and exerts some elbow grease will burn about four calories for every minute spent cleaning, says Blake. Scrub for 30 minutes and you could work off approximately 120 calories, the same number in a half-cup of vanilla frozen yogurt. And your surroundings will sparkle!

36 Make one social outing this week an active one. Pass on the movie tickets and screen the views of a local park instead. Not only will you sit less, but you'll be saving calories because you won't chow down on that bucket of popcorn. Other active date ideas: Plan a tennis match, sign up for a guided nature or city walk (check your local newspaper), go cycling on a bike path, or join a volleyball league or bowling team.

Birthday Cake
or Petits Fours?

Answer: *Petits fours.*
Give one petit four to every guest at the
party. That way, not only will you have
built-in portion control, but it's ever so
much easier to send any uneaten ones
home with a guest, says Susie Galvez,
author of *Weight Loss Wisdom.*

37 Order the smallest portion of everything. If you're ordering a sub, get the 6-inch sandwich. Buy a small popcorn, a small salad, a small hamburger. Studies find we tend to eat what's in front of us, even though we'd feel just as full on less.

38 Switch from regular milk to 2%. If you already drink 2%, go down another notch to 1% or skim milk. Each step downward cuts the calories by about 20 percent. Once you train your taste buds to enjoy skim milk, you'll have cut the calories in the whole milk by about half and trimmed the fat by more than 95 percent.

39 Take a walk before dinner. You'll do more than burn calories—you'll cut your appetite. In a study of 10 obese women conducted at the University of Glasgow in Scotland, 20 minutes of walking reduced appetite and increased sensations of fullness as effectively as a light meal.

40 Substitute a handful of almonds in place of a sugary snack. A study from the City of Hope National Medical Center found that overweight people who ate a moderate-fat diet containing almonds lost more weight than a control group that didn't eat nuts. Really, any nut will do.

41 Eat a frozen dinner. Not just any frozen dinner, but one designed for weight loss. Most of us tend to eat an average of 150 percent more calories in the evening than in the morning. An easy way to keep dinner calories under control is to buy a pre-portioned meal. Just make sure that it contains only one serving. If it contains two, make sure you share.

42 Don't eat with a large group. A study published in the *Journal of Physiological Behavior* found that we tend to eat more when we eat with other people, most likely because we spend more time at the table. But eating with your significant other or your family, and using table time for talking in between chewing, can help cut down on calories—and help with bonding in the bargain.

43 Watch one less hour of TV. A study of 76 undergraduate students found the more they watched television, the more often they ate and the more they ate overall. Sacrifice one program (there's probably one you don't *really* want to watch anyway) and go for a walk instead. You'll have time left over to finish a chore or gaze at the stars.

44 Get most of your calories before noon. Studies find that the more you eat in the morning, the less you'll eat in the evening. And you have more opportunities to burn off those early-day calories than you do to burn off dinner calories.

45 Close out the kitchen after dinner. Wash all the dishes, wipe down the counters, turn out the light, and, if necessary, tape closed the cabinets and refrigerator. Late-evening eating significantly increases the overall number of calories you eat, a University of Texas study found. Stopping late-night snacking can save 300 or more calories a day, or 31 pounds a year.

46 Sniff a banana, an apple, or a peppermint when you feel hungry. You might feel silly, but it works. When Alan R. Hirsch, M.D., neurological director of the Smell & Taste Treatment and Research Foundation in Chicago, tried this with 3,000 volunteers, he found that the more frequently people sniffed, the less hungry they were and the more weight they lost—an average of 30 pounds each. One theory is that sniffing the food tricks the brain into thinking you're actually eating it.

47 Order wine by the glass, not the bottle. That way you'll be more aware of how much alcohol you're downing. Moderate drinking can be good for your health, but alcohol is high in calories. And because drinking turns off our inhibitions, it can drown our best intentions to keep portions in check.

48 Watch every morsel you put in your mouth on weekends. A University of North Carolina study found people tend to consume an extra 115 calories per weekend day, primarily from alcohol and fat.

49 Stock your refrigerator with low-fat yogurt. A University of Tennessee study found that people who

cut 500 calories a day *and* ate yogurt three times a day for 12 weeks lost more weight and body fat than a group that only cut the calories. The researchers concluded that the calcium in low-fat dairy foods triggers a hormonal response that inhibits the body's production of fat cells and boosts the breakdown of fat.

50 Order your dressing on the side and then stick a fork in it—not your salad. The small amount of dressing that clings to the tines of the fork are plenty for the forkful of salad you then pick up.

51 Brush your teeth after every meal, especially after dinner. That clean, minty freshness will serve as a cue to your body and brain that mealtime is over.

52 Serve individual courses rather than piling everything on one plate. Make the first two courses soup or vegetables (such as a green salad). By the time you get to the more calorie-dense foods, like meat and dessert, you'll be eating less or may already be full (leftovers are a good thing).

53 Passionately kiss your partner 10 times a day. According to the 1991 *Kinsey Institute New Report on Sex,* a passionate kiss burns 6.4 calories per minute. Ten minutes a day of kissing equates to about 23,000 calories—or eight pounds—a year!

54 Add hot peppers to your pasta sauce. Capsaicin, the ingredient in hot peppers that makes them hot, also helps reduce your appetite.

55 Pack nutritious snacks.
Snacking once or twice a day helps stave off hunger and keeps your metabolism stoked, but healthy snacks can be pretty darn hard to come by when you're on the go. Pack up baby carrots or your own trail mix made with nuts, raisins, seeds, and dried fruit.

56 When you shop, choose nutritious foods based on these four simple rules:
▶ Avoid partially hydrogenated oil.
▶ Avoid high-fructose corn syrup.
▶ Choose a short ingredient list over long; there will be fewer flavor enhancers and empty calories.

▶ Look for two or more grams of fiber per 100 calories in all grain products (cereal, bread, crackers, and chips).

57 Weed out calories you've been overlooking: spreads, dressings, sauces, condiments, drinks, and snacks.
These calories count, whether or not you've been counting them, and could make the difference between weight gain and loss.

58 When you're eating out with friends or family, dress up in your most flattering outfit. You'll get loads of compliments, says Susie Galvez, author of *Weight Loss Wisdom,* which will be a great reminder to watch what you eat.

REMINDER

 Fast Results
These are bits of advice that deliver benefits particularly quickly—in some cases, immediately!

 Easy Gains
These are tips that give the biggest value for the least amount of effort.

 Super Effective
These are tips proven to be particularly effective through scientific research or widespread usage by experts.

Greater Energy

26 WAYS TO FIND YOUR GET UP AND GO AFTER IT HAS GOTTEN UP AND GONE

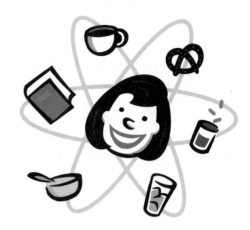

Find yourself dive-bombing the couch by midafternoon? Feeling more sluggish than a hungover sloth? Envying the boundless energy of your kids or grandchildren—or even your on-the-go next-door neighbor? Don't blame your age; blame your lifestyle. A low-energy lifestyle leaves you with low energy. A high-energy lifestyle leaves you with lots of energy. For most people, it's that simple.

Indeed, with just a few easy changes to your daily routine, we guarantee that the seemingly permanent imprint of your backside on the La-Z-Boy will rise up and vanish, along with your inertia. Your friends and family may start asking what you're taking. Tell them nothing, except some good Stealth Health advice.

1 **Nurse a coffee throughout the day.** If you need a quadruple shot of espresso just to bring your eyelids to half-mast in the morning, you may be driving yourself deeper and deeper into a low-energy rut. Compelling research from Brigham and Women's Hospital, Harvard Medical School, and other institutions finds that frequent *low* doses of caffeine—the amount in a quarter-cup of coffee—were more effective than a few larger doses of caffeine in keeping people alert.

2 **Lighten your glycemic load.** Foods with a low glycemic load—like beans, bran cereal, brown rice, whole wheat bread, and nuts—have less impact on your blood sugar than foods with a high glycemic load—like white rice, spaghetti, potatoes, cornflakes, and sugary juices and drinks. Eating more low-glycemic-load foods will help you keep your blood sugar steady and avoid the lightheadedness and "shakes" associated with blood sugar drops, which usually follow spikes.

3 **If you have dried rosemary in your kitchen, crush a small handful** and take a whiff or three. The herb's intense woody fragrance is known to herbalists as an invigorating stimulant.

4 **Once a day, go for a 10-minute "thank you" walk.** As you walk, focus your thoughts on what you feel most thankful for. After the walk, make a mental

note of how you feel. "This simple technique combines the power of gratefulness with the positive effects of walking and exercise, flooding your brain with happy neurotransmitters and endorphins. It's a simple yet powerful exercise that energizes the mind and body and builds mental and physical muscle," says Jon Gordon, a professional speaker, energy coach, and author of *Become an Energy Addict*.

5 **When you find yourself thinking a negative thought, picture a stop sign.** Then either push the thought out of your mind or replace it with a positive one. "Negative feelings take a lot of mental energy," says Kathleen W. Wilson, M.D., an internal medicine specialist and author of *When You Think You Are Falling Apart*. "Whenever possible, avoid unnecessary self-criticism. Stop blaming yourself for past events that you cannot change, and know that you deserve the same level of consideration and mercy as others."

6 **Drink two glasses of icy water.** Fatigue is often one of the first symptoms of dehydration, and if all you've sipped all day is coffee and soft drinks, it's quite likely you're dehydrated. Plus, the refreshing coldness will serve as a virtual slap in the face.

7 **Soak a washcloth in icy water and place it over your face.** The icy coolness of the washcloth will quickly rejuvenate your facial muscles and eyes. It likely will lift your spirits as well.

8 **Get enough iron.** Constantly dragging yourself around? You could have iron-deficiency anemia, a common cause of fatigue. Iron is essential for producing hemoglobin, which carries oxygen to your body's cells, where it is used to produce energy. Good food sources of iron are red meat, iron-fortified cereal, green leafy vegetables, and dried beans. You may also need a supplement; check with your doctor.

9 **When someone asks you to do something, say, "Let me check my schedule and I'll get back to you."** This gives you time to think about the request and decide if it's something you *really* want to do, or simply an energy-sucking waste of your time.

10 **Have your thyroid checked.** If it's not producing enough thyroid hormone, it could be making you feel tired and run-down. A simple blood test will tell. Other symptoms of low thyroid are dry skin, weight gain, constipation, and feeling cold.

11 **Create a "just say no" notebook.** Overextending yourself, especially to do tasks you don't really enjoy, stalls out your energy engines. If you don't want to bake for another bake sale or help that friend with a home improvement project, say so. Need an excuse? Keep some in a notebook. Include legitimate reasons—you're reserving time for your daily walks, for instance.

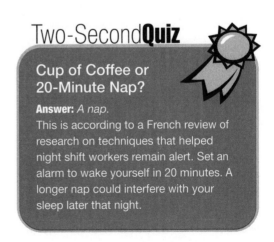

Two-Second**Quiz**

Cup of Coffee or 20-Minute Nap?

Answer: *A nap.*
This is according to a French review of research on techniques that helped night shift workers remain alert. Set an alarm to wake yourself in 20 minutes. A longer nap could interfere with your sleep later that night.

12 **List all the people you're angry with and write each a letter of forgiveness.** Stewing over past events only drains your energy. "Try to accept others for who they are and don't expend a lot of effort on changing them," says Dr. Wilson. Oh, and you don't have to send the letter. Simply writing it is enough.

13 **Soak up a little sun in winter.** Have all the energy of a hibernating bear in the winter? Make a point of getting outside for 30 minutes to an hour during the day. The natural light can improve your energy level and help fight seasonal affective disorder—also known as the winter blahs.

14 **In the hour before bedtime, turn off the TV, put away your work, and relax with a good book,** some needlepoint, or a crossword puzzle. Take a warm bath and listen to soothing music. This ritual will help you fall asleep more quickly and experience a more restful slumber, resulting in more energy the following day.

15 **Turn off CNN for one week.** Depressing television news of murders, fires, and terrorism can quickly drain your mental reserves. If you're a news junkie, try this experiment for one week: Stop reading your newspaper and watch only one television news program a day (or none if you can stand it). Notice how you feel at the end of the week. If you feel more energetic and peaceful, stick to your new habit.

16 **Create a mail-sorting center.** Clutter is not only distracting, it's frustrating and energy-wasting. (How many times have you scoured the house for lost keys or bills that were right in front of you?) To keep track of your bills and other mail, buy an open file box or hanging files from an office supply store. Place it in your kitchen and use it to sort your mail into categories such as "bills," "receipts," and "letters." "When you know where your bills are, you can pay them on time, thus reducing frustration and stress," says Audrey Thomas, an organizational consultant and author of *The Road Called Chaos.*

17 **Breathe in new energy.** Sit in a chair with a straight back. Place your hands over your stomach and breathe into your tummy so that your hands rise and fall with your breath. Imagine you are inhaling a white light that fills your body with vital energy. Do this for five full breaths. Then, as you inhale, tighten the muscles that connect your shoulders and neck, pulling your shoulders up toward your ears. "When you have inhaled all you can and your shoulders are snug around your ears, hold your breath for just a second," says Karl D. La Rowe, a licensed clinical social worker and mental health investigator in Oregon. "Then exhale as you release the tension and your breath in one big whoosh—as if you were releasing the weight of the world from your shoulders. Repeat until you feel clear, refreshed, and revitalized."

18 **Make a list of everything you're looking forward** to in the next month. Do this every month when you pay your rent or mortgage. Simply building more anticipation into your life helps stoke your energy.

19 **Get your energy vitamins.** Research at the University of California at Berkeley found that the amino acid L-carnitine and the antioxidant alpha-lipoic acid can boost both memory and energy, possibly by improving the way body cells produce energy. Bruce Ames, Ph.D., one of the study authors and a professor of biochemistry and molecular biology at Berkeley, says you can consume the right amount of both nutrients by taking a daily multivitamin and eating a well-balanced diet rich in colorful fruits and vegetables.

20 Eat something crunchy. Pretzels, carrots, and other crunchy foods make your jaw work hard, which can wake up your facial muscles, helping you feel more alert.

21 Chew a piece of peppermint or spearmint gum. You'll get a burst of energy from the invigorating flavor and scent, not to mention the physical act of chewing (it's hard to chew if you're asleep).

22 Eat every four hours. It's much better to continually refuel your body before it hits empty than to wait until you're in the danger zone and then overdo it. So every four hours (except, of course, when you're sleeping), have a mini-meal or snack. A mini-meal might be a handful of roasted peanuts, a hard-boiled egg or slice of lean luncheon meat, and a sliced apple. Nonfat yogurt sprinkled with flaxseeds makes a great snack.

23 Stay still. You wouldn't think stillness would lead to energy, but often, that's just what you need to create your second wind. Simply sit for 10 minutes in a comfortable chair and stare out the window. Let your mind drift wherever it wants to go. Some might call this meditation. We just call it "being," something we're often too frenzied to remember to do.

Two-SecondQuiz

Yoga or Aerobic Exercise?

Answer: *Either.*
In a study of patients with multiple sclerosis, yoga and stationary cycling improved energy levels to the same degree. Just pick one and do it!

24 Or stretch. Stand up, get on your toes, and lift your fingertips as close as you can to the ceiling. Keep the stretch expanding for several seconds, feeling it in your calves, your abdomen, your shoulders, your arms, your fingers. After a few seconds, relax, take a few deep breaths, and do it again. By doing this, you activate almost every muscle you have, sending oxygen-rich blood throughout your body.

25 Eat a bowl of all-bran cereal. It contains 792 milligrams of phosphorous, an important mineral that the body needs to metabolize carbohydrates, fat, and protein so they can be used as energy, Heck, it will do you a lot more good than those greasy chips from the vending machine!

26 Make a list of every relationship in your life and rank how those relationships make you feel, from 1 (terrible) to 5 (fabulous). Bad relationships are known energy sappers. Take note of the relationships that don't add any positive energy, and develop plans to adroitly remove yourself from them.

Monitor Your Health

16 WAYS TO DO IT WITHOUT A DOCTOR

We're all for getting regular checkups and blood tests. But that's not to say that in between visits you should close your eyes and cross your fingers that all's still well. The fact is that while your doctor may see you once or twice a year, you live in your body every single day, and that makes you the best judge of your own health—if you know what cues to look for. Here are 16 ways to play doctor detective.

1 **Every evening, think PERF.** Essentially, there are four things you should monitor every day to make sure you are living healthy: the amount of vegetables and fruits you ate that day (**P**roduce); whether you walked and were active (**E**xercise); whether you got at least 15 minutes of laughter and fun time for yourself (**R**elaxation); and whether you got enough beans, grains, and other high-fiber food in your diet (**F**iber). If you can say you did well on all four of these, you lived a very healthy day. If you can say you do well on these on most days, your life begins to look a lot longer and healthier.

2 **Monitor your sleepiness.** There are three good ways to tell if you are getting enough sleep. First, do you require an alarm clock to wake up most mornings? Second, do you become drowsy in the afternoon to the point that it affects what you are doing? Third, do you doze off shortly after eating dinner? If the answer to any of these is yes, you need

more sleep for good health. And if you *are* getting enough sleep and still have these troubles, you should talk with your doctor about your low energy. A healthy, well-rested person should wake up refreshed without the aid of an alarm clock each morning, not be overly drowsy during the day, and still have some energy left over for after-dinner activity.

3 **Check your hairbrush.** If your hair is falling out, ask your doctor to check your levels of blood ferritin, an indication of how much iron your body is storing. Some studies suggest that low levels may be related to unexplained hair loss. Thyroid disease is another fairly common cause.

4 **Keep a mental color chart of the color of your urine.** Sure, it sounds gross, but at least you don't have to pee into a cup to do it. Your urine should be a clear, straw color; if it's dark or has a strong smell, you may not be getting enough

226

fluids. If it continues dark colored even after you increase your liquid intake, follow up with your doctor. Bright yellow urine? Chalk it up to the B vitamins in your multivitamin.

5 **Check your heartbeat after you exercise.** A study published in the *Journal of the American Medical Association* found that women who had poor heart rate recovery, or HRR, after exercise had twice the 10-year risk of having a heart attack as those who had normal HRR. To test your HRR after regular strenuous activity, count your heartbeats for 15 seconds, then multiply by four to get your heart rate. Then sit down and wait two minutes before checking again. Subtract the second number from the first. If it's under 55, then your HRR is higher than normal and you should follow up with your doctor.

6 **Measure your height every year after you turn 50.** This is especially important for women as a way of assessing posture and skeletal health. A change in stature can be as informative as a change on a bone density test in terms of assessing your overall bone health. Don't skip the bone density test, though: It picks up bone loss before your height changes.

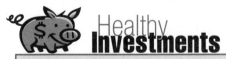

Healthy Investments

A Home Blood Pressure Monitoring Test

A study published in the *Journal of the American Medical Association* found that monitoring your blood pressure at home can save money and give your doctor valuable insight into your risk of hypertension.

7 **If you have diabetes, play footsies every day.** By yourself, that is. This form of footsies consists of examining your feet carefully for any blisters, fungus, peeling skin, cuts, or bruises. Because people with diabetes often have some nerve damage in extremities like the feet, these daily self-examinations are critical clues to how well you're monitoring your blood sugar and if you might have nerve damage.

8 **Guys only: check down below.** Believe it or not, it's even more important that men conduct a testicular self-examination than women conduct a breast self-exam. Catching testicular cancer early is the best way to beat it. The Testicular Cancer Resource Center recommends following these steps every month to become familiar with what's normal so you can recognize if anything feels wrong:

▸ Stand in front of a mirror. Check for any swelling on the scrotal skin.
▸ Examine each testicle with both hands. Place the index and middle fingers under the testicle with the thumbs placed on top. Roll the testicle gently between the thumbs and fingers—you shouldn't feel any pain when doing the exam. Don't be alarmed if one testicle seems *slightly* larger than the other.
▸ If you find a lump on your testicle, see a doctor, preferably a urologist, right away. The abnormality may only be an infection, but if it is testicular cancer, it will spread without treatment. Any free-floating lumps in the scrotum that aren't attached to a testicle are not testicular cancer. Still, it's smart to get checked.

9 **Take the fall test.** If you have osteoporosis, you are at great risk if you fall. So take this simple self-test developed

by Joseph Lane, M.D., and his colleagues at the Hospital for Special Surgery in New York City. Time yourself standing on one leg. Do it in shoes or barefoot, but don't hold on to anything. Try it on both legs (one at a time) three times. A normal 80-year-old should be able to stand without difficulty for at least 12 seconds, says Dr. Lane. If your best leg time is less than 12 seconds, or you wobble back and forth, you have poor balance and should talk to your doctor or physical therapist about exercises to improve it.

10 **Check your blood pressure every six months,** either at home with a home blood pressure cuff, at the drugstore, or at a health fair or screening. If the top number is over 120 and the bottom number is higher than 80, wait a day, then check it again. If it's still high, follow up with your doctor.

11 **Check your cholesterol once a year either with a home kit,** which is available at most drugstores, or at a health fair or screening. If your total cholesterol is over 150 mg/dl, follow up with your doctor.

12 **Check the pulse in your feet once every three to six months** to monitor the circulation in your legs. There are two pulses you should be able to find: one near the middle of the top of your foot (called the dorsalis pedis), and the other right behind the big bony lump on the inside of your ankle (called the posterior tibialis). Of the two, the posterior tibialis is more important because it's more consistently in the same place. If the pulses become weak or hard to find, follow up with your doctor, especially if you have any leg pain when walking.

13 **Get naked every two to three months.** Then, with a significant other (or *very* close friend) conduct a head-to-toe skin exam looking for any new moles, changed moles, suspicious spots, or rashes. Make sure to check your scalp, between your toes and fingers, and even on the underside of your arms. If you find anything worrisome, follow up with a dermatologist. Do the ABCD test when checking moles:

- **Asymmetry:** The two halves don't match
- **Border irregularity:** The edges are jagged
- **Color:** It's not uniform
- **Diameter:** It's more than one-quarter inch wide

14 **Go over your toenails once a month.** Look for early signs of fungal infection or in-grown toenails; both are best treated early.

15 **For women only: Conduct a breast self-exam every month just after your period, or, if you're post-menopausal, on the first of the month.** The American Cancer Society provides the following instructions:

- Lie down and place your right arm behind your head.
- Use the finger pads of your three middle fingers on your left hand to feel for lumps in the right breast. Use overlapping dime-size circular motions of the finger pads to feel the breast tissue.
- Use three different levels of pressure to feel all the breast tissue. Light pressure is needed to feel the tissue closest to the skin; medium pressure to feel a little deeper; and firm pressure to feel the tissue closest to the chest and ribs.

- Move around the breast in an up-and-down pattern starting at an imaginary line drawn straight down your side from the underarm and moving across the breast to the middle of the breastbone (sternum). Check the entire breast area going down until you feel only ribs and up to the neck or collarbone (clavicle).
- Repeat the exam on your left breast, using the finger pads of the right hand.
- While standing in front of a mirror with your hands pressing firmly down on your hips, look at your breasts for any changes of size, shape, contour, or dimpling. (Pressing down on the hips contracts the chest wall muscles and enhances any breast changes.)
- Examine each underarm while sitting up or standing and with your arm only slightly raised so you can easily feel in this area. Raising your arm straight up tightens the tissue in this area and makes it very difficult to examine.

If you find any changes, see your doctor right away.

16 **Know your body mass index, or BMI.** This measure has become particularly popular to gauge the health of your weight, because it relates weight to

Two-Second **Quiz**

Weight or Waist Size?

Answer: *Waist size.*
Turns out that the circumference of your waist is a better predictor of heart disease risk than your body mass index. The reason is that it is belly fat—not the fat on thighs or buttocks—that poses the most danger to your heart and arteries. Research shows that for women, health risk begins to rise with a waist circumference above 31 inches; over 35 inches is a serious threat. For men, risk rises above 37 inches; over 40 inches is a serious threat. When you measure, wrap a tape measure around your skin at mid-abdomen, at or near the belly button. Keep it snug, but not tight—and don't suck in your gut.

height. A normal BMI is 18.5 to 24.9. A BMI of 25 to 30 puts you in the overweight category, increasing your risk for numerous diseases and health conditions. A BMI above 30 means you are obese, a formal medical condition recognized by the federal government and most insurers. To figure your BMI, go to www.cdc.gov/nccdphp/dnpa/bmi/.

Preventing Colds and Flu

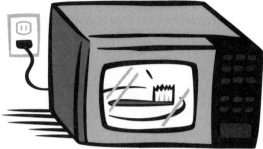

23 WAYS TO STAY HEALTHY YEAR-ROUND

Chances are, when you're burrowed under the covers with a box of tissues by your bedside, you turn even greener with envy thinking of those people who seem to never get sick. Want to be one of them? We can't promise you'll never get hit with another cold or suffer another bout of the flu, but you can increase your odds of staying well with these strategies. If you do get sick, we've also included some tips for getting better faster.

While colds won't kill you, they can weaken your immune system to the point that other, more serious, germs can take hold in your body. Just think how many times your cold turned into bronchitis or a sinus infection. And given that the average American adult suffers two to three colds a year, that's a lot of opportunities for serious illness—and just as many to prevent one! There's even more incentive to prevent the flu: Every year in the United States about 200,000 people are hospitalized and 36,000 die from the flu or its complications.

1 Wash your hands and wash them often. The Naval Health Research Center conducted a study of 40,000 recruits who were ordered to wash their hands five times a day. The recruits cut their incidence of respiratory illnesses by 45 percent.

2 Wash your hands twice every time you wash them. When Columbia University researchers looked for germs on volunteers' hands, they found one handwashing had little effect, even when using antibacterial soap. So wash twice if you're serious about fending off colds.

3 Use this hand-drying strategy in public restrooms. Studies find a shockingly large percentage of people fail to wash their hands after using a public restroom. And every single one of them touches the door handle on the way out. So after washing your hands, use a paper towel to turn off the faucet. Use another paper towel to dry your hands, then open the door with that paper towel as a barrier between you and the handle. It sounds nuts, but it's an actual recommendation from the Centers for Disease Control to protect you from infectious diseases like cold and flu.

4 Carry hand sanitizer with you. Colds are typically passed not from coughing or kissing (although those are two modes of transmission) but from hand-to-hand or hand-to-object contact, since most cold viruses can live for hours on objects. You then put your hand in or near your mouth or nose, and voilà! You're sick. Carry hand sanitizer gel or sanitizing towelettes with you and you can clean your hands anytime, even if the closest water supply is 100 miles away. It works. One study of absenteeism due to infection in elementary schools found schools using the gel sanitizer had absentee rates from infection nearly 20 percent lower than those using other hand-cleaning methods.

5 Use your knuckle to rub your eyes. It's less likely to be contaminated with viruses than your fingertip. This is particularly important given that the eye provides a perfect entry point for germs, and the average person rubs his eyes or nose or scratches his face 20-50 times a day, notes Jordan Rubin, Ph.D., author of the book *The Maker's Diet.*

6 Run your toothbrush through the microwave on high for 10 seconds to kill germs that can cause colds and other illnesses. You think it gets your teeth clean—and it does. But once you're done brushing, your toothbrush is a breeding ground for germs. Sterilize it in the microwave before you use it, or store it in

Two-Second Quiz

Hot Wash or Cold Wash?

Answer: *Hot.*
A government study found that using hot water for white laundry reduced infectious disease risk by about a third. That means setting your washing machine between 178°F and 194°F.

hydrogen peroxide (rinse well before using), or simply replace it every month when you change the page on your calendar and after you've had a cold.

7 Get a flu shot every fall. The Centers for Disease Control recommends flu shots for anyone 50 years old or older, residents of long-term care facilities, people of any age who have chronic medical problems (heart or lung disease, asthma, diabetes, etc.), pregnant women, and people whose immune systems have been weakened (by cancer, AIDS, or other causes). Also, people who work or live with a high-risk person should get a flu shot so they don't spread the flu. Of course, anyone who just wants to avoid the flu should also get one. Hate shots? Ask for the nasal spray vaccine.

8 Stop blaming yourself when things go wrong at work. Believe it or not, blaming yourself makes you more likely to catch a cold! At least, that's what researchers found when they studied more than 200 workers over three months. Even those who had control over their work were more likely to begin sneezing if they lacked confidence or tended to blame themselves when things went wrong. Researchers expect such attitudes

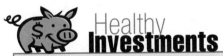

Healthy Investments

A Paper Cup Dispenser
Put one in the bathroom *and* kitchen to cut down on germ transfer during cold season.

make people more stressed on the job, and stress, as you know, can challenge your immune system.

9 Put a box of tissues wherever people sit. Come October, buy a 6- or 12-pack of tissue boxes and strategically place them around the house, your workplace, your car. Don't let aesthetics thwart you. You need tissues widely available so that anyone who has to cough or sneeze or blow his nose will do so in the way least likely to spread germs.

10 Leave the windows in your house open a crack in winter. Not all of them, but one or two in the rooms in which you spend the most time. This is particularly important if you live in a newer home, where fresh circulating air has been the victim of energy efficiency. A bit of fresh air will do wonders for chasing out germs.

11 Lower the heat in your house 5 degrees. The dry air of an overheated home provides the perfect environment for cold viruses to thrive. And when your mucous membranes (i.e., nose, mouth, and tonsils) dry out, they can't trap those germs very well. Lowering the temperature and using a room humidifier helps maintain a healthier level of humidity in the winter.

12 Speaking of which, buy a hygrometer. These little tools measure humidity. You want your home to measure around 50 percent. A consistent measure higher than 60 percent means mold and mildew may start to set in your walls, fabrics, and kitchen; lower than 40 percent and the dry air makes you more susceptible to germs.

13 Sit in a sauna once a week. Why? Because an Austrian study published in 1990 found that volunteers who frequently used a sauna had half the rate of colds during the six-month study period than those who didn't use a sauna at all. It's possible that the hot air you inhale kills cold viruses. Most gyms have saunas these days.

14 Inhale air from your blow-dryer. It sounds nuts, we know. But one study conducted at Harvard Hospital in England found that people who breathed heated air had half the cold symptoms of people who inhaled air at room temperature. Set the dryer on warm, not hot, and hold it at least 18 inches from your face. Breathe in the air through your nose for as long as you can—20 minutes is best.

15 Take a garlic supplement every day. When 146 volunteers received either one garlic supplement a day or a placebo for 12 weeks between November and February, those taking the garlic were not only less likely to get a cold, but if they did catch one, their symptoms were less intense and they recovered faster.

16 Eat a container of yogurt every day. A study from the University of California-Davis found that people who ate one cup of yogurt—whether live culture or pasteurized—had 25 percent fewer colds

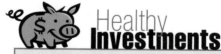

Healthy Investments

A T-Fal Electric Kettle

This kettle boils a teapot of water in under a minute. Great for immune-bolstering teas, to make a quick cup of soup when you're sniffling, or even to heat a pot of water and use as a steamer to open clogged sinuses.

than non-yogurt eaters. Start your yogurt eating in the summer to build up your immunity before cold and flu season starts.

17 Once a day, sit in a quiet, dim room, close your eyes, and focus on one word. You're meditating, a proven way to reduce stress. And stress, studies find, increases your susceptibility to colds. In fact, stressed people have up to twice the number of colds as non-stressed people.

18 Scrub under your fingernails every night. They're a great hiding place for germs.

19 Change or wash your hand towels every three or four days during cold and flu season. When you wash them, use hot water in order to kill the germs.

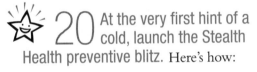 **20** At the very first hint of a cold, launch the Stealth Health preventive blitz. Here's how:

▶ Suck on a zinc lozenge until it melts away. Then suck another every two waking hours. Or use a zinc-based nasal spray such as Zicam.
▶ Take one 250-milligram capsule of the herb astragalus twice a day until you are better.
▶ Cook up a pot of chicken soup.
▶ Roast garlic in the oven (drizzle whole clove with olive oil, wrap in tinfoil, roast for an hour at 400°F), then spread the soft garlic on toast and eat.

Studies find that all either reduce the length of time you suffer with a cold or help prevent a full-blown cold from occurring.

21 Wipe your nose—don't blow. Your cold won't hang around as long, according to a University of Virginia study. Turns out that the force of blowing

not only sends the gunk out of your nose into a tissue, but propels some *back* into your sinuses. And, in case you're curious, they discovered this using dye and X rays. If you need to blow, blow gently, and blow one nostril at a time.

22 Sneeze and cough into your arm or a tissue. Whoever taught us to cover our mouths when we cough or sneeze got it wrong. That just puts the germs right on our hands, where you can spread them to objects—and other people. Instead, hold the crook of your elbow over your mouth and nose when you sneeze or cough if a tissue isn't handy. It's pretty rare that you shake someone's elbow or scratch your eye with an elbow, after all.

23 Don't pressure your doctor for antibiotics. Colds and flu (along with most common infections) are caused by viruses, so antibiotics—designed to kill bacteria—won't do a thing. They can hurt, however, by killing off the friendly bacteria that are part of our immune defenses. If you've used antibiotics a lot lately, consider a course of probiotics—replacement troops for friendly bacteria.

Reduce Your Risk of Heart Disease and Stroke

30 SIMPLE SOLUTIONS

Between 1950 and 2000, the death rate from heart disease in the United States plummeted nearly 70 percent, and the death rate from stroke nearly 80 percent. Seems like pretty good news! But this silver lining has a bit of cloud stuffed inside it.

True, we're dying of heart attack and stroke less often, but we're still getting cardiovascular disease just as often. In fact, some factors that put us at risk, such as obesity and diabetes, have become *more* common.

We're dying less often because of the technological and pharmacological advances of modern medicine. But is your idea of a healthy future being pulled back from the brink by bypass surgery? Needing a personal secretary to keep track of your medications? Better living through angioplasty?

We thought not. Far preferable is avoiding cardiovascular disease altogether. It can take some work to convert a high risk for heart disease into a low risk. But we're here to tell you that it *can* be done! You know the mission we're on: putting the power of stealth at the service of your health. Add up these small changes to your daily routine, and you've got a powerful dose of heart disease prevention—no coronary care units or intra-aortic balloon pumps required!

1 **Ride your bike 20 minutes a day.** You can handle that, can't you? When German researchers had 100 men with mild chest pain, or angina, either exercise 20 minutes a day on a stationary bike or undergo an artery-clearing procedure called angioplasty, they found that a year after the angioplasty, 21 men suffered a heart attack, stroke, or other problem compared to only 6 of the bikers. Just remember that if you already have angina, you should only begin an exercise program under medical supervision.

2 **Eat a piece of dark chocolate several times a week.** Believe it or not, several small studies suggest dark chocolate could be good for your heart! The beneficial effects are likely due to chemicals in chocolate called flavonoids, which help arteries stay flexible. Other properties of the sweet stuff seem to make arteries less likely to clot and prevent the "bad" cholesterol, LDL, from oxidizing, making it less likely to form plaque. Dark chocolate is also rich in magnesium and fiber. But steer clear of milk chocolate,

which is high in butterfat and thus tends to raise cholesterol.

3 **Have a beer once a day.** A study published in the *Journal of Agricultural and Food Chemistry* found that men who drank one beer a day for one month lowered their cholesterol levels, increased their blood levels of heart-healthy antioxidants, and reduced their levels of fibrinogen, a protein that contributes to blood clots. Of course, red wine might be even better (see Tip 3 on page 241). Choose either beer or wine—not both.

4 **Take a B vitamin complex every morning.** When Swiss researchers asked more than 200 men and women to take either a combination of three B vitamins (folic acid, vitamin B_6, and vitamin B_{12}) or a placebo after they had surgery to open their arteries, they found that levels of homocysteine, a substance linked to an increased risk of heart disease, were 40 percent lower in those who took the vitamins. The placebo group had no change. Plus, the vitamin group had wider-open blood vessels than those taking the sugar pill.

5 **Tape-record yourself at night.** If you hear yourself snoring (or if your sleeping partner has been kicking you a lot), make an appointment with your doctor. You may have sleep apnea, a condition in which your breathing stops hundreds of times throughout the night. It can lead to high blood pressure and other medical problems, and even increase your risk for heart attack and stroke.

6 **Go to bed an hour earlier tonight.** A Harvard study of 70,000 women found that those who got less than seven hours of sleep had a slightly higher risk of

Two-Second**Quiz**

Egg McMuffin or Cantaloupe With Yogurt?

Answer: *Fruit and yogurt.*
That's an easy one. A study from the State University of New York found that within an hour of eating a large, high-fat, high-carb breakfast, your body starts making inflammatory chemicals associated with heart disease.

heart disease. Researchers suspect lack of sleep increases stress hormones, raises blood pressure, and affects blood sugar levels. Keep your overall sleeping time to no more than nine hours, however. The same study found women sleeping nine or more hours had a slightly *increased* risk of heart disease.

7 **Eat fish at least once a week.** Have it grilled, sautéed, baked, or roasted—just have it. A study published in the *Journal of the American Medical Association* in April 2002 found that women who ate fish at least once a week were one-third less likely to have a heart attack or die of heart disease than those who ate fish only once a month. Other studies show similar benefits for men. Another major study found regular fish consumption reduced the risk of atrial fibrillation—rapid, irregular heartbeat—a major cause of sudden death.

8 **Eat a high-fiber breakfast cereal at least four times a week.** In a study published in the *American Journal of Clinical Nutrition* in September 1999, Harvard University scientists found that women who ate 23 grams of fiber a day—mostly from cereal—were 23 percent less

likely to have heart attacks than those who consumed only 11 grams of fiber. In men, a high-fiber diet slashed the chances of a heart attack by 36 percent.

9 Sprinkle one ounce of ground flaxseed on your cereal or yogurt every day. This way you'll be getting about 2 grams of omega-3 fatty acids, healthy fats that numerous studies find help prevent heart disease and reduce your risk of dying suddenly from heart rhythm abnormalities.

10 Make fresh salad dressing with one tablespoon of flaxseed oil. It packs a whopping 7 grams of omega-3 fatty acids, which, as we've just mentioned, are a great way to improve your overall heart health.

11 Drink at least two cups of tea a day. Black or green, it doesn't seem to matter. At least, that's the result of a Dutch study that found only 2.4 percent of 5,000 healthy Rotterdam residents who drank two or more cups of tea a day had a heart attack within six years, compared with 4.1 percent of those who never drank tea. Another major analysis of 17 studies on tea drinkers found three cups a day could slash the risk of a heart attack by 11 percent.

12 Stir a handful of hazelnuts into a vegetable-and-chicken stir-fry. Just 1.5 ounces of these healthy nuts a day can reduce your risk of cardiovascular disease. Another hazelnut idea: Crush them and use to coat fish or chicken, then bake.

A Strong Case for Fish Oil

Consider, for a moment, the Eskimos of Alaska and their indigenous cousins in Canada and Russia. These hardy souls survive on diets of nearly pure fat, and yet they tend to be completely free of heart disease. How in the world is this possible? The answer is fish oil.

Every medical journal on heart health brings, it seems, another study demonstrating the cardiovascular benefits of the oil—specifically, its omega-3 fatty acids, a type of polyunsaturated fat found in few foods other than fish and flaxseed. A primary reason it's so healthy: omega-3s are a natural anti-inflammatory. In recent years, scientists have discovered that inflammation within our arteries—triggered in response to damage done by plaque, high blood pressure, and free radicals—is a major cause of heart disease. While inflammation is a healing response, in your blood vessels it only causes further damage, leaving them stiffer and working at far less then optimal capacity. Omega-3s cause this type of inflammation to recede.

There's more. Omega-3 fatty acids also seem to make blood less sticky so it's less likely to form clots that can block blood flow and trigger a heart attack. They also seem to affect heart rhythm, keeping it more regular and reducing your risk of sudden death caused by arrhythmia, or erratic heartbeat, a major cause of death from coronary artery disease. And they lower levels of triglycerides, blood fats linked with heart disease.

Bottom line: Get more omega-3 fatty acids into your body, either through foods or supplements. Ideas for doing this are throughout this book. Plus, here are the fish with the largest amounts of this crucial nutrient (amounts are per 3.5 ounces of fish):

- Mackerel: 2.6 grams
- Atlantic herring: 1.7 grams
- Chinook salmon: 1.5 grams
- Fresh albacore tuna: 1.5 grams
- Anchovies: 1.4 grams

13 Include beans or peas in four of your dishes every week. Researchers at Tulane University found that people who followed this advice slashed their risk of heart disease by 22 percent compared to those who ate fewer legumes.

14 Have sex tonight. It counts as physical activity, which, of course, is good for your heart. And that may be why University of Bristol researchers found that men who have sex at least twice a week are less likely to have a stroke or other cardiovascular problems than men who have it less often. As the researchers put it: "Middle-aged men should be heartened to know that frequent sexual intercourse is not likely to result in a substantial increase in risk of strokes, and that some protection from fatal coronary events may be an added bonus." Women probably stand to benefit too. Yeah, baby!

15 Take a baby aspirin every day. University of North Carolina researchers found that the tiny tablet slashes the risk of heart disease by nearly a third in people who have never had a heart attack or stroke but who were at increased risk (because they smoked, were overweight, had high blood pressure, or had some other risk factor). Just double-check with your doctor that there's no reason for you *not* to take aspirin daily.

16 Eat 15 cherries a day. Studies find the anthocyanins (plant chemicals) that give cherries their scarlet color also work to lower levels of uric acid in blood, a marker for heart attacks and stroke. Cherries out of season? Try sprinkling dried cherries on your salad or substituting a cup of cherry juice for orange juice in the morning.

17 Eat one cup of beans per day. Do that and you'll be getting at least 300 micrograms of folate. A study from Tulane in New Orleans found people who consumed at least that much folate slashed their risk of stroke 20 percent and their risk of heart disease 13 percent more than those who got less than 136 mcg per day of the B vitamin. Not into beans? Try an orange (55 mcg), spinach (58 mcg in 1 cup raw spinach) romaine lettuce (62 mcg in 1 cup), or tomatoes (27 mcg in 1 cup). Since January 1998, wheat flour has been fortified with folic acid, the synthetic form of folate, adding an estimated 100 mcg per day to the average diet.

18 Eat an orange every day. Or drink a glass of orange juice. Oranges, as you know, are a great source of vitamin C. Studies suggest diets high in this vitamin may reduce your risk of stroke, especially if you smoke. Tired of oranges? Substitute a bowlful of strawberries, a serving of brussels sprouts or broccoli, or a chopped red bell pepper, all excellent sources of vitamin C.

19 Skip the soda and have orange juice instead. The reason has to do with inflammation, the body's response to damage or injury. Chronic inflammation, linked to heart disease, is significantly affected by what you eat. For instance, researchers at the State University of New York found that drinking glucose-sweetened water triggered an inflammatory response in volunteers, but drinking the same calories in a glass of orange juice didn't. They theorize that the anti-inflammatory effects of vitamin C and various flavonoids in juice may provide some protection. Choose 100 percent juice instead of drinks that are mostly sweetened, flavored water. Other studies on orange juice find it can increase blood levels of heart-protective folate almost 45 percent and reduce levels of heart-damaging homocysteine by 11 percent.

20 Drink an 8-ounce glass of water every two hours. A study from Loma Linda University in California found that women who drank more than five glasses of water a day were half as likely to die from a heart attack as those who drank less than two. This is likely due to the fact that maintaining good hydration keeps blood flowing well; dehydration can cause sluggish blood flow and increase the risk of clots forming. Water works best when it comes to improving blood flow; soda is worthless.

21 Cook with ginger or turmeric twice a week. They have anti-inflammatory benefits, and inflammation is a major contributor to heart disease.

22 Go to the loo whenever you feel the urge. Research at Taiwan University found that a full bladder causes your heart to beat faster and puts added stress on coronary arteries, triggering them to contract, which could lead to a heart attack in people who are vulnerable.

23 Ask for next Monday and Friday off. Researchers at the University of Pittsburgh analyzed data on more than 12,000 middle-aged men from the Fram-

---

Just for Women

Tell a woman that she's more likely to die of a heart attack or stroke than of breast cancer and she might not believe you. A 2003 survey of 204 women with heart disease found that many considered their condition "a man's disease." Not so. Cardiovascular disease, which causes heart attacks, stroke, and heart failure, is actually the leading cause of death in women. One in 10 women ages 45-64 and one in five women ages 65 or older has some form of heart disease. So follow these Stealth Healthy gender-based tips:

● **Remember who comes first: you.** A New York Presbyterian Hospital study found that women rate poor self-esteem as the primary reason for not making changes to improve their cardiovascular health.

Remember: If you're not around, it won't matter what you *used* to do for others!

● **Meditate or simply go into a dark, quiet room for 20 minutes when you get home from work.** Stress harms the heart directly and also indirectly— by preventing you from making lifestyle changes that could help your heart. And in a woman's life, the stress of work is simply compounded by the stress of home. Give yourself a time-out period between your two worlds—it will do you a whole heart-healthy heaping bit of good.

● **Ask your doctor to give you a treadmill exercise test—*not* an electrocardiogram.** A study of nearly 3,000 women found treadmill exercise tests clearly identified women at risk for death from heart disease. The study also found a measure

of decreased blood flow on electrocardiogram readings called ST-segment depression, used to diagnose hidden heart disease in men, didn't accurately identify women with hidden heart disease.

● **Listen to your body.** Don't assume that if you're not having crushing chest pain you're not having a heart attack. Symptoms of a heart attack in women can include extreme weakness or a feeling similar to indigestion. So pay attention to your body. Surveys of women who have had heart attacks find they may exhibit some unique symptoms in the month before the attack, such as feeling unusually fatigued, having problems sleeping, having indigestion, and weakness in their arms.

ingham Heart Study and found that those who took regular vacations sliced their risk of death from heart disease by a third. And no, taking along the cell phone, laptop, and a briefcase full of papers will not help you achieve the stress-reducing effects of a vacation that, in turn, reduces your risk of heart disease.

24 Drive with the windows closed and the air conditioning on.

This reduces your exposure to airborne pollutants, which a Harvard study found reduces something called "heart rate variability," or the ability of your heart to respond to various activities and stresses. Reduced heart rate variability, also called HRV, has been associated with increased deaths among heart attack survivors as well as the general population.

25 Keep a bottle of multivitamins on your kitchen counter and

make the pills a regular addition to breakfast. After six months of taking daily multivitamins, participants in one study had significantly lower levels of a protein connected with inflammation than those who didn't take a vitamin.

26 Call a friend and arrange dinner.

A study published in the journal *Heart* in April 2004 found that having a very close relationship with another person, whether it's with a friend, lover, or relative, can halve the risk of a heart attack in someone who has already had a heart attack.

27 Pay attention to the basics.

Two major studies published in the summer of 2003 found that nearly everyone who dies of heart disease, including heart attacks, had at least one or more of the con-

ventional risk factors, such as smoking, diabetes, high blood pressure, or high cholesterol levels. You can find dozens of tips on lowering your blood pressure, reducing your cholesterol, stabilizing your blood sugar, and quitting smoking throughout *Stealth Health*.

28 Along with exercising every day, take a supplement

containing the amino-acid L-arginine and the antioxidant vitamins C and E. A study published in the *Proceedings of the National Academy of Sciences* found that while moderate exercise alone reduced the development of atherosclerosis, or hardening of the arteries, adding L-arginine and the vitamins to the mix boosted the effects astronomically. The two—exercise and the supplements—have a synergistic effect in enhancing production of nitric oxide, which protects against a variety of heart-related problems.

29 If you find you're having trouble getting out of bed in the

morning, have lost interest in your normal activities, or just feel really blah, call your doctor. You may be depressed, and untreated depression significantly increases your risk for a heart attack.

30 Go to the pound this weekend and adopt a dog.

Okay, so there's nothing very stealthy about a bounding, barking canine. But the power of furry friends to improve heart health is proven. Not only will a dog force you to be more active (think about all the extra walking you'll be doing), but the companionship and unconditional affection a pooch provides has been shown to reduce the risk of heart attack and other cardiovascular problems.

Lower Your Cholesterol

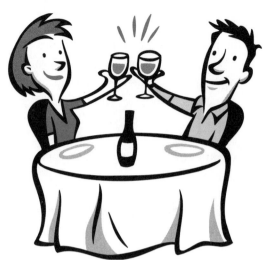

18 WAYS TO GET THE NUMBERS DOWN

No doubt you've heard it a thousand times by now: Heart disease is the number one killer among both men and women. And about half of all adults in American have cholesterol levels that are too high—which means there's a good chance yours are. If you haven't had them checked lately, don't ignore it any longer.

Cholesterol, the naturally occurring waxy substance produced by your body, isn't a bad thing—unless you have too much of the bad kind. Then it contributes to the formation of artery-clogging plaque, increasing your risk of heart disease and stroke.

Bad kind? That's right. You have two main types of cholesterol: Low-density lipoprotein, or LDL (the "bad" cholesterol), and high-density lipoprotein, or HDL (the "good" cholesterol). LDL carries cholesterol into your arteries, and HDL carries it away to your liver. Needless to say, the less LDL and the more HDL you have the better. Beyond that basic fact, other details matter too, like the size of your LDL particles. Smaller, denser LDL particles are more dangerous because it's easier for them to burrow into artery walls.

If you have high cholesterol, your doctor may put you on cholesterol-lowering medication. But even if he does, pay special attention to the tips in this chapter. Because research suggests that by eating the right foods, getting enough exercise, and generally taking good care of yourself, you could slash your risk of dying from heart disease by an incredible 80 percent.

1 **Drink two glasses of orange juice every morning.** But make it Minute Maid's Heart Wise or another brand spiked with the same kind of cholesterol-lowering plant sterols found in margarine spreads like Benecol. When researchers at the University of California-Davis asked 72 men and women with mildly high cholesterol to drink either Heart Wise or regular OJ, those drinking the sterol-fortified juice found their total cholesterol levels dropped 7 percent (an average of 13 points) and levels of "bad" LDL cholesterol dropped 13 percent (an average of 8 points). Those who drank regular juice had no changes. But maybe they weren't drinking enough: Another study, this one from the University of Western Ontario, found that three glasses a day of orange juice—any orange juice—for four weeks raised HDL levels 21 percent and improved the ratio of good to bad cholesterol by 16 percent.

2 Eat six or more small meals a day. A large study of British adults found that people who ate six or more times a day had significantly lower cholesterol than those who ate twice a day, even though the "grazers" got more calories and fat! In fact, the differences in cholesterol between the two groups were large enough to reduce the grazers' risk of coronary heart disease 10-20 percent. Just make sure those six meals are truly small.

3 Quaff a glass of wine every evening with dinner. Studies find a daily glass of wine or beer a day can boost levels of HDL cholesterol. Make the wine a red one—red wines are 3-10 times higher in plant compounds called saponins believed to be responsible for much of wine's beneficial effects on cholesterol.

4 Fix all your sandwiches on whole grain bread. Simply cutting back on simple carbs like white bread and eating more complex carbs, like whole grain bread and brown rice, can increase HDL levels slightly and significantly lower triglycerides, another type of blood fat that contributes to heart disease.

5 Use paper filters when brewing your coffee and skip the espresso. Two substances found in brewed coffee, kahweol and cafestol, increase cholesterol levels. But paper filters trap these compounds, so they're only a problem if you drink espresso or use coffeemakers without filters.

6 Use olive oil in your homemade salad dressing tonight. A Baylor College of Medicine study found that diets rich in the kind of monounsaturated fat found in olive oil reduced LDL cholesterol

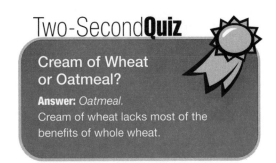

Two-Second Quiz

Cream of Wheat or Oatmeal?

Answer: *Oatmeal.* Cream of wheat lacks most of the benefits of whole wheat.

in people with diabetes or metabolic syndrome—a cluster of risk factors including low HDL, high insulin levels, and overweight—just as well as following a low-fat diet.

7 Sip a cup of black tea every four hours. Government scientists found that three weeks of drinking five cups a day of black tea reduced cholesterol levels in people with mildly high levels.

8 Add half a tablespoon of cinnamon to your coffee beans (ground or whole) before starting the pot. A Pakistani study found that 6 grams cinnamon a day (about ½ tablespoon) reduced LDL cholesterol in people with type 2 diabetes nearly 30 percent and cut total cholesterol 26 percent.

Get Tested in the Fall

Belonging in the "believe it or not" category, researchers from the University of Massachusetts Medical School in Worcester found that cholesterol levels in healthy adults were higher in the fall and winter than in the spring and summer— as much as 18 points higher. Why? We tend to have greater blood volume in the spring and summer, which will reduce cholesterol levels. So if you got tested in July and had a normal test, check again at Thanksgiving.

9 **Have oatmeal for breakfast every morning.** There's a reason oat manufacturers are allowed to boast about the grain's cholesterol-lowering benefits: Plenty of research has proved them. Rich in a soluble fiber called beta glucan, oatmeal can drop your LDL 12-24 percent if you eat 1½ cups regularly. Choose quick-cooking or old-fashioned oats over instant.

10 **This week, have a few glasses of cranberry juice every day** (cut it with seltzer or water so you get less sugar). Cranberries are rich sources of anthocyanins, flavonols, and proanthocyanidins, plant chemicals that prevent LDL cholesterol from oxidizing, a process that makes it more likely to stick to artery walls. These chemicals also keep red blood cells from getting too sticky. An added bonus: They initiate a complex chemical reaction that helps blood vessels relax. Plus (the part you were waiting for) they decrease LDL cholesterol levels. Not only that, but University of Scranton researchers reported that three glasses of cranberry juice a day can raise HDL levels up to 10 percent.

11 **Eat a grapefruit every other day.** Grapefruits are particularly high in pectin, a soluble fiber that can help reduce

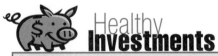

Healthy Investments

A Crockpot

Terrific for easy cooking of bean-based soups and stews high in cholesterol-lowering soluble fiber. Slow cookers are also perfect for preparing lean cuts of meat, which are healthier due to their low fat content, but also tougher for the same reason.

cholesterol levels. Grapefruits interfere with the absorption of several medications, however, so check with your doctor first. Other good sources of pectin include apples and berries.

12 **Use honey in your tea instead of sugar, and honey instead of jam on PB&J sandwiches.** A study from Dubai in the United Arab Emirates found total and LDL cholesterol levels dropped in healthy people after they drank a solution containing honey, but not after they drank solutions containing glucose or artificial honey. After 15 days of the honey drink, participants' HDL levels rose and homocysteine levels dropped. Homocysteine is an amino acid linked to an increased risk of heart disease, stroke and peripheral vascular disease (reduced blood flow to the hands and feet).

13 **Pop edamame as a snack.** Just half a cup contains nearly 4 grams fiber, not to mention the soy isoflavones in these soybeans. Consumption of both has been linked to lower cholesterol. Edamame are now available in the frozen food section of the supermarket.

14 Pour soy milk over your morning cereal. A Spanish study of 40 men and women found that those who drank about two cups of soy milk a day for three months reduced their LDL cholesterol levels an average of eight points and increased their HDL levels an average of four points. Just make sure you buy soy milk fortified with calcium.

15 Whip up a batch of guacamole this evening. Several studies find that eating one avocado a day as part of a healthy diet can lower your LDL as much as 17 percent while raising your HDL.

16 Spend 10 minutes a day doing strength-training exercises. You don't have to do these at a gym—push-ups, squats, leg lifts, hip extensions—they all count. And they count when it comes time to count your cholesterol levels: A study in the *British Journal of Sports Medicine* found that strength training lowered total cholesterol 10 percent and LDL cholesterol 14 percent among women who worked out for 45–50 minutes three times a week. If you can't manage that amount, start with 10 minutes a day, six days a week, and gradually work up.

17 Have a glass of purple grape juice every day. Rich in cholesterol-lowering flavonoids, grape juice is the perfect drink, particularly if you don't like red wine.

18 Spread your bagel with Benecol, not butter. This cholesterol-lowering spread contains sterols, natural plant compounds that block your body's absorption of the cholesterol in the foods you eat.

Cholesterol by the Numbers

Don't let your doctor get away with just telling you your cholesterol is high. Ask for details and a breakdown of HDL and LDL, as well as the ratio between the two. Here's what the numbers mean:

Total cholesterol	Category
Less than 200	Desirable
200-239	Borderline high
240 and above	High

LDL level	Category
Less than 100 mg/dl	Optimal
100-129 mg/dl	Near optimal
130-159 mg/dl	Borderline high
160-189 mg/dl	High
190 mg/dl and above	Very high (risky)

HDL level	Category
Less than 40 mg/dl	Low (risky)
40-50 mg/dl	Average (neutral)
60 mg/dl and above	High (protective)

Ratio of total cholesterol to HDL	Category
4.5:1	Good for men
4:1	Good for premenopausal women
3.5:1	Ideal for all

Lowering Blood Pressure

20 WAYS TO GO BEYOND LOW-SODIUM

You can't see it, you can't feel it, and unless you get checked, you won't even know you have it. That makes high blood pressure, or hypertension, a quiet killer, one that slowly damages your blood vessels, heart, and eyes while simultaneously increasing your risk of heart disease, stroke, dementia, and kidney disease. High blood pressure results in stiff, inflexible arteries that are virtual magnets for cholesterol and other blood components that form the gunk known as plaque. If you already have this gunk, blood rushing past at high force is just what it takes to nick the "cap" off mounds of plaque, setting the dominoes in motion for a heart attack.

One in five Americans have high blood pressure, and nearly a third don't know they have it. Many of the rest of us are at risk, as blood pressure slowly creeps up with age. Regardless of where your blood pressure lies along the spectrum, the following tips will help lower it if it's high, and keep it from rising if it's where it should be—guaranteed. In addition, see "Cutting Back on Salt," page 121, for 24 more Stealth Healthy ways to lower blood pressure through reduced sodium intake.

1 **Every morning, take a brisk 15-minute walk.** Amazingly, you don't need a lot of exercise to make a difference in your blood pressure. When Japanese researchers asked 168 inactive volunteers with high blood pressure to exercise at a health club for different amounts of time each week for eight weeks, blood pressure dropped almost as much in those who exercised 30-90 minutes a week as in those who exercised more than 90 minutes a week.

2 **Write "take medication" on your calendar every day.** Twenty-five percent of the time, when your blood pressure hasn't dropped after you've started medication, the reason is that you forgot to take your pills.

3 **Buy a home blood pressure kit.** A study in the *Journal of the American Medical Association* found that home blood pressure testing provides a better overall picture of blood pressure than measurement in a doctor's office. In the study, office measurement failed to identify 13 percent of patients who had high blood pressure only in the office but not at home (called "white-coat hypertension"). It also failed to identify 9 percent of people who had high blood pressure at home but not in the doctor's office. Another study, this one

presented at the 2004 European Society of Hypertension meeting, found that people who monitored their blood pressure at home had lower overall blood pressure than those who only had their pressure taken at the doctor's office. A good home blood pressure kit costs under $100, a small price to pay for peace of mind.

4 Sprinkle 2 tablespoons flaxseed over your yogurt in the morning and mix 2 tablespoons into your ice cream, spaghetti sauce, or other food later in the day. One small study found that adding 4 tablespoons of the crunchy stuff significantly lowered systolic blood pressure (a strong predictor of heart disease) in postmenopausal women with a history of heart disease. Flaxseed is rich in many nutrients and in fiber. Its effects on blood pressure are likely due to its high content of omega-3 fatty acids.

5 Substitute tea for your morning (and afternoon and evening) coffee. An Australian study found that every one-cup increase in daily tea consumption decreased systolic blood pressure (the top number) two points and diastolic pressure one point. The benefits ended after four cups, however.

6 Dip your chips into guacamole. Why? Avocados have more blood-pressure-lowering potassium than any other fruit or vegetable, including bananas. We should get about 4.7 grams a day of potassium, but most Americans get just half this amount.

7 Turn to dark chocolate when your sweet tooth asserts itself. Unlike milk chocolate, dark chocolate is rich in flavonoids that keep your arteries flexible,

preventing the increases in pressure that come with stiffer blood vessels. That's thought to be one reason for the normal blood pressure of a tribe of Panamanian Indians who eat a high-salt diet but also consume massive amounts of cocoa. In addition, a study published in the *Journal of the American Medical Association* found that three ounces of dark chocolate a day helped to lower blood pressure in older people with isolated systolic hypertension (a type of high blood pressure in which only the upper number of a pressure reading is high). Other good sources of flavonoids include tea and wine, as well as many fruits and vegetables.

Choosing a Home Blood Pressure Kit

The number of kits available has jumped, so how do you know which is the best? Here's a key test finding: Finger or wrist devices are extremely sensitive to position and body temperature and do not measure blood pressure very accurately, reports the American Academy of Family Physicians (AAFP). They are also more expensive (upward of $100) than other monitors. The AAFP has this advice about features to look for in a home blood pressure monitor:

- Get the right-size cuff. Ask your doctor, nurse, or pharmacist to tell you the cuff size you need for your arm. Blood pressure readings will be wrong if your cuff is the wrong size.

- Make sure you can read the numbers on the monitor.

- If you are using a stethoscope, you must be able to hear heart sounds through it.

- At least once, bring the cuff to your doctor's office and compare the readings on your cuff and the professional model. If they agree, you know you can trust yours.

8 Snack on roasted soybeans. These make a crunchy, nutrient-packed munch that's as yummy as any bag of chips. Studies show that people with high blood pressure can lower their systolic readings by an average of 10 points by eating one ounce of roasted soybeans (also called soy nuts) a day for two weeks. The beans are available at some supermarkets, as well as specialty and health food stores. Just look for unsalted beans.

9 Flavor your food with lots of ground pepper. Why? Pepper is a strong, dominant flavor that can help you reduce your interest in salt. In fact, your tongue is easily trained away from its salt addiction. When you switch to low-salt foods, your meals may taste bland for a couple of days. Bring in the pepper. And if that doesn't appeal to you, try garlic, lemon, ginger, basil, or other big-punch flavors you like. After a week, your old favorite foods will taste dreadfully oversalted and your blood pressure will be singing your praises.

10 Eat a banana or a quarter of a cantaloupe at each breakfast. That's because both are rich in potassium. Potassium is sometimes called the "un-salt" because if you don't get enough of it, your blood pressure is likely

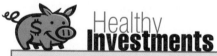

Healthy Investments

A Yoga Video

The stress-reducing and blood-pressure-lowering benefits of practicing yoga are well documented. A video is a great way to introduce yourself to this ancient practice in the privacy of your own home, with just a minimal investment.

to rise. It's easy to slide potassium into your diet. Other high-potassium foods include spinach, lima beans, sweet potatoes, and the aforementioned avocados.

11 Eat a handful of dried apricots every afternoon. Like bananas, apricots are a particularly good source of potassium. Plus they have lots of fiber, loads of iron, and oodles of beta-carotene. The drying process actually increases the concentration of these nutrients, all of which are good for your circulatory system. And as a snack, dried apricots are low in calories: roughly eight total just 100 calories. Look for an unsulfured brand.

12 Park in the Outer Mongolia of the parking lot. All you need is an extra 4,000 to 5,000 steps a day and you could lower your blood pressure 11 points! At least, that's what researchers from the University of Tennessee found when they tracked postmenopausal women.

13 Hold hands with your partner for 10 minutes. That's all it took in a University of North Carolina study to keep blood pressure steady during a stressful incident. Oh, and a brief hug afterward. You can handle that, can't you?

14 **Sleep with earplugs tonight.** Studies suggest that being exposed to noise while you're sleeping may increase your blood pressure as well as your heart rate, so block out the noise.

15 **Drink a glass of OJ every morning and another at night.** That's all it took in a Cleveland Clinic study to lower systolic blood pressure an average of 7 percent and diastolic blood pressure an average of 4.6 percent. Praise the high levels of potassium in orange juice.

16 **Go to the pound and adopt a pet.** One study found that a pet helped control blood pressure changes in people with hypertension as much as the hypertension drug Zestril.

17 **Think about how you've been sleeping lately.** Waking up tired? Partner complaining you snore a lot? Talk to your doctor. You may have a condition called sleep apnea. Studies find that half of the people who have the condition, in which you stop breathing dozens or even hundreds of times during the night, also have hypertension.

18 **Find (and eliminate) at least one hidden source of salt a day.** For instance, did you know that many breakfast cereals contain sodium? Who needs salt in their cereal? Find a brand that's sodium-free.

19 **Spend five minutes a day sitting in a quiet room repeating this mantra: "One day at a time."** Meditation is a known stress-relieving technique, with numerous studies attesting to its ability to lower blood pressure. Other good mantras include: "I'm doing the right thing," "This, too, shall pass," "Breathe," and "Calm, calm, calm."

20 **Stock your medicine chest with these supplements** and take them daily: Garlic, fish oil, calcium, CoQ_{10}. All have blood-pressure-lowering properties. Just check with your doctor first.

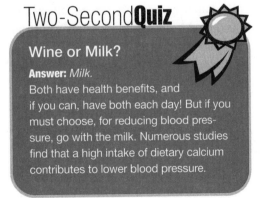

Two-SecondQuiz

Wine or Milk?

Answer: *Milk.*
Both have health benefits, and if you can, have both each day! But if you must choose, for reducing blood pressure, go with the milk. Numerous studies find that a high intake of dietary calcium contributes to lower blood pressure.

Stabilizing Your Blood Sugar

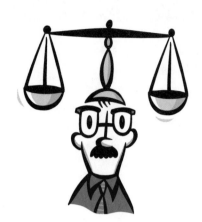

20 TIPS FOR STABLE, STEADY GLUCOSE LEVELS

Blood sugar, or glucose, has emerged as one of the most studied and discussed health topics around. There are many reasons why. The most obvious is that diabetes, a disease reaching epidemic proportions today, is linked directly to blood sugar levels. In recent years, researchers have also linked blood sugar to heart disease, memory problems, even fertility problems. Plus, with the emergence of low-carb diets, Americans have learned that there is a connection between high blood sugar and gaining weight.

All this scary talk of blood sugar and body chemistry is intimidating to many people. But it needn't be so; blood sugar isn't really that complicated. In a nutshell: Much of the food you eat is converted to blood sugar, which is used by the cells of your body for energy. Too much (or little) glucose in your bloodstream leads to complications. Your blood sugar levels are linked primarily to two things: the types and amounts of food you eat, and your body's ability to create and use insulin, a hormone that transports blood sugar into your body's cells.

Whether you already have diabetes, or are overweight, or just want to prevent future health problems, here are 20 Stealth Healthy ways to make sure your blood sugar and insulin levels are as healthy as can be. In addition, look to "Cutting Down on Sugar," page 111, as well as the other Stealth Healthy cooking chapters for more ideas for stable blood sugar counts.

 1 Drink a cup of skim milk and eat eight ounces of nonfat yogurt a day. A study of 3,000 people found that those who were overweight, but ate a lot of dairy foods, were 70 percent less likely to develop insulin resistance (a precursor to diabetes) than those who didn't. Turns out lactose, protein, and the fat in dairy products improves blood sugar by filling you up and slowing the conversion of food sugars to blood sugar.

2 Buy bread products that have at least three grams of fiber and three grams of protein per serving. They'll slow absorption of glucose and decrease possible insulin spikes, says J. J. Flizanes, a nutritionist and owner of Invisible Fitness in Los Angeles. Plus, the hearty dose of fiber and protein will keep your stomach feeling satisfied longer.

3 **Serve up a spinach salad for dinner.** Spinach is high in magnesium, which a large study suggests can help prevent the development of type 2 diabetes. One study in women found higher intakes of magnesium (also found in nuts, other leafy greens, and fish) reduced diabetes risk about 10 percent overall, and about 20 percent in women who were overweight. Another great source of magnesium? Avocados.

4 **Sprinkle cinnamon over your coffee, yogurt, cereal, and tea.** Researchers from Pakistan (where cinnamon reigns) had volunteers with type 2 diabetes take either one, three, or six grams of cinnamon or a placebo for 40 days. Those taking the fragrant spice saw their blood glucose levels drop 18-29 percent depending on how much cinnamon they took.

5 **Eat soba noodles for dinner one night a week.** The "Japanese pasta" is made from buckwheat, a grain that lowered blood glucose levels 12-19 percent in one well-controlled study on rats. Sure, you're not a rat, but buckwheat is an excellent source of fiber, and the evidence on fiber and blood glucose improvement is unimpeachable. Add a helping of buckwheat pancakes every Sunday and get double the benefits.

6 **Include a glass of wine with your dinner.** One study found women who had a drink of wine a day cut their risk of diabetes in half compared to teetotalers. Not a wine lover? The study found the same effects for beer. But cork the wine bottle once dinner is over. An Australian study found that drinking a glass of wine immediately after eating can result in a sudden drop in the insulin in your blood, meaning the glucose from your meal hangs around longer, eventually damaging arteries.

7 **Munch on baked chips.** Made without the saturated fat found in fried foods, baked chips—tortilla, potato, vegetable, or soy—are an excellent substitute when you're craving something crunchy and salty. The reason you want to avoid the saturated fat is simple: University of Minnesota scientists evaluated 3,000 people and found those with the highest blood levels of saturated fats were twice as likely to develop diabetes.

8 **Walk eight blocks a day.** That's all it took in one large study from the Centers of Disease Control and Prevention to slash the risk of dying from diabetes by more than one-third. Believe it or not, if you walk eight blocks a day, you'll have covered six miles by the end of the week, making you nearly 40 percent less likely to die from all causes and 34 percent less likely to die from heart disease, the leading cause of death in people

Healthy Investments

A Vegetarian Cookbook

Learn to use beans and lentils as alternatives to meat for some of your dinners. These foods are high in quality protein, but also rich in soluble fiber—which can help improve blood sugar and insulin levels, help with weight control, and lower cholesterol!

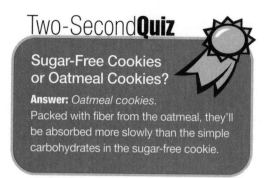
with diabetes. The reason? Walking makes your cells more receptive to insulin, which leads to better control of blood sugar. It also raises levels of "good" HDL cholesterol. See "Walking," page 154, for great ways to motivate yourself to walk.

9 Rent a comedy and watch it after dinner. A Japanese study found that people with diabetes who laughed soon after eating (while watching a comedy) had significantly lower blood sugar levels than those who listened to a boring lecture. The connection held even for those without diabetes.

10 Have half a grapefruit with breakfast tomorrow morning. Researchers from the Scripps Clinic in San Diego had 50 obese patients eat half a grapefruit with each meal for 12 weeks and compared them to a group that didn't eat any. Those patients who ate the grapefruit lost an average of 3.6 pounds. They also had lower levels of insulin and glucose after each meal, suggesting a more efficient sugar metabolism.

11 Add at least one day a week of resistance training. You'll build more muscle than you will by walking, and the more muscle mass you have, the more efficiently your body burns glucose and the less hangs around in your blood.

12 Add a cup of decaffeinated coffee if you simply must have that doughnut. British researchers found that combining decaf with simple sugars (like those in doughnuts, cakes, and cookies) reduces the blood sugar spike such sweets create. Regular coffee didn't have the same benefit. The reason? While plant chemicals in coffee slow the rate at which your intestines absorb sugar, caffeine delays sugar's arrival in muscles, keeping it in the bloodstream longer.

13 Dish out your breakfast, lunch, and dinner, but then divide each meal in half. Eat half now, then the other half in a couple of hours. Eating several small meals rather than three large meals helps avoid the major influx of glucose that, in turn, results in a blood sugar surge and a big release of insulin.

14 Don't skip a meal. First off, your blood sugar drops like a rock when you're starving (hence the headache and shakiness). Second, when you do eat, you flood your system with glucose, forcing your pancreas to release more insulin and creating a dangerous cycle.

Do**Three**Things

If you were to do only three things to maintain healthy blood sugar levels and prevent diabetes, here is what doctors recommend. Together, they can slash your risk of the disease by nearly 60 percent:

1. **Lose weight.** Seven or eight pounds is all it takes.

2. **Be physically active.** Thirty minutes a day is all you need.

3. **Add more fiber** to your diet by eating vegetables, fruits, whole grains, nuts, seeds, beans, and lentils regularly.

Two-Second **Quiz**

Cut Carbs or Cut Fat?

Answer: *Neither.*
It's more important to make sure you choose the *right* carbs and the *right* fats. Carbs from sugary foods and white breads and pasta raise blood sugar, while "good" carbs—whole grains, fruits, vegetables, beans, lentils, nuts, and seeds—help stabilize it. Similarly, some fats—the saturated fats in meats and full-fat dairy and trans fats such as hydrogenated oils—are bad for your health, while the polyunsaturated and monounsaturated oils in nuts, seeds, olives, avocados, and fish reduce the risk of diabetes.

15 **Go to bed at 10 p.m. and don't wake up until 6 a.m.** Adjust accordingly so you're getting a consistent eight hours. Numerous studies find that sleep deprivation has a dramatic effect on your blood sugar and insulin levels. If you need help falling (and staying) asleep, see "The Sleep Routine," page 79, for 24 tips for better rest.

16 **Ask your partner if you snore.** Harvard researchers found that women who snored were more than twice as likely as those who didn't to develop diabetes—regardless of weight, smoking history, or family history of diabetes. If you do snore, see your doctor. You may have a physical problem, or you may simply need to lose some weight and change the way you sleep.

17 **Spend 10 minutes a day tensing and then relaxing each muscle** in your body, from your toes to your eyes. This technique is called progressive muscle relaxation, and a study of 100 people with high blood sugar levels found stress relief efforts like this significantly improved their blood sugar levels. For other stress relieving advice, see "Defusing Stress," page 290.

18 **Eat half a cup of beans a day.** These high-fiber foods take longer to digest, so they release their glucose more slowly. Studies find just half a cup a day can help stabilize blood sugar and insulin levels.

19 **Toast a handful of walnuts, chop, and sprinkle over your salad.** Walnuts are great sources of monounsaturated fat, which won't raise your blood sugar as many other foods do. And some researchers suspect this fat even makes cells more sensitive to insulin, helping combat high blood sugar.

20 **Sprinkle powdered psyllium seed over your salad, yogurt, and scrambled eggs.** Mix it into meat loaf; stir it into sauces. Studies find the high-fiber seed may help lower elevated blood sugar.

Preventing Cancer

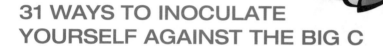

31 WAYS TO INOCULATE YOURSELF AGAINST THE BIG C

Consider this number: 10 million. That's how many cases of cancer are diagnosed worldwide each year. Now consider this number: 15 million. That's how many cases of cancer the World Health Organization estimates will be diagnosed in the year 2020—a 50 percent increase—if we don't get our act together.

Most cancers don't develop overnight or out of nowhere. Cancer is largely predictable, the end result of a decades-long process, but just a few Stealth Healthy changes in your daily life can significantly reduce your risk. Here are 31 great tips.

1 Serve sauerkraut at your next picnic. A Finnish study found that the fermentation process involved in making sauerkraut produces several other cancer-fighting compounds, including ITCs, indoles, and sulforaphane. To reduce the sodium content, rinse canned or jarred sauerkraut before eating.

2 Eat your fill of broccoli, but steam it rather than microwaving it. Broccoli is a cancer-preventing superfood, one you should eat frequently. But take note: A Spanish study found that microwaving broccoli destroys 97 percent of the vegetable's cancer-protective flavonoids. So steam it, eat it raw as a snack, or add it to soups and salads.

3 Toast some Brazil nuts and sprinkle over your salad. They're a rich form of selenium, a trace mineral that convinces cancer cells to commit suicide

and helps cells repair their DNA. A Harvard study of more than 1,000 men with prostate cancer found those with the highest blood levels of selenium were 48 percent less likely to develop advanced disease over 13 years than men with the lowest levels. And a dramatic five-year study conducted at Cornell University and the University of Arizona showed that 200 micrograms of selenium daily—the amount in two unshelled Brazil nuts—resulted in 63 percent fewer prostate tumors, 58 percent fewer colorectal cancers, 46 percent fewer lung malignancies, and a 39 percent overall decrease in cancer deaths.

4 Pop a calcium supplement with vitamin D. A study out of Dartmouth Medical School suggests that the supplements reduce colon polyps (a risk factor for colon cancer) in people susceptible to the growths.

5 **Add garlic to everything you eat.** Garlic contains sulfur compounds that may stimulate the immune system's natural defenses against cancer, and may have the potential to reduce tumor growth. Studies suggest that garlic can reduce the incidence of stomach cancer by as much as a factor of 12!

6 **Sauté two cloves of crushed garlic in 2 tablespoons of olive oil,** then mix in a can of low-sodium, diced tomatoes. Stir gently until heated and serve over whole wheat pasta. We already mentioned the benefits of garlic. The lycopene in the tomatoes protects against colon, prostate, and bladder cancers; the olive oil helps your body absorb the lycopene; and the fiber-filled pasta reduces your risk of colon cancer. As for the benefits of all of these ingredients together: They taste great!

7 **Every week, buy a cantaloupe at the grocery store and cut it up after you put away your groceries.** Store it in a container and eat several pieces every morning. Cantaloupe is a great source of carotenoids, plant chemicals shown to significantly reduce the risk of lung cancer.

8 **Mix half a cup of blueberries into your morning cereal.** Blueberries rank number one in terms of their antioxidant power. Antioxidants neutralize free radicals, which are unstable compounds that can damage cells and lead to diseases including cancer.

9 **Learn to eat artichokes tonight.** Artichokes are a great source of silymarin, an antioxidant that may help prevent skin cancer. To eat these delicious veggies, peel off the tough outer leaves on the bottom, slice the bottom, and cut off the spiky top. Then boil or steam until tender, about 30-45 minutes. Drain. Dip each leaf in a vinaigrette or garlic mayonnaise, then gently tear the fibrous covering off with your front teeth, working your way inward to the tender heart. Once there, gently scoop the bristles from the middle of the heart, dip in a little butter or lemon juice, and enjoy!

10 **Coat barbecue food with a thick sauce.** Grilling meat can create a variety of cancer-causing chemicals. But researchers from the American Institute for Cancer Research found that coating the meat with a thick marinade and thereby preventing direct contact with the charring flames reduced the amount of such chemicals created. Another tip: Precook your meat in the oven and then throw it on the grill to finish.

11 **Every time you go to the bathroom, stop by the kitchen or water cooler for a glass of water.** A major study published in *The New England Journal of Medicine* in 1996 found that

Two-Second **Quiz**

Pap Smear Before or After Your Period?

Answer: *Before.*

The best time is between days 10 and 20 of your menstrual cycle, says Mack Barnes, M.D., a gynecologic oncologist at the University of Alabama at Birmingham. This is the ideal time to evaluate the cervix and uterus cells under a microscope, ensuring the most accurate results possible, he says.

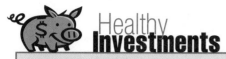

Healthy Investments

A Pepper Grinder

But don't fill it with pepper. Instead, fill it with organic flaxseed. This makes it easy to add a sprinkle of the disease-fighting seeds (which contain important phytochemicals, fiber, and omega-3 fatty acids) to cereal, yogurt, soups, and stews. Studies find ground flaxseed reduces levels of hormones linked to breast cancer.

men who drank six 8-ounce glasses of water every day slashed their risk of bladder cancer in half. Another study linked the amount of water women drank to their risk of colon cancer, with heavy water drinkers reducing their risk up to 45 percent.

12 **Take up a tea habit.** The healing powers of green tea have been valued in Asia for thousands of years. In the West, new research reveals that it protects against a variety of cancers as well as heart disease. Some scientists believe that a chemical in green tea called EGCG could be one of the most powerful anticancer compounds ever discovered.

13 **Have a beer tonight.** Beer protects against the bacterium *Helicobacter pylori*, known to cause ulcers and possibly linked to stomach cancer. But don't overdo it. Drinking more than one or two alcoholic drinks a day may increase your risk of mouth, throat, esophageal, liver, and breast cancer.

14 **Throw some salmon on the grill tonight.** Australian researchers studying Canadians (go figure) found those who ate four or more servings of fish per week were nearly one-third less

likely to develop the blood cancers leukemia, myeloma, and non-Hodgkin's lymphoma. Other studies show a link between eating fatty fish (salmon, mackerel, halibut, sardines, and tuna, as well as shrimp and scallops) with a reduced risk of endometrial cancer in women. Ah, those amazing omega-3s at it again!

15 **Take a multivitamin every morning.** Many studies suggest getting the ideal levels of vitamins and minerals can improve your immune system function and help prevent a variety of cancers.

16 **Get about 15 minutes of sunlight on your skin each day.** You've heard of the sunshine vitamin, vitamin D haven't you? Turns out we've been so good at heeding advice to slather on sun lotion and avoid the sun's rays that many of us aren't getting enough of this valuable nutrient. Researchers find that getting too little vitamin D may increase your risk of multiple cancers, including breast, colon, prostate, ovarian, and stomach, as well as osteoporosis, diabetes, multiple sclerosis, and high blood pressure.

If You Must Eat Hamburgers...

Flip them every minute. One study found that turning hamburgers every minute reduced the amount of carcinogens that result from frying 75-95 percent. Another hamburger tip: Add red or white wine plus a tablespoon of sugar to the meat before you shape it into patties. Adding sugar to your meat with red or white wine reduces the carcinogens in grilled or fried hamburgers. Onions also seem to have a similar effect. Of course, we'd rather see you choose turkey or salmon burgers; fatty meats like ground beef contribute to cancer risk on their own.

The best source? Exposure to UVB rays found in natural and artificial sunlight. About 15 minutes a day ought to do it. Avoid overexposure, of course. That can *increase* your risk for cancers of the skin. You can also get vitamin D in your calcium supplement if you choose a supplement that contains both.

17 **Carry a shot glass in your beach bag.** Then fill it with sunscreen and rub it all over your body. A shot glass holds about 1.5 ounces, which is how much sunscreen dermatologists estimate you need to protect yourself from the cancer-causing UV rays of the sun. Repeat every two hours.

18 **Cut a kiwifruit in half, then scoop out the flesh** with a spoon. Now eat! Kiwi is a little hand grenade of cancer-fighting antioxidants, including vitamin C, vitamin E, lutein, and copper. You can also rub a couple of cut kiwifruit on a low-fat cut of meat as a tenderizer.

19 **Use a condom and stick to one partner.** The more sexual partners a woman has, the greater her risk of contracting human papillomavirus, or HPV, which causes cervical cancer. Having an unfaithful husband also increases her risk.

20 **Cut out high-fat animal protein.** A Yale study found that women who ate the most animal protein had a 70 percent higher risk of developing non-Hodgkin's lymphoma, while those who ate diets high in saturated fat increased their risk 90 percent. So switch to low-fat or nonfat dairy, have poultry or fish instead of beef or pork, and use olive oil instead of butter.

Two-Second Quiz

Fresh Tomatoes or Tomato Sauce?

Answer: *Tomato sauce.* Tomatoes are rich in lycopene, an antioxidant believed to reduce the risk of prostate cancer and possibly several other cancers. But only cooking releases the lycopene from tomato cell walls so our bodies can absorb it. What's more, lycopene is fat-soluble, meaning your body is better able to absorb and use it when you get it with a bit of fat—such as the olive oil found in most tomato sauces.

21 **Have your partner feed you grapes.** They're great sources of resveratrol, the cancer-protecting compound found in wine, but don't have the alcohol of wine, which can increase the risk of breast cancer in women. Plus, the closeness such an activity engenders (we hope) strengthens your immune system.

22 **Sprinkle scallions over your salad.** A diet high in onions may reduce the risk of prostate cancer 50 percent. But the effects are strongest when they're eaten raw or lightly cooked. So try scallions, Vidalia onions, shallots, or chives for a milder taste.

23 **Make a batch of fresh lemonade or limeade.** A daily dose of citrus fruits may cut the risk of mouth, throat, and stomach cancers by half, Australian researchers found.

24 **Take a 30-minute walk every evening after dinner.** That's all it takes to reduce your breast cancer risk, according to a study from the Fred

Hutchinson Cancer Research Center in Seattle. Turns out that moderate exercise reduces levels of estrogen, a hormone that contributes to breast cancer. When 170 overweight, couch potato women ages 50-75 did some form of moderate exercise for about three hours a week, levels of circulating estrogen dropped significantly after three months. After a year, those who lost at least 2 percent of their body fat had even greater decreases in estrogen. Another study linked four hours a week of walking or hiking with cutting the risk of pancreatic cancer in half. The benefits are probably related to improved insulin metabolism due to the exercise.

25 **Buy organic foods.** They're grown without added pesticides or hormones, both of which can cause cellular damage that may eventually lead to cancer.

26 **Learn to love dandelions.** Using commercial pesticides on your lawn may increase your risk of cancer, since most contain pesticides such as 2,4-D (linked to non-Hodgkin's lymphoma) and MCPP (associated with soft-tissue cancers). Plus, pesticides used solely on lawns don't have to go through the same rigorous testing for long-term health effects as those used on food. And, as *E/The Environmental Magazine* noted in a 2004 article, no fed-

In**Perspective**

Annual Screenings

Okay, so making an appointment with your doctor, sitting in a waiting room leafing through magazines, and possibly undergoing some uncomfortable tests may not be the stealthiest ways to avoid cancer, but they are among the best ways to ensure that if you *do* have cancer, it's caught at the treatable stage. Here's what most health-care organizations recommend in terms of regular screenings:

- **Skin.** Get an annual skin examination, preferably from a dermatologist.

- **Breast.** Women should have yearly mammograms starting at age 40.

- **Cervical.** All women should begin cervical cancer

screening about three years after they begin having vaginal intercourse, but no later than age 21. Get screened every year with the regular Pap test or every two years using the newer liquid-based Pap test until you reach age 30. At that point, if you've had three normal Pap test results in a row (and have no special risk factors for cervical cancer) you can get screened every two to three years with either the conventional (regular) or liquid-based Pap test.

- **Colon and rectal cancer.** Beginning at age 50, follow one of these five screening strategies (make the decision with your doctor):

  1. A yearly fecal occult blood test (FOBT)

  2. A flexible sigmoidoscopy every 5 years
  3. A yearly FOBT plus flexible sigmoidoscopy every 5 years (better than either test alone)
  4. A double-contrast barium enema every 5 years
  5. A colonoscopy every 10 years

- **Prostate cancer.** Beginning at age 50, men should have a prostate-specific antigen (PSA) blood test and a digital rectal examination every year. Men who are at high risk should begin testing at age 45. This group includes African American men and men with a strong family history of one or more first-degree relatives (father, brothers) who were diagnosed at an early age.

eral studies have assessed the safety of lawn-care chemicals in combination, the way most are sold.

27 **Buy clothes that don't need to be dry-cleaned.** Many dry cleaners still use a chemical called perc (perchloroethylene), found to cause kidney and liver damage and cancer in animals repeatedly exposed through inhalation. Buying clothes that don't require dry cleaning, or hand washing them yourself, can reduce your exposure to this chemical. If you must dry-clean your clothes, take them out of the plastic bag and air them outside or in another room before wearing.

28 **Choose cucumbers over pickles, fresh salmon over lox.** Studies find that smoked and pickled foods contain various carcinogens.

 29 **Switch from french fries and potato chips to mashed potatoes and pretzels.** A potential cancer-causing compound called acrylamide forms as a result of the chemical changes that occur in foods when they're baked, fried, or roasted. Not surprisingly, many foods with the greatest amounts of acrylamide are also some of the worst-for-you foods, such as french fries, potato chips, and baked sweets. Although the results aren't final yet, Michael Jacobson, Ph.D., executive director of the Center for Science in the Public Interest, estimates acrylamide causes between 1,000 and 25,000 cancers per year. His agency has petitioned the Food and Drug Admin-istration to set limits on the amount of acrylamide foods can contain. The FDA is studying the issue.

30 **Go for a spray-on tan.** They're available in most tanning salons these days and, unlike tanning beds, there's no evidence that they increase your risk of skin cancer.

31 **Call up your bowling pal and hit the lanes.** A study from the State University of New York at Stony Brook found that men with high levels of stress and those with less satisfying contacts with friends and family members had higher levels of prostate-specific antigen (PSA) in their blood, a marker for the development of prostate cancer.

REMINDER

 Fast Results
These are bits of advice that deliver benefits partic-ularly quickly—in some cases, immediately!

 Easy Gains
These are tips that give the biggest value for the least amount of effort.

Super Effective
These are tips proven to be particularly effective through scientific research or wide-spread usage by experts.

Greater Lung Power

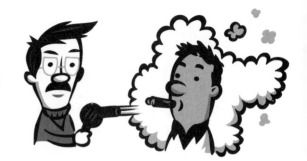

18 WAYS TO BREATHE EASIER

If you want to be able to blow out all the candles on your cake when you're 75 (assuming your family dares to put a candle for every year) not to mention climb three flights of stairs without needing oxygen, now is the time to take action. What, you're wondering, could you possibly do beyond quitting smoking to get your bellows in better shape? Plenty. Although quitting smoking tops our list, we also found another 18 tips that will have you doing less huffing and puffing and protect your lungs from damage and disease. In addition, read about proper breathing technique on page 293, part of the discussion on managing stress.

1 **Have a heart-to-heart with your bed partner.** Key question to ask: Do I snore? If the answer is yes, make an appointment with a sleep specialist and get checked for sleep apnea. The condition, in which you stop breathing dozens or even hundreds of times during the night, can actually damage your lungs nearly as much as smoking. Fortunately, it's treatable.

2 **Make several trips downstairs to the basement every day.** The kind of exercise that makes your heart beat faster, like climbing stairs, riding a bike, or walking briskly, is very important for keeping your heart and lungs in good shape. For instance, studies find that walking about 15 minutes at a time, three to four times a day, improved breathing in people with emphysema, a lung disease.

3 **Pop a fish-oil supplement every morning.** Most airway problems, including asthma, are related to inflammation. Omega-3 fatty acids, which are the main ingredient in fish-oil supplements, reduce inflammation.

4 **Breathe from your belly for at least five minutes every day.** This kind of breathing, called diaphragmatic breathing, involves training and strengthening your diaphragm so it requires less effort to take in each breath. To do it, inhale deeply through your nose, filling your lungs from the bottom up. If you're doing it right, your stomach will pooch out. Exhale and repeat.

5 **Expand your chest like a cocky rooster.** To help your chest expand and boost your lung capacity, lie on the floor with your knees bent and your feet flat on

the floor. Place your hands behind your head and bring your elbows together so they're nearly touching. As you inhale, slowly let your elbows drop to the sides so your arms are flat on the floor when your lungs are full. As you exhale, raise your elbows again.

6 **Read the fine print on household cleansers.** Some products, like oven cleaner, can be toxic if inhaled. And if the instructions say to open a window or use in a well-ventilated space, follow them, says Kevin Cooper, M.D., a Virginia Commonwealth University Medical Center pulmonologist.

7 **Enforce a no-smoke zone in your house.** And avoid smoky bars and smoking areas in restaurants. It doesn't seem fair, but secondhand smoke you breathe from these sources can damage your lungs just as much as the smoke from your own cigarette.

8 **Wear a face mask or even a gas mask** when working around toxic dust or fumes. "Occupational exposure is a major hazard to lung health," Dr. Cooper says. Even simple household tasks like sanding paint could send damaging fragments into your lungs, he says.

9 **Work in 10-20 crunches a day.** Your abdominal and chest muscles allow you to suck air in and out. Strengthen them, and if you're also practicing your deep breathing, you'll have the breath power of a professional opera singer (or at least close).

10 **Take your medicine and listen to your doctor if you have asthma.** There's some pretty good evidence that people with asthma eventually develop

chronic obstructive pulmonary disease, or COPD, a lung disease that strikes people 65 and older. There's also evidence that keeping your asthma under control with medication and lifestyle changes can prevent the disease from developing.

11 **Make spaghetti sauce tonight, tomato and basil salad tomorrow night, and roasted tomatoes over the weekend.** British researchers found that people who ate tomatoes three times a week had improved lung function and experienced less wheeziness and fewer asthma-like symptoms.

12 **Look on the bright side.** So the stock market is down; at least the bond market is up. When Harvard researchers followed 670 men with an average age of 63 years for eight years, they found those who were more optimistic had much better lung function and a slower rate of lung function decline than the pessimists in the bunch.

13 **Get at least seven servings of fruits and vegetables a day.** A 1998 study found that high amounts of antioxidants found in such

foods, including vitamin C, vitamin E, selenium, and beta-carotene, meant better lung function—even in smokers! Look at several of the chapters in "Stealth Healthy Cooking," page 86 for clever ways to sneak more fruits and vegetables into your diet.

14 Have a glass of wine tonight. Drinking wine, particularly white wine, both in the recent past and over your lifetime, seems to help your lungs. It has to be wine, though. Researchers found no such correlation when they looked at the effects of other forms of alcohol. Researchers aren't certain why, but suspect it may be due to high levels of antioxidants in wine that protect cells from the damage from smoke and air pollution.

15 Brush your teeth twice a day and floss after every meal. Seems the state of your gums makes a difference when it comes to your lungs. Researchers at the State University of New York in Buffalo found patients with periodontal, or gum, disease were 1½ times more likely to also have COPD. Plus, the worse the gum disease, the worse the lung function, suggesting a direct correlation between the two.

16 Say no to dessert. There's a direct link between what you weigh and the health of your lungs. Having extra weight makes your respiratory muscles work harder and less efficiently, researchers found in a 2004 study. This, in turn results in short-

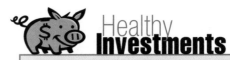

Healthy Investments

A Spirometer

This little device, commonly used in hospitals to prevent lung collapse from underuse when patients are bedridden, is the equivalent of the carnival game in which you hit a strike pad with an oversized mallet to ring a bell. Only this is no game, and you do the work by breathing, rather than swinging a mallet. Blow into the tube, and see how high you can raise the ball. This is a good test of your lung function, but also a great way to exercise the muscles of breathing—maybe while you're watching TV. You can find spirometers in medical supply stores.

ness of breath, which makes it hard to exercise, which makes it hard to lose the weight ... You can break out of this depressing cycle by following our tips in "Losing Weight," page 213.

17 In hot, dry, or very cold weather, or in dusty or polluted air, breathe in through your nose and out through your mouth. Our nasal passages are designed to filter the air and regulate its temperature and humidity. If you breathe in through your mouth, everything—dust, coldness, etc.—goes straight on into the lungs.

18 Take it easy when pollution or ozone levels are in the red zone. The more you exert yourself, the more you have to breathe through your mouth to take in larger volumes of air. This, in turn, means less filtering of the air during some very dangerous air quality times.

Greater Mobility

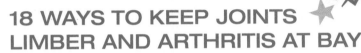

18 WAYS TO KEEP JOINTS LIMBER AND ARTHRITIS AT BAY

If you've ever crawled out of bed in the morning aching as if you'd played a mean game of rugby in your sleep, heard your knees creaking as you descended the stairs, required three ibuprofen before you could bend over to tie your shoes, and/or received an embroidered sampler with the words "My Back Hurts" for your birthday, then this chapter is for you.

Making some simple changes in your diet and daily activities—even the way you sit—coupled with taking a few key supplements a day can save a lot of wear and tear on your joints and ligaments as well as reduce your pain. Here's a starting lineup of tips that help you where you hurt.

1 Sip a cup of green tea in the morning. Polyphenols called catechins in green tea prevent arthritis in mice and significantly reduce cartilage damage in humans.

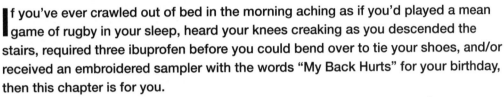

2 When you sit, keep both feet on the ground. Crossing your legs cuts off your blood circulation and pulls your back out of alignment.

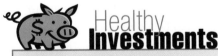

Healthy Investments

A Pair of Walking Poles

A study from the University of Washington and the Steadman-Hawkins Sports Medicine Foundation found they help you move faster while sparing wear and tear on your joints. Since you're moving faster, you're burning more calories.

3 Switch over to spicy foods when your arthritis flares. Spices such as cayenne pepper, ginger, and turmeric contain compounds that reduce swelling and block a brain chemical that transmits pain signals. So head to the bookstore for some Mexican, Indian, and Thai cookbooks, or keep a bottle of hot sauce on your table at all times.

4 Empty out (or better yet, have someone else empty them for you) any cabinet or shelf below waist level. You'd be surprised how much unnecessary bending people do to get at those low places, says Howard Pecker, M.D., an orthopedic surgeon in Rahway, New Jersey. He gives this advice to all his patients with arthritis. They tell him it makes their lives much less painful. Just fill the empty cabinets with less-used items,

like the turkey roaster that only comes out at Thanksgiving.

5 **Use a wrist rest to keep your wrists straight, not to rest your wrists on.** Resting your wrists on the pad when typing can compress soft tissues—such as tendons, nerves, and blood vessels—in your forearms, reducing blood flow to your wrists and fingers, says Peter W. Johnson, Ph.D., assistant professor of environmental health at the University of Washington in Seattle. This, in turn, can increase pressure in the carpal tunnel located inside your wrists and ultimately lead to nerve damage. Instead, use the pad only for support during typing breaks. Even then, most experts recommend resting the palms of your hands, rather than your wrists, on the pad to reduce the risk of injury, he says.

6 **Keep a small rubber ball on your desk and in your car.** Every time you get up to go to the bathroom (at work) or hit a red light (in the car) squeeze the ball 20 times on each hand. This helps strengthen your hands and improve flexibility.

Two-Second**Quiz**

Heat or Ice for Injuries?

Answer: *Ice.*
Use ice in the first 24 hours after injury to reduce inflammation and fluid buildup. But for chronic injuries, like a sore back, arm, or knee, use heat. By increasing circulation, heat makes muscles and tendons more pliable while aiding joint movement.

Do**Three**Things

If you do only three things for back pain, doctors concur that these make the most sense:

1. **Get up and go.** The old idea of lying around when your back hurts just makes things worse. As soon as the acute stage of back pain is over, you need to get up and move. Walking is great. So are stretching exercises.

2. **Make sure you're sleeping on the right mattress.** One study of 313 men with low back pain found those who slept on a medium-firm mattress were twice as likely to get some pain relief. If your mattress is more than 10 years old, it's time to go mattress shopping.

3. **Wear soft-soled shoes with low heels.** High heels throw your entire body out of alignment, contributing not only to back pain but also to knee and hip pain and injuries as well, not to mention what they do to your feet.

7 **Wash your dishes by hand and give the dishwasher the night off.** The combination of warm, running water and light exercise, requiring complex movement of the wrist and hand, is an effective and low-cost way of rehabilitating the hand and wrist after injury or surgery, says B. Sonny Bal, M.D., assistant professor of orthopedic surgery at the University of Missouri School of Medicine in Columbia. It will also keep your wrists and hands flexible with good blood circulation if you have arthritis or other painful problems.

8 **Prevent tennis elbow by icing your arm after play.** The easiest way, says Scott Herron, M.D., who directs the sports medicine department at the Advanced Orthopaedic Surgery Center in

Temecula, California, is to put water in a Styrofoam cup before you start playing, freeze it, then peel back the top of the cup to expose the ice. Now you can hold the ice against your arm without freezing your hand off. If, however, the tennis elbow arrives despite the ice, try this exercise: Bend your arm at 90 degrees, keeping your elbow at your side, palm facing up. Hold this pose for 5-10 seconds, then slowly lower your arm. Do this 10 times.

9 Enhance the range of motion in your wrist with this exercise. Slowly bend your wrist backward and forward, holding for a 5-second count in each position, suggests Dr. Herron. Do three sets—10 times for each hand—twice a day.

10 Always bend from the knees, not the back, when lifting. Also, keep the weight you're carrying close to your body, as if you were carrying a baby. This puts less strain on your back.

11 On long drives, pull over every hour, get out of the car, and walk around for five minutes, stretching like a cat. Your back will thank you later.

12 For back relief, get on your hands and knees (on a padded surface) and round your back like a scared cat. Hold for five seconds, then let your stomach relax and sag for five seconds. Do two sets of 10 each anytime you've been sitting for more than an hour.

13 Crunch your way through 20 modified sit-ups every morning. These strengthen the abdominal muscles while stretching and relaxing the back,

says Dr. Herron. To do a modified sit-up, bend your knees or place your feet on a small stool or chair as you complete the crunch.

14 Serve up some pickled herring for breakfast or lunch. This fish is rich in omega-3 fatty acids, shown to reduce inflammation and alleviate pain from arthritis and other joint diseases.

15 Play a video game, read the latest Dan Brown book, or watch a Lord of the Rings movie when your joints are hurting. Researchers find that concentrating on what you're doing, whether leisure activities or work, distracts you from your pain.

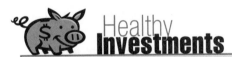

Healthy Investments

A Bottle of Glucosamine/Chondroitin

Even the most conservative orthopedic surgeon admits that this supplement, derived from animal products, can not only provide pain relief, but may even slow the degeneration of cartilage. Glucosamine doesn't fight pain right away the way drugs like ibuprofen do. But over time, it becomes an effective pain reliever and anti-inflammatory. More important, it can actually help repair damaged cartilage—something ibuprofen can't do at all. In fact, drugs like ibuprofen may even interfere with normal cartilage repair. So if you have pain and need relief right away, use a drug like ibuprofen for prompt pain relief, but start glucosamine at the same time. After about a month, you should be getting enough pain relief from the glucosamine to stop the ibuprofen. Then continue the glucosamine indefinitely for its anti-inflammatory and cartilage-repairing effects.

16 Wear tight-fitting gloves at night. They help reduce swelling and fluid accumulation in the night so your hands don't ache when you wake up.

 17 Take these super supplements:

▸ **Ginger extract twice a day.** Researchers from the University of Miami found ginger significantly reduced knee pain in patients with osteoarthritis of the knee, as well as improved how the knee worked. Turns out ginger has some anti-inflammatory effects, just like ibuprofen.

▸ **Fish–oil capsules.** A British study found that 86 percent of people with arthritis who took cod liver oil had far fewer enzymes that cause cartilage damage compared to those who got a placebo. Plus, they had far fewer pain-causing enzymes. Cod liver oil is a fish oil, so your basic fish-oil supplement will do fine.

▸ **Vitamin E containing pure alpha-tocopherols.** A German study found taking 1,500 IU of vitamin E every day reduced pain and morning stiffness and improved grip strength in people with rheumatoid arthritis as well as prescription medication.

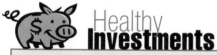
Healthy Investments

A Session With an Ergonomic Expert

Whether you work at home or in an office, whether you have to pay for it yourself or your employer will foot the bill, it's worth it to make sure your desk is at the right height, your mouse is in the right position, and your keyboard is centered properly.

▸ **Glucosamine/chondroitin.** See the Healthy Investments item for more on this topic.

18 Quit smoking. Smoking reduces your circulation and that, according to a study in the medical journal *Spine*, increases your risk for back pain and slows healing.

Proper Sleeping Positions

If you're waking up sore and achy every morning and your mattress is new, you may need to re-evaluate how you're sleeping, says Scott D. Boden, M.D., director of the Emory Spine Center in Atlanta. Lying flat on your back forces your spine into an unnatural position, which can strain your muscles, joints, and nerves. "Your spine isn't meant to be straight," he says. "It has three natural curves: one in your lower back, one in the middle of your back, and one near your neck." His advice:

● Lie on your side in the fetal position with your knees bent and a pillow tucked between your legs. This will take the most stress off your back.

● If you must sleep on your back, prop a big, fluffy pillow under your knees to reduce the pressure on the sciatic nerve in your lower back.

● Use a small pillow or a rolled-up towel under your neck as long as it doesn't push your chin too far forward.

● Don't sleep on your stomach. Sleeping facedown can exaggerate the arch at the base of your spine and cause strain. Our advice? Sew or tape a tennis ball to the front of your nightgown or nightshirt. We guarantee your stomach-sleeping days will be over.

Stronger Bones

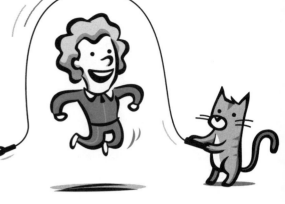

28 WAYS TO HELP PREVENT OSTEOPOROSIS

Drink your milk! Surely you remember your mother admonishing you with those words when you were a kid. And she was absolutely right: Kids who drink plenty of milk (or get plenty of calcium from other sources) grow up to have less risk of osteoporosis, the disease that causes bones to become thin and brittle.

It appears that not many of us listened very well to Mom; annually, osteoporosis accounts for about 700,000 spine fractures, 300,000 hip fractures, about 250,000 wrist fractures, and 300,000 fractures at other sites. One out of two women over 50 and one in eight men over 50 will have an osteoporosis-related fracture at some point.

Even if you're not a kid anymore, there's plenty you can do to protect yourself. From upping your calcium intake to getting the right exercise, here are the 28 best ways to protect your 206 bones. Pay special attention to this advice if you are over age 50, have a family history of osteoporosis, or are a woman who has gone through menopause, because your bones may be more vulnerable.

1 Add almonds to everything. They're packed with bone-strengthening calcium. Just an ounce, about a handful, of the sweet nuts provides 70 mg calcium. Try them toasted and sprinkled over salad or yogurt, ground and mixed into meat or turkey for meat loaf or meatballs, used in place of pine nuts for homemade pesto, or as a topping for ice cream or frozen yogurt.

2 Drain a can of sardines, mash the fish with a tablespoon of low-fat mayonnaise, add some salt and pepper, and spread over whole wheat crackers. Another packed-with-calcium food, sardines (the kind with the bones) make a great substitute for tuna. Pair this snack

with a glass of milk and your bones have got it made!

3 Stash calcium supplements everywhere. If you're like most people, between the vitamins, supplements, and medications you may be taking every day, a calcium supplement—best taken *twice* a day—is apt to be forgotten. So stash them all over the place. Put a bottle in the glove compartment of your car. Keep one on your desk at work. Slip a roll of Tums (a great source of calcium) in your purse or pocket. Put a bottle in full view on your kitchen counter. Calcium is best absorbed in two doses of 500 or 600 mg taken at least three hours apart. Choose a brand that has vitamin D, too, which your body needs in order to use the calcium.

4 **Drink one cup of tea a day.** That's all it took in a study of 1,256 women ages 65-76 to increase their bone density 5 percent. That translates to a 10-20 percent reduction in fracture risk! Another study found that among more than 1,000 Chinese men and women, those who regularly drank tea (usually green tea) had denser bones than those who didn't.

5 **Make two glasses of water a day mineral water.** Mineral water contains calcium, and a study published in *Osteoporosis International* in 2000 found that your body absorbs the mineral just as well from water as it does from milk. Make sure the water is labeled "mineral water," not "spring water."

6 **Do 12-16 squats every day just before you get into bed.** Squats are particularly beneficial for your hips, which are especially prone to fracture. Pretend you're about to sit in a chair, only there's no chair behind you. As you "sit," try to lower yourself enough so that your thighs are parallel or nearly parallel to the floor, but don't let your knees extend beyond your toes.

7 **Jump rope for 10 minutes every day.** It's one of the best all-around exercises for building bone. You can even find jump ropes that measure not only the number of jumps you complete, but how many calories you burn. Be careful when you start, though. This exercise requires coordination, and if your bones already happen to be thin, the last thing you want to do is fall.

8 **Turn your face up to the sun every day when you walk** to and from your car. Aim for about 15 minutes a day of sun exposure, without sunscreen. That's how much your body needs to make vitamin D, the "sunshine vitamin" important to bone health. And exposure to sunlight enhances mood because sunlight affects levels of the hormone melatonin. Too little sun can result in a form of depression known as seasonal affective disorder, or SAD. Studies find that women who are prone to depression are also more likely to have lower bone density.

9 **Try some coleslaw or stuffed cabbage rolls for dinner once a week.** Cabbage is rich in vitamin K, a vitamin that helps turn on a bone-building protein called osteocalcin.

10 **Ride your bike off-road this weekend.** A study published in the journal *Bone* found that cyclists who spent part of their time off-road had above-

Two-Second**Quiz**

Cheese or Calcium Tablets?

Answer: *Cheese.*
A study of preteen girls found those getting 3.5 ounces of low-fat cheese a day increased their total bone mass more than girls who took calcium tablets containing the same amount of calcium. Researchers speculate the calcium in the cheese is better absorbed. Still, there *is* a trade-off. The cheese has calories and saturated fat, the supplements none. So we advocate plenty of nonfat dairy in your diet, occasional cheese as a treat, and a calcium supplement as an insurance policy.

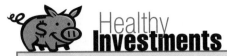

average bone density, while those who stuck to the streets had slightly below-average bone density. They speculate that the bouncing you do over rough terrain helps stimulate bone growth.

11 Roast a butternut squash tonight. Butternut squash is high in calcium (about 10 percent of the daily value in a one-cup serving). Slice open, scoop out the seeds, then spray the top with butterless cooking spray and sprinkle with brown sugar and cinnamon. Roast until soft, about 45-60 minutes, and scoop out the flesh. Voilà! Osteoporosis fighter in a veggie.

12 Order your pizza topped with sardines and spinach. Not only is it delicious (come on, give it a try), but you'll get a ton of bone-protecting calcium in every bite.

13 Pop four dried figs for a midafternoon snack. Dried figs are a great source of calcium. Sprinkle a cup of diced figs over your yogurt, and you'll meet more than half your daily calcium needs.

14 Sip water or iced tea instead of soda. A study out of Tufts University in Boston found that women who drank at least one 12-ounce cola every day for four years had up to 5 percent lower bone mineral density than women who drank fewer than one a week. All the women were drinking the same amount of milk, so researchers think the phosphoric acid in soda affects the body's absorption of calcium.

15 Figure out how much sodium you're consuming a day to see if you need more calcium. If you're at or below 2,100 milligrams of sodium (slightly less than the recommended limit) you're probably okay with about 1,200 mg calcium a day. But if you're getting more sodium than that—and most Americans do—increase your calcium intake. An Australian study found that the more sodium 124 postmenopausal women urinated (an indication of how much they took in) the more bone they lost in their hips (where their bone density was measured). You don't have to analyze your pee; just take a day and pay attention to all the processed foods you eat (where most sodium is found). Add up the milligrams to get a sense of where you are, sodium-wise. By the way, if you're using the saltshaker, one teaspoon contains 2,000 mg sodium.

16 Take the right kind of calcium at the right time. Calcium citrate, for instance, is absorbed more easily on an empty stomach, so take it before meals. Calcium carbonate, the cheapest and most common type of supplement, is absorbed best when taken with food, particularly acidic foods such as citrus juice or fruit.

17 Hang room-darkening shades in your bedroom. You'll sleep much better without ambient light, and sleep is important for bone. Much of bone remodeling, in which old bone is replaced

Swimming or Walking?

Answer: *Walking.*
While swimming is a great exercise for your lungs and heart, it doesn't do anything for your bones, because there's little resistance in water.

women who didn't walk at all. Walking briskly, you should be able to cover two miles in 30 minutes; walk for 30 minutes just four days a week and you'll get the 7.5 miles in. Add an extra day, though, just for good measure!

19 Start a vegetable and flower garden this spring.

Researchers at the University of Arkansas in Fayetteville found yard work (and weight training) were highly associated with reducing the risk for osteoporosis in 3,310 women ages 50 and older. Turns out that pushing a lawn mower, thrusting a shovel into the ground, lifting heavy wheelbarrows filled with mulch, raking, leaning, carrying, and pulling weeds are all great weight-bearing exercises. So which would you rather do? Lift weights in some stinky gym, or dig in the dirt to plant and harvest your own ruby-red tomatoes?

by new, occurs at night during sleep. If you're not sleeping enough, just when do you think your body is going to have the time to perform this valuable job?

18 Walk for 30 minutes a day.

Most women lose 3-6 percent of their bone mass every year during the five years before and after menopause. But women who regularly walked (about 7.5 miles a week) took four to seven years longer to lose the same amount of bone as

20 Add nonfat powdered milk to soups, casseroles, baked goods and drinks.

It's an easy, unobtrusive way to sneak more calcium into your diet, particularly if you don't like drinking milk. Here's a great recipe that does just that:

Oatmeal Banana Chocolate Chip Cookies

1 medium ripe banana
⅓ cup fat-free powdered milk
⅓ cup dark brown sugar
5 tablespoons Smart Balance spread
2 tablespoons unsweetened applesauce
2 eggs (organic omega-3)
1½ cups rolled oats
½ cup all-purpose flour
¼ cup slivered almonds
¼ teaspoon baking soda
1½ cups semi-sweet chocolate chips (Ghirardelli)

1. Preheat oven to 360°F. Grind the almonds in a coffee grinder to a fine powder.
2. Place first five ingredients in the bowl of an electric mixer and beat until fluffy and creamy. Add eggs and beat again until smooth. The dough will seem liquid and not compact, but that's okay—that's how it's supposed to be.
3. Add in rolled oats, flour, ground almonds, and baking soda and beat until well blended. Mix in chocolate chips. Bake in preheated oven 10-12 minutes.

21 Learn to cook with yogurt.

Many cultures, particularly Indian, use yogurt every day in cooking. Here are two great recipes that take advantage of this flexible food that's also high in calcium:

Crispy Multigrain Chicken Tenders   Serves 4

1 pound boneless, skinless chicken breasts
¾ cup fat-free plain yogurt
3 tablespoons orange juice concentrate
½ teaspoon garlic powder
½ teaspoon salt
3 cups multigrain cereal (Nature's Path Heritage)
¼ cup oat bran flour
Quick spray of olive oil

1. Wash and pat dry the chicken; cut into one-inch chunks.
2. Mix yogurt, orange juice concentrate, garlic powder, and salt in a large bowl. Add chunks of chicken to the yogurt mixture, coating each piece thoroughly, and store in refrigerator for at least 30 minutes (you can make this the night before—it will be even more tender).
3. Place multigrain cereal with oat bran flour and a pinch of salt in another bowl and crumble up with your fingers (you can also grind the cereal in a food processor if you prefer a finer texture).
4. When ready to bake, preheat the oven to 425°F. Take the yogurt-coated chicken out of the fridge. Dip each piece in the cereal mixture and place on a baking sheet covered with parchment paper lightly sprayed with olive oil. Discard extra cereal and extra yogurt.
5. Give a quick olive oil spray over all the pieces. Bake in preheated oven until golden and crisp, 10-12 minutes.

Baked Chicken in Creamy Mustard Sauce

If you are lucky enough to have leftovers, this makes a great sandwich for the next day's lunch.

1 pound boneless, skinless chicken breasts
3 tablespoons Dijon mustard
¼ cup plain, nonfat yogurt
½ cup dry vermouth
⅓ cup fat-free chicken broth
¼ cup fat-free buttermilk
1 tablespoon grainy mustard
⅛ teaspoon black pepper

1. Preheat oven to 375°F.
2. Wash and pat dry the chicken. Mix the Dijon mustard with the yogurt and coat the chicken with it. Cover and refrigerate for at least 30 minutes (this step can be done the night before).
3. When ready to bake, arrange the chicken in a shallow baking dish that can also go on top of the stove. Mix ¼ cup vermouth with the chicken broth in a measuring cup and pour around the chicken. Bake for approximately 10 minutes, turning the chicken over once, and bake until just tender, an additional 10-15 minutes (do not overcook).
4. When ready, take the chicken breasts out of the baking dish and set them aside on a plate.
5. Place baking dish with the cooking "juices" on the stovetop over medium-high heat and pour in remaining vermouth. Bring to a boil and whisk in the buttermilk and grainy mustard. Lower heat and cook for a few minutes while stirring until well blended and creamy.
6. Place the chicken back in the baking dish, spoon the creamy sauce over it, and turn the heat off. Serve immediately with fresh ground pepper.

22 Lick a fat-free Fudgsicle. What better way to get 40 grams of calcium with only 43 calories?

23 Choose brown over white rice tonight and every night. It's got three times the calcium.

24 Serve up a shrimp stir-fry tonight. Or dine on scallops or crab. Shellfish (along with dairy and meat) is rich in vitamin B$_{12}$, in which men and women 65 and older may be deficient. Low levels can result in faster bone loss, studies find.

25 Sign up for a t'ai chi class at your local community center or YMCA. Several studies found t'ai chi cut the risk of falling nearly in half and cut the rate of fractures even in people who had falls, notes Joseph Lane, M.D., chief of the metabolic bone disease service at the Hospital for Special Surgery in New York City. Ideally, you should practice t'ai chi for 10–15 minutes at a time, once or twice a week, to gain the benefit.

26 Make a container of nonfat yogurt a daily snack. With 216 milligrams of calcium, you're well on your way to your daily allowance.

27 Get your calcium in unexpected places, like calcium-fortified orange juice, calcium-fortified cereals, and frozen yogurt. Okay, you probably knew there was calcium in frozen yogurt, but the bone benefits should go a long way toward assuaging any guilt over lapping up this delectable dessert.

28 Steam up a bowl of edamame this evening. Just five minutes is all it takes to prepare these delicious soy-beans. Sprinkle with a bit of sea salt and pop the beans into your mouth as a before-dinner snack. The science is still evolving, but it seems that the natural plant estrogens in soy help strengthen bone the same way our own hormones do.

Stronger Libido, Better Sex

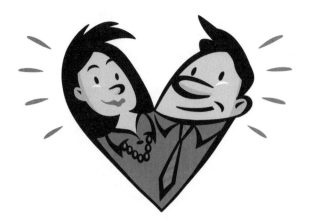

31 WAYS TO GET THERE

Your mom probably never told you this, but it's true: Sex is good for you! (Tell *that* to your spouse tonight.) Plenty of studies show it: Regular sex increases immunity from viruses, relieves stress, and even helps protect the health of a man's prostate gland by emptying fluids held there. It also triggers the release of chemicals that improve mood and ease pain.

Your doctor probably never told you this, but it's also true: Most people can and should have sex well into old age! While menopause in women does affect sexual drive and function somewhat, there is no reason healthy men or women can't experience sexual pleasure at any stage in life. Sure, the nature and intensity of the sex may change, but the love and pleasure don't!

If your sex drive has stalled out, you have good reasons to rev it back up again. You don't need jumper cables or even little blue pills. Just try a couple of these Stealth Health tips and we guarantee your engine will be turning over again in no time.

1 **Have sex tonight!** Having intercourse regularly helps to keep your sex drive in high gear by increasing the production of testosterone, which is the hormone mainly responsible for libido in both men and women.

2 **Men: If you smoke, ask your doctor to prescribe you the nicotine patch.** Why? Because it's scientifically proven that smoking can clog the blood vessels in the penis in the same way it clogs the arteries in your heart. Ever heard a better reason to quit?

3 **Go write a list of all the medicine you're taking, then check for party poopers.** More than 200 medications can cause erection problems and diminished sex drive, including drugs used to treat high blood pressure, heart disease, depression, and stomach problems. Check the Internet or ask your pharmacist or doctor if any of the drugs on your list could be culprits. Of course, you can't stop taking a drug you need, but you can talk to your doctor about possibly changing the brand, dose, or timing of your medication.

4 Spend tonight planning a steamy vacation. Even if you don't go, spending time together picturing where you'd go, looking at photos on the Web, and imagining yourself in some tropical paradise will be enough of a libido booster to get you to bed—early. Plus, it's a lot more stimulating to talk about than why your teenager is failing geometry.

5 Women: Practice Kegel exercises. You know what Kegels are—they're the squeezing exercises your doctor told you to do after pregnancy or because you were having a bit of a problem with leaking urine. What Doc probably didn't tell you is that they're also great for strengthening the pubococcygeus muscle, essential for orgasm. To do Kegels, take note of the muscle you use to stop urinary flow, then practice contracting that muscle, gradually releasing it. Work up to 20 contractions three times a day.

6 Men: Start taking supplements of ginkgo biloba every day. The herb promotes better blood flow, getting more blood to the brain and...other organs. It doesn't take much imagination to figure out how that might help you! Follow the instructions on the bottle, but check with your doctor first.

7 Make pesto and serve it over pasta tonight. Pesto contains pine nuts, great sources of arginine, the precursor for nitric oxide, a main ingredient in drugs like Viagra. Arginine helps open blood vessels so blood flow improves.

8 Go to the movies with your partner, sit in the back row, and neck like you used to when you were a teenager. You'll be combining the forbidden with

the frustrating—a sure bet to get your juices flowing.

9 Every time you pass your partner, reach out and touch or kiss him or her. Don't allow these moments to go beyond the kiss or hug. Simply increasing the amount of physical contact you have with your partner will help with desire.

10 Sprinkle 1 tablespoon wheat germ on every cup of yogurt and every bowl of cereal you eat. Wheat germ's rich in zinc, which is important to the production of that all-important hormone, testosterone. You can also get your fill of zinc in beef, eggs, and seafood—especially oysters!

11 When you're at a party or out in public with your partner, take a moment to stare at him/her across the room as if you were still wooing one another. Sex falls out of a relationship when you take one another's presence for granted. So don't!

12 Rent an erotic video and watch it with your partner. Use the time to talk about what you like and don't like during sex (and before and after).

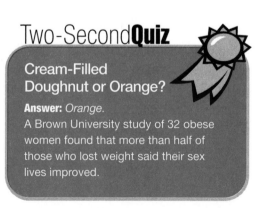

Two-Second **Quiz**

Cream-Filled Doughnut or Orange?

Answer: *Orange.*
A Brown University study of 32 obese women found that more than half of those who lost weight said their sex lives improved.

13 **Read a sexy "bodice ripper" out loud to your partner.** Play-act the parts of the ravishing heroine and her handsome, yet dangerous lover.

14 **Open your eyes when you kiss and when you are, um, intimate.** Looking into your partner's eyes during such times sends an incredible message of trust and honesty.

15 **Say exactly what's on your mind—sexually, that is.** If you're watching your husband pull out the tree stump in the backyard and you get a certain weakness in your legs watching the sweat roll off his back, tell him. If the sight of your wife comforting your teenage son after his first-ever girlfriend dumped him makes you glad all over again that you married her, tell her. Simply expressing how everyday things make you feel deepens your intimacy when said out loud.

16 **Pretend you've just met.** Remember that weak in the knees, shivers-up-your-back feeling you used to get when you first met? You can have that again. Call her and ask her out on a date. Dress up for lunch with him. Buy new underwear.

17 **Create your own intimate rituals.** No, we're not talking about sex. But what about waking him up with a steaming cup of coffee instead of the alarm every morning? What about having a hot bath ready for her in the evening? How about a special dinner out every Tuesday—when most couples are zoned out in front of the TV? Or massaging her feet while you watch a DVD with a big bowl of popcorn? The key is consistency. These are not things you do just once, but over and over again until

they become like a secret language between the two of you.

18 **Get a massage.** Or a pedicure, or a facial, or whatever makes you feel better about *yourself.* If you take care of your own body, you're much more likely to be able to enjoy it. Another good way to take care of yourself is exercise. A side benefit for both men and women: better blood flow to crucial organs.

19 **Turn the timer on for 15 minutes and talk to him (or her)** about anything other than kids, money problems, or work annoyances. Tell him about the dream you had last night. The cute teenager you saw at the diner who reminded you of yourself when you were in high school. The great presentation you made today and how it made you feel. When the timer goes off, it's your partner's turn.

20 **Go away for a couple of days— by yourself.** While you're away, make a list of all the things you love and like about your partner. Close your eyes and picture yourself making love. Call him/her and have an erotic phone conversation. By the time you get home, you'll be so greedy for each other that the front hall will look like a king-size mattress.

21 **Send the kids away and stay home together.** Make love in a different part of the house. It can be as steamy as in your bathtub or as romantic as on a blanket in front of your fireplace.

22 **Before you go to bed, take a few minutes to write out a to-do list** and a list of your worries. This gets rid of the worries that can often interfere with your ability to relax and become aroused.

Two-Second**Quiz**

23 Spend an hour with your partner touching every part of his/her body—but you can't use your hands. Use other parts of your body (including your imagination) instead. Conversely, caress one another *only* with your hands touching every part of the body except the genital zones. This can remove any pressure you might feel to "get right to it" after a hectic day on the job and is a wonderful way, at least for the woman, to relax and escape from the daily grind and transition from her other (oh-so-non-sexual) roles.

24 Open up a dozen oysters. After all, Casanova is said to have had 50 oysters every morning off the breast of a young woman in the bathtub—so they have to be good for something. Actually, as you read a few tips ago, oysters are loaded with zinc, critical for production of testosterone, the sex hormone in both men and women.

25 Stop at one (or two) drinks at the most. A small amount of alcohol can set the mood; more can drown the flame of desire, or lessen your ability to see your desire through.

26 Go purchase at least one item of sexy lingerie. Okay, this is for the ladies...but the feel of soft silk against your skin will help wake up those sensuality nerve endings. And who knows what will happen when *that* happens?

27 Re-create your favorite sexy scene in a movie. You know the ones—the lobster scene in *Flashdance*. The ice scene in *9½ Weeks*. Mena Suvari's cheerleading routine in *American Beauty,* Clark Gable carrying Vivien Leigh up the stairs in *Gone With the Wind*, the pottery scene in *Ghost*, the part in The *Bridges of Madison County* when Meryl Streep and Clint Eastwood dance in her kitchen. Whew!

28 Create a romance CD for him (or her). Have it playing when your partner returns home. Light a few scented candles while you're at it. Who knows what might ensue?

29 Tell your partner two things you love about him/her every day. Love, affection, and mutual respect are the bases for a steamy sex life.

30 Call your partner at work. Tell him or her in no uncertain terms what you would like to do when he or she gets home. Another option: Set up a private e-mail account and e-mail the message.

31 Do something physical together, like skiing, a long country walk, a stroll along a beach, canoeing. Such activities let you see one another in a different light, creating a sense of physical vitality that readily translates into intimacy.

Combating Allergies

20 WAYS TO STOP BEING SNEEZY

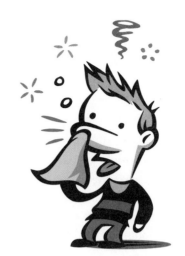

If the drip, sniff, sneeze, and itch of allergies have you thinking of buying stock in the company that makes Kleenex, dry your eyes and prepare to take action. You're going to wage battle inside your house and even inside your body to reduce the number of allergy attacks you suffer and minimize those so-annoying symptoms. Allergies may not be life-threatening, but they're nothing to sneeze at either. Here are 20 of the best ways to protect yourself. Plus, turn to "Cleaning," page 74, for more on safe, healthy ways to purge your home of allergens.

1 Choose chicken instead of beef. A two-year study of 334 adults with hay fever and 1,336 without found those who had the most trans oleic acid in their diets, a form of monounsaturated fat found primarily in meat and dairy products, were nearly three times as likely to have hay fever as those who ate the least. Don't worry, olive oil is okay; although it's got a lot of oleic acid, it's not the "trans" form.

2 Pop a fish-oil supplement every morning after you brush your teeth. A study of people with allergic asthma (asthma caused by allergies) found those who took daily fish-oil supplements for a month had lower levels of leukotrienes, chemicals that contribute to the allergic reaction.

3 Turn on the AC. Air conditioners remove mold-friendly moisture and filter allergens entering the house. Just make sure to clean or change the filters often or you'll just make things worse.

4 Eat one kiwifruit every morning. They're rich in vitamin C, which acts as a natural antihistamine. Some studies link low levels of C with allergies. When your allergies are flaring up, consider taking a vitamin C supplement.

5 Steam vacuum your furniture and carpets and include a solution of disodium octaborate tetrahydrate (DOT), a boron-based product, in the water. A 2004 study published in the journal *Allergy* found DOT cut dust mite populations and their associated allergen levels to undetectable levels for up to six months.

6 Take 250 milligrams of quercetin three times a day. This natural supplement is a potent anti-inflammatory flavonoid, and it is widely used in natural medicine practices to fight allergies.

7 Clean out your gutters and make sure they're not clogged. Clogged gutters can result in water seeping into the house, leading to mold growth, which can exacerbate allergies. Next time it rains, check your gutters. If you see water leaking out of end caps, flowing on the outside, or dripping behind them, it's time to get out the ladder.

8 Always run the exhaust fan and/or leave the window and door open when taking a shower or bath. Another option is to run a small portable fan (away from water sources) during and after showers. Again, you're trying to keep surfaces dry and prevent the growth of mold. Also, check to see that the vent on the outside of your house where the exhaust exits isn't blocked by leaves.

9 Wash the shower curtain in hot water and bleach every month. Or use a shower liner that you can replace every couple of months for just a few bucks.

10 Keep your thermostat set above 65°F in the winter. If you set it too low, you're encouraging the growth of mold in damp air. The heat dries out the air, preventing mold growth. Of course, too-dry air can also irritate your lungs and sinuses. The perfect humidity in a home is around 50 percent.

11 Wash all your bedding in very hot water every week. It's the best way to kill those pesky microscopic dust mites that love your bed even more than you do.

12 Follow your dryer vent and make sure it's vented to the outside. For every load of laundry you dry, 20 pounds of moisture has to go somewhere! If your dryer is vented to the garage or basement, you're just asking for mold buildup.

13 Clean the tray under the fridge with a bleach solution and sprinkle with salt. The tray is a veritable mold magnet. Adding salt reduces the growth of mold and bacteria. Also, clean under the refrigerator occasionally; food can become trapped there, become moldy, and the mold spores are blown into the kitchen every time the compressor kicks in.

14 Water your plants sparingly and put pebbles on top of the dirt to discourage mold spores from getting into the air. Overwatering houseplants can contribute to the growth of mold. Also, water might leak through the plant onto the carpet.

15 Spend this weekend decluttering. Throw out or give away coats and other clothing you haven't used in the past year. Put sports equipment in the garage or basement where it belongs. Slip shoes into hanging shoe bags. When you finish, you should be able to see all your closets' floors and back

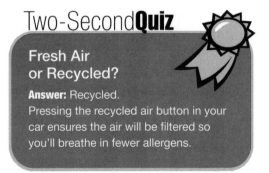

Two-Second**Quiz**

Fresh Air or Recycled?

Answer: Recycled.
Pressing the recycled air button in your car ensures the air will be filtered so you'll breathe in fewer allergens.

walls. Now give everything a good vacuum and you'll have significantly reduced the amount of dust in your house.

16 Keep your bedroom door shut so your dog and/or cat can't get in. Let him bark or meow. You spend more time in your bedroom than any other room of the house, and this keeps down cat and dog dander, to which many people are allergic.

17 Choose a doormat made of synthetic material. Doormats made of natural material (wicker, etc.) can break down and become excellent feeding grounds for mites, mold, and fungus, and then get tracked into the house. Wash all mats weekly.

18 Clean all dead insects from your porch lights. As they decompose, they can become an allergen source.

19 Put a shelf by the front door for shoes and encourage your family and guests to remove their shoes before entering to reduce the amount of dust, mold, and other allergens tracked in. Keep some soft slippers in a basket by the front door for people who don't want to walk around in their stocking feet.

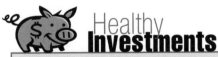

Healthy Investments

Hard-Surface Flooring

Okay, this is an expensive one. But it's worth it. Carpets are breeding grounds for dust mites and mold, and do a wonderful job of capturing animal dander and pollen—only to release it every time you vacuum or even just walk on it. Wood, tile, or laminate floors are the best for people with allergies.

Herbal Allergy Remedies

Before there was Claritin, there was **butterbur**, a herbaceous plant whose extracts have been used to treat allergies and asthma for centuries. In modern times, a study comparing it to the prescription allergy drug Zyrtec (cetirizine) found people taking either one had the same level of improvement in their symptoms, but those taking Zyrtec were more likely to report drowsiness.

Other herbs that have some scientific support behind them include **chamomile** and **peppermint** (try them both as teas), **grapeseed extract,** and **stinging nettle** (make sure you're not allergic to the weed). Remember: Always check with your health-care professional or pharmacist before taking any alternative remedies if you're already taking prescription or over-the-counter medications.

20 Read labels and avoid foods that contain the additive monosodium benzoate. An Italian study found that monosodium benzoate triggered allergy-like symptoms, including runny, stuffy nose, sneezing, and nasal itching, in adults without allergies. The preservative is often found in juices, pie fillings, pickles, olives, and salad dressings.

Improving Your Vision

24 WAYS TO SEE CLEARLY FOREVER

They are two of your most precious possessions, but chances are, you take your eyes for granted. Most of us do. But think for a second what life would be like without being able to gaze on your grandchild or your flower garden or even navigate the kitchen without incident. Prevent Blindness America, a nonprofit organization dedicated to vision issues, estimates that 50,000 people lose their sight needlessly every year and that 80 million Americans are at risk of eye diseases that can lead to low vision and even blindness.

The good news: The most common diseases—age-related macular degeneration (ARMD), cataracts, glaucoma, and dry eye disease—are all preventable to some extent. Read on to see (pun intended) how you can get Stealth Healthy protection for your peepers. Before we go any further, we have to tell you that the first step, if you smoke, is to stop. Smoking increases your risk of cataracts, glaucoma, dry eyes, and age-related macular degeneration.

1 **Mix a cup of blueberries with a cup of yogurt for breakfast this morning.** Blueberries are one of the richest fruit forms of antioxidants, and a study published in *The Archives of Ophthalmology* found that women and men who ate the greatest amount of fruit were the least likely to develop age-related macular degeneration (ARMD), the leading cause of blindness in older people.

2 **Spread bilberry jam on your morning toast.** Or take a bilberry supplement every morning. The berries contain compounds called anthocyanosides, which may protect the retina against macular degeneration.

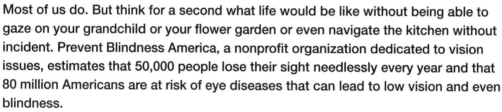

3 **Have spinach twice a week.** Could be a spinach quiche, steamed spinach, or maybe Tuscan spinach—sautéed in some olive oil with garlic and raisins. Regardless, be sure to get your spinach. Studies find that lutein, a nutrient that is particularly abundant in spinach, may prevent age-related macular degeneration and cataracts. Ideally, get your lutein in combination with some form of fat (olive oil works great) for the best absorption.

4 Cook with red onions, not yellow. Red onions contain far more quercetin, an antioxidant that is thought to protect against cataracts.

5 Aim your car vents at your feet—not your eyes. Dry, air-conditioned air will suck the moisture out of eyes like a sponge. Aim the vents in your car away from your eyes, or wear sunglasses as a shield. Dry eyes can be more than an inconvenience; serious dryness can lead to corneal abrasions and even blindness if left untreated.

6 Move your computer screen to just below eye level. Your eyes will close slightly when you're staring at the computer, minimizing fluid evaporation and the risk of dry eye syndrome, says John Sheppard, M.D., who directs the ophthalmology residency program at Eastern Virginia Medical School in Norfolk, Virginia.

7 Take a multivitamin every day. Make it a habit, like brushing your teeth. A major study suggested that if every American at risk for age-related macular degeneration took daily supplements of antioxidant vitamins and zinc, more than 300,000 people could avoid ARMD-associated vision loss over the next five years. Other studies find that women who took vitamin C supplements for at least 10 years were 77 percent less likely to show initial signs of cataracts than those who took no supplemental C. So take a multi with at least 150 mg vitamin C, or take a separate C supplement.

8 Walk at least four times a week. Some evidence suggests that regular exercise can reduce the intraocular pressure, or IOP, in people with glaucoma. In one study, glaucoma patients who walked briskly four times per week for 40 minutes lowered their IOP enough so they could stop taking medication for their condition. It's also possible—although there's no proof yet—that walking could also reduce your overall risk of developing glaucoma.

9 Eat fish twice a week. A study from Harvard researchers presented at the 2003 Association for Research in Vision and Ophthalmology's annual meeting evaluated the diets of 32,470 women and found those who ate the least amount of fish (thus getting the least amount of omega-3 fatty acids) had the highest risk of dry eye syndrome. Even tuna fish (yes, the kind that comes in a can) protected against the syndrome. If you can't stand fish, or are worried about mercury consumption, try fish-oil supplements to get your omega-3s.

10 Twice a week, walk away from greasy or sweet snacks. A 2001 study found that people whose diets were high in omega-3 fatty acids and low in omega-6 fatty acids (found in many

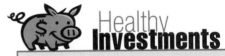

Healthy
Investments

Sunglasses

Make sure they are close-fitting, preferably wraparound, and block 99-100 percent of UVA and UVB rays. Step outside while wearing them before you buy to make sure they do a good job of blocking glare and yet aren't too dark. To save money if you need prescription sunglasses, have your optician or optometrist darken the lenses on an existing pair of glasses, or buy a pair of drugstore sunglasses and then have lenses made for those less-expensive frames.

fat-filled snack foods like commercially prepared pie, cake, cookies, and potato chips) were significantly less likely to develop ARMD than those whose diets were high in omega-6 fatty acids and low in omega-3 fatty acids. In fact, if your diet was high in omega-6 at all—even if you still ate plenty of fish—the protective effects of the omega-3 fatty acids disappeared.

11 **Have sweet potatoes for dinner tonight.** Since they are rich in vitamin A, these sweet spuds can help improve your night vision.

12 **Turn down the heat in your house.** Heat dries out the air, which, in turn, dries out your eyes. In the winter, you might also try adding some humidity with a humidifier or even bunching a lot of plants together in the room in which you spend the most time.

13 **Wear sunglasses whenever you leave the house.** When researchers examined the relationship between exposure to sunlight and cataracts or ARMD in Chesapeake Bay fishermen, they found that fishermen who protected their eyes from the harsh glare of the sun and its damaging UV rays were significantly less likely to develop these conditions than those who went bare-eyed. Wear the sunglasses even when it's not sunny out, says Dr. Sheppard. They protect your eyes from the drying effects of wind. See "Healthy Investments," on page 279, for tips on choosing the right sunglasses.

14 **Wear a broad-brimmed hat along with your sunglasses.** A wide-brimmed hat or cap will block roughly 50 percent of the UV radiation

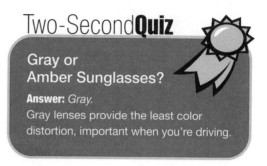

Two-Second Quiz

Gray or Amber Sunglasses?
Answer: *Gray.*
Gray lenses provide the least color distortion, important when you're driving.

and reduce the UV radiation that may enter your eyes from above or around glasses.

15 **Pick some Southern greens for dinner tonight.** Because they are high in lutein and zeaxanthin, greens like collards and kale (delicious when lightly steamed with a splash of hot pepper vinegar) may reduce your risk of developing both cataracts and ARMD, and may even slow progression of these diseases once they've begun. Both have strong antioxidant properties, which may help repair some of the damage that contributes to both conditions.

16 **Roast some fresh beets for an eye-saving side dish.** Beets get their deep red color from phytochemicals called anthocyanins, powerful antioxidants that protect the smaller blood vessels in your body, including those in your eyes.

17 **Switch to "lite" salt or use spices and herbs instead of salt.** Studies find that high-salt diets increase your risk of certain types of cataracts, so stay away from the salty stuff. And while you're de-salting your diet, don't forget the salt in processed foods. Check labels for "no-salt" or "no-sodium," or "low-salt" or "low-sodium" tags when buying canned and other prepared foods.

18 Dab an essential oil of jasmine, peppermint, or vanilla on your arm and sniff. Jasmine, says scent researcher Alan R. Hirsch, M.D., of the Chicago-based Smell and Taste Treatment Research Foundation, increases the beta waves in the frontal lobes of your brain, promoting wakefulness and enabling you to focus better and see things more acutely. All three scents stimulate the limbic system in your brain, which, in turn, stimulates the rods in your eyes, which help you see in dim light.

19 When you're working or reading, set your alarm to beep every 30 minutes. Use this as a reminder to look up and away from your computer or book to some distant point for 30 seconds. This helps prevent eye fatigue and eyestrain.

20 Check your blood pressure every month. You can do this yourself with a home blood pressure kit, at the doctor's office, or at the pharmacy. The two leading causes of blindness in the United States are high blood pressure and diabetes, both of which damage blood vessels. For more on controlling blood pressure, turn to page 244. For more on maintaining healthy blood sugar levels, check out page 248.

21 Replace your mascara every three months and other eye makeup once a year. Eye makeup is a great repository for bacteria, which can easily be transferred to your eyes and cause infections.

22 Use eye makeup remover every night before going to bed. This prevents small pieces of mascara from winding up in your eye and possibly scratching your cornea.

23 Wear goggles when you're doing carpentry or even yard work. Debris in the eye can lead to corneal abrasions, which can ultimately damage your vision. Also use protective goggles when you're swimming to protect your eyes from the chlorine.

24 Use a fresh towel every time you wipe your face. Sharing face towels is a great way to get conjunctivitis, the infection also known as pinkeye.

Improving Your Hearing

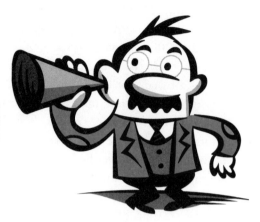

18 WAYS TO HEAR A PIN DROP

If you spent your youth hanging out at rock concerts or mowing lawns without ear protection, chances are you're paying for it now with a bit of age-related hearing loss. Do visiting family members casually mention that your TV is blaring? Do you keep asking people to repeat themselves? You're not alone. Roughly one-third of Americans over 60, and 40-50 percent of those 75 and older, have hearing loss. And plenty of younger adults have it as well, thanks to the rock-and-roll era. (Want objective input on your hearing? Schedule a hearing test with a licensed audiologist, recommended every couple of years from age 50 on. Check out the American Academy of Audiology at www.audiology.org to find a professional near you.)

Unfortunately, once you lose your hearing, you can't get it back without help from hearing aids. Here's how to protect what you have left:

1 **Go for a hike in the woods.** Not only will the silence help you focus better on sounds, but researchers find that physically fit people tend to have better hearing than those who aren't in good shape. The reason? Aerobic exercise brings more oxygen into your system and improves blood flow to your ears.

2 **Scoop up the guacamole at your next picnic.** Guacamole is rich in magnesium. Studies find low levels of magnesium might make you more suscep-tible to noise-induced hearing loss.

3 **Switch to decaf coffee and low-sodium soups.** Caffeine appears to interfere with blood flow to the ear, while salt can lead to fluid retention, which can cause swelling in the functional

organs of the ear. Plus, studies find that people with high blood pressure are more likely to have age-related hearing loss than those with normal pressures.

4 **Quit smoking and stay away from other smokers.** A study published in the *Journal of the American Medical Association* found that the more exposure you receive to cigarette smoke, the more likely you are to experience age-related hearing loss.

5 **Wear earplugs when you use the weed whacker or go to the shooting range.** Although it's only common sense that the deafening blast from a shotgun would affect your hearing, several studies back this up, finding that recreational firearm use can lead to marked high-frequency hearing loss. Other studies

find significantly increased hearing loss in people who pursue woodworking as a hobby, or ride motorcycles, snowmobiles, and other off-road vehicles.

6 **Sip a beer or glass of wine, but don't overdo it.** Believe it or not, moderate drinking can protect against age-related hearing loss. But excessive amounts may actually contribute to hearing loss.

7 **Brush your teeth at least twice a day and floss after every meal.** For some reason, there's a connection between the number of teeth you've lost and your hearing, with researchers finding that the more teeth you still have in your mouth in old age, the better your hearing. No, dentures don't count!

8 **Serve a whole grain bread and split-pea soup for lunch.** Whole grains and legumes are great sources of B vitamins, which studies find protect the neurons and blood vessels connected to the cochlea, the tiny bone found in your inner ear. Also, one study published in *The American Journal of Clinical Nutrition* found that women with hearing problems had low blood levels of vitamin B_{12} and folate.

9 **Drink a glass of skim milk every morning.** The calcium and vitamin D found in milk are critical for keeping the bones in your ear, especially the cochlea, healthy. One study of 70 healthy women found that those with hearing loss had much lower spinal density (a measure of bone strength) and calcium intake than women with normal hearing.

10 **Bake a sweet potato for dinner tonight.** A wonderful source of vitamin A, it can also help your hearing because, according to animal studies, too little of this nutrient may increase the inner ear's sensitivity to noise, thus potentially increasing the risk of noise-induced hearing loss.

11 **Tape a tennis ball into the back of your partner's PJs (use duct tape).** It's a great way to prevent snoring. Some people who really saw wood produce about as much noise as a chain saw, or so it seems. Over time, that noise can damage your ears. Another option: Send the snoring one to the couch.

12 **Wear your seat belt and drive defensively, not aggressively.** That way you're less likely to get into an accident, which means your airbags are less likely to inflate. British researchers find that inflating airbags are loud enough to contribute to hearing loss. Additionally, head trauma is a major cause of hearing loss.

13 **Get five servings of veggies a day.** When researchers explored the connection between a variety of lifestyle factors and sudden deafness in 109 patients,

Two-Second Quiz

Turn Up the Sound or Move Closer?

Answer: *Move closer.*

Also, listen more closely. Any effort you can make to listen at quieter levels should help to preserve hearing, says Suzanne Hasenstab, Ph.D., director of audiology and professor of otolaryngology at Virginia Commonwealth University in Richmond. If you cannot comfortably hear another person talking to you in the same room within six feet, the TV is probably too loud.

comparing their deaf patients to those with normal hearing, they found those who ate the most fresh veggies had the lowest risk of sudden deafness. You can find lots of easy ways to sneak more vegetables into your diet starting on page 91.

 14 Ask your doctor to clean out the wax in your ears. That's often all that's needed to improve your hearing. Just don't try it yourself; sticking pointed objects into your ear canal is a no-no. If you want to de-wax at home, try wax-softening ear drops, sold at drugstores. Follow up with some forceful squirts of warm water from a bulb syringe (also sold in drugstores) to get the softened wax out.

How Loud Is Too Loud?

The National Institute on Deafness and Other Communication Disorders (NIDCD) notes that exposure of just one minute to sounds of 110 decibels or higher can damage your hearing. No more than 15 minutes of unprotected exposure is recommended for noises of 100 decibels, as well as several hours exposure to noises of 90 decibels or higher. Here's the decibel level of some common noises:

- 140 decibels: rock concerts, firecrackers
- 120 decibels: boom cars, snowmobiles
- 110 decibels: chain saw
- 100 decibels: woodshop
- 90 decibels: lawn mower, motorcycle
- 80 decibels: city traffic noise
- 60 decibels: normal conversation
- 40 decibels: refrigerator humming
- 20 decibels: whispered voice
- 0 decibels: threshold of normal hearing

---

15 Go to bed and rest when you have a cold. That gives your body the strength it needs to fight off the infection and reduces the risk that the cold will develop into something more serious, like an upper respiratory tract infection or ear infection, which can eventually affect your hearing.

16 Make earplugs a regular part of your wardrobe. Keep a pair in your purse, in your car, in the garage with the gardening tools, and by the lawn mower, suggests Suzanne Hasenstab, Ph.D., director of audiology and professor of otolaryngology at Virginia Commonwealth University in Richmond. So if you're cutting the grass, find yourself in the car next to someone blaring the bass, or realize too late that the live music is a little too live, you're always prepared to protect your hearing.

17 Have a friend stand next to you while you're plugged into your iPod (or Walkman or other musical device). If your friend can hear the sound through your earphones, says Dr. Hasenstab, you've got the volume turned up too loud.

18 Try a ginkgo biloba supplement. Some studies suggest the herb might not only help with ringing in the ears, or tinnitus, but may also help treat some types of hearing loss by improving blood flow to the ears. The herb takes weeks to work, so be patient.

Sharpen Your Sense of Smell and Taste

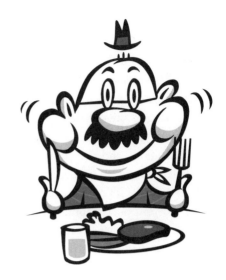

20 SENSIBLE STRATEGIES

We all know that feeling of having a bad taste in our mouth, or the way a stuffy nose makes even the most fragrant garlic pizza taste like cardboard. But did you know that our sense of smell and taste naturally declines as we age? Often the change is so gradual you barely notice it. That wouldn't be a problem, except that it can affect your health—studies find people with impaired ability to smell and taste tend to follow less healthful diets. It also puts you in danger: Your sense of smell serves as an early warning system for things like rotten food and gas leaks.

Here's how to sustain smell and taste so that every bite (and sniff) tells you what you need to know:

1 **Serve food that looks like itself.** Forget fancy-schmancy presentation. If you're serving fish, keep it looking like a fish. Your sense of taste is stronger if your brain can connect what you're eating with how it looks.

2 **Put on your seat belt.** A common cause of loss of smell (which then directly affects taste) is automobile accidents, even low-speed crashes, says Alan Hirsch, M.D., neurological director of the Smell and Taste Treatment and Research Foundation in Chicago. Any impact can shift the brain within your skull, tearing delicate nerve fibers that connect your nose to your brain.

3 **Go for a brisk, 10-minute walk or run.** Our sense of smell is higher after exercise. Researchers suspect it might be related to additional moisture in the nose.

4 **Drink a glass of water every hour or so.** Dry mouth—whether due to medication or simply dehydration—can adversely affect your sense of taste, says Evan Reiter, M.D., an otolaryngologist at Virginia Commonwealth University's Eye & Ear Specialty Center in Richmond.

5 **Shuck a dozen oysters.** Among their other benefits, oysters are one of the highest food sources of zinc, and zinc

deficiencies contribute to a loss of smell as well as taste.

6 **Make a list of any medicines you're taking** and ask your doctor about their effect on smell and taste. Hundreds of medications affect taste and smell, including statins, antidepressants, high blood pressure medications, and chemotherapy drugs like methotrexate, also used to treat rheumatoid arthritis. If your meds are on the list, talk to your doctor about possible alternatives or lower doses. Don't, however, stop taking your medication or cut your dosage on your own.

7 **Stub out that cigarette and make it your last.** Nothing screws up the smell receptors in your nose and the taste receptors on your tongue like cigarettes. Long-term smoking can even permanently damage the olfactory (a.k.a., sniffing) nerves in the back of your nose.

8 **Eat only when you are hungry.** Our sense of smell (and thus taste) is strongest when we're hungriest.

9 **Humidify your air in the winter.** Our sense of smell is strongest in the summer and spring, says Dr. Hirsch, most likely because of the higher moisture content in the air.

10 **Eat in a restaurant or with other people.** Dr. Hirsch calls this the "herd response." He cites studies that find that eating in the presence of other people makes food taste better than eating alone.

11 **Stay away from the diaper pail and other stinky smells.** Prolonged exposure to bad smells (like the sewer plant up the road) tends to wipe out your ability to smell, says Dr. Hirsch. So if you must be exposed to such odors on a prolonged basis, wear a mask over your nose and mouth that filters out some of the bad smells.

12 **Add spices to your food.** Even if your sense of smell and taste has plummeted, you should still retain full function in your "irritant" nerve, which is the nerve that makes you cry when you cut an onion, or makes your eyes water when you taste peppermint or smell ammonia. So use spices like hot chili powder to spice up your food.

13 **Blow your nose and clean it out with saline spray.** A simple thing, but it can help, because a blocked nose means blocked nerve receptors.

14 **Chew thoroughly and slowly.** This releases more flavor and extends the time that the food lingers in your mouth so it spends more time in contact with your taste buds. Even before you start chewing, stir your food around. This has the effect of aerating the molecules in the food, releasing more of their scent.

Two-Second**Quiz**

Airline Food or Bring Your Own Food?

Answer: *Bring your own food.* And put some hot peppers on whatever you bring. The dry air of an airplane affects your sense of smell and taste, making anything you eat while aloft taste worse. That's one reason airline food is often heavily salted and sugared—to compensate for the blandness.

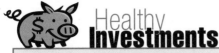

Healthy Investments

A Neti Pot or Sinus Irrigator

These are particularly useful if you're subject to recurrent sinusitis. Clearing out your sinuses not only improves your sense of smell, but can also help get rid of the bad taste in your mouth that often comes with a sinus infection.

15 Stick to one glass of wine or beer. Dr. Hirsch's research finds the sense of smell declines as blood alcohol levels rise.

 16 Eat a different food with every forkful. Instead of eating the entire steak at once, then moving on to the potato, take a bite of steak, then a bite of potato, then a bite of spinach, etc. Recurrent new exposures to the scent will keep your olfactory nerves from getting bored, thus enhancing your taste buds.

17 Make an appointment with an allergist. Stop trying to treat recurrent allergies or runny nose with over-the-counter products. See an expert.

There are a range of lifestyle changes and medications that can have you breathing clearly (thus improving your sense of smell and taste) in just a week or so.

18 Reset your taste for sugar and salt by cutting them out for at least a week. Processed foods have so much sugar and salt that you'll practically stop tasting them if you eat these foods often. Try this experiment: Check the salt content of your favorite cereal, and if it's more than 200 mg sodium per serving, switch to a low-sodium brand for two weeks. Once you switch back, you'll suddenly taste all the salt you were overlooking. Same goes for sugar.

19 Avoid very hot foods and fluids. They can damage your taste buds.

20 Try sniff therapy. It is possible to train your nose (and brain) to notice smells better. Start by sniffing something with a strong odor for a couple of minutes several times a day. Do this continually for three or four months and you should notice your sense of smell getting stronger—at least where that particular item is involved, says Dr. Hirsch.

REMINDER

 Fast Results
These are bits of advice that deliver benefits particularly quickly—in some cases, immediately!

Easy Gains
These are tips that give the biggest value for the least amount of effort.

 Super Effective
These are tips proven to be particularly effective through scientific research or widespread usage by experts.

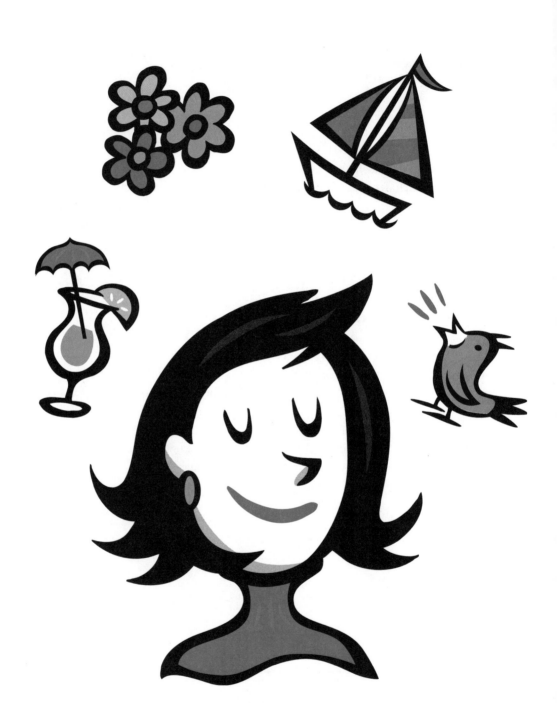

PART SIX

Stealth Healthy

MENTAL RELIEF

Attitudes can harm, and attitudes can heal—science has proved both beyond question. For better health, here's how to replace stress and worry with calm and happiness.

Defusing Stress
37 Ways to Calm Down Fast

Defusing Anger
25 Ways to Release
Your Emotional Steam

Dealing With Anxiety
17 Ways to Stay Settled

Depression
17 Ways to Banish the Blues

Dealing With Guilt
22 Tips for a Cleaner
Conscience

**Dealing With the
Uncontrollable**
13 Ways to Maintain
a Healthy Perspective

**Enhancing Your
Sense of Humor**
19 Ways to Bring Out
the Laughter Inside You

Improving Memory
27 Tricks to Keep Your
Brain In Shape

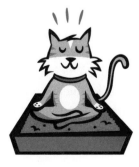

Defusing Stress

37 WAYS TO CALM DOWN FAST

It's 4:45 p.m., when your dimwit boss (who, by the way, is 20 years your junior) orders you to finish a lengthy task before you leave. As you're doing a slow burn over that, the phone rings. It's your 19-year-old son hitting you up for money to cover his car payment—again. Never mind that the car he drives is flashier and more expensive than anything you've ever owned. When you finally drag home at 7 p.m., you discover your spouse is out with friends and didn't bother to leave any dinner. As you open the mail over your can of soup, you get sideswiped by a 401(k) statement devastated by a tumbling stock market. At this rate, you'll be lucky if you can retire at 93.

Let's face it. Some days it seems as if life throws you stress left, right, up, and down. It can drain your energy, destroy your good mood, and challenge your outlook. Those are the obvious mental repercussions. But science has shown that stress is not merely a metaphysical thing. We have discovered that stress causes your body to release hormones that raise blood pressure, speed up your heart and breathing, halt digestion, cause a surge in blood sugar, and more. When stress is ongoing—such as the stress caused by money problems, bad relationships, or an overburdensome job—this constant physical reaction can significantly raise your risk of colds, diabetes, heart disease, back troubles, and almost every other major health concern. Indeed, stress is emerging as one of the principal contributors to poor health in modern countries.

There's more. On a daily basis, stress often leads to unhealthy habits. A really bad day pushes you to the nearest doughnut or ice-cream store. It saps your willingness to exercise or eat well or have fun. It causes you to tune out the world, to sit in front of the television and ignore your relationships.

And yet stress can be relatively easy to manage. All it takes is a mental commitment to it—and an open mind. Old-fashioned thinkers scoff at things like deep breathing, positive thinking, and guided imagery. Some are also put off by the openness and public display of emotions involved in some stress-relief methods. But these are scientifically proven to work, doctors endorse and recommend them, and the benefits are fast and real. These Stealth Healthy approaches to stress management work. Give several a try.

1 Embrace the number one truth about stress: Only you create it. Stress isn't defined as a large workload, a difficult child, or a rise in terrorism. Stress is *your physical and mental reaction* to these external stimuli. Remember the truism about alcoholism? The one that says admitting you are an alcoholic is more than 50 percent of the cure? The same is true for stress: Embracing the fact that stress is your reaction to external stimuli—and not the stimuli themselves—is half the battle toward managing it. You can't change a crazy world. But you can learn to handle it with humor, humility, and hope. Not coincidentally, virtually every stress-relief method that follows is about how to improve your reaction to external factors.

2 Give your partner a hug every day before work. It's so simple, yet so often overlooked when you're trying to make your lunch, find your shoes and keys, and get on the highway before rush-hour gridlock. Research from the University of North Carolina at Chapel Hill found that the few seconds it takes to hug your partner can help you remain calm as chaos unfolds around you.

3 Buy yourself flowers once a week and display them prominently on your desk. Women who sat near a bouquet of flowers were more relaxed during a typing assignment than women who didn't have flowers, according to a Kansas State University study of 90 women.

4 Take a deep breath and then try to see yourself in someone else's shoes. As for your dimwit boss and others who seem to try to annoy you, know that they are probably experiencing just as much inner turmoil as they are creating around them, says Jay Winner, M.D., a family physician, stress-management teacher in Santa Barbara, California, and author of *Stress Management Made Simple: Effective Ways to Beat Stress for Better Health.* "When people are rude, they are usually suffering in one way or another," says Dr. Winner.

5 Use the otherwise stressful time of waiting in line as a chance to relax. When you make a split decision about which line of cars to pull behind at a tollbooth or which line of carts to stand behind at the grocery store, chances are some *other* line will move more quickly. In the worst-case scenario, one of the customers in front of you needs not one, but two price checks—and then comes up short on cash and must void out some of the items the clerk just rang up. Rather than sending your stress hormones into the stratosphere as you steam over your bad luck, think about how busy you usually are and recognize the time—in reality, usually just a few minutes—as a gift in which you can just relax, says Dr. Winner.

Healthy Investments

The Shoulder Triggerpoint Pillow

The weight of this pillow, which fits around your shoulders and neck, relaxes hunched shoulders, relieving muscle tension. Put it on at the end of a stressful day to soothe away muscle tension and transition more smoothly—and calmly—to home life. It is available from Mother Earth Designs (call 800-344-2072 or visit their Web site at www.motherearthpillows.com).

"As you wait, think about things in life for which you are grateful, meditate on your breath, talk to one of the other customers, or look at a magazine."

6 **Develop a ritual in the morning that focuses on calmness, beauty, people who support you,** or anything that helps you feel a sense of peace. You might, for example, spend a few moments reminding yourself of your blessings. Joan Lang, M.D., chair of the department of psychiatry at Saint Louis University School of Medicine, says she finds daily balance each morning by making a mental note to do something spiritual, something nurturing for herself and for someone else, and something physical. Your ritual might involve sitting outside (weather permitting), taking in your surroundings, and appreciating the sounds of the birds and the sights of sun glistening off the leaves and grass. If you can't sit outdoors, go to a room in your home that you find calming. Settle down, take a few deep breaths, and call to mind three people or things that make your life worth living. As your inner gratitude builds, pledge to commit one small act during the day that will help someone else—either someone

you know or a perfect stranger—experience this same inner gratitude.

7 **Twice a day, breathe deeply for three to five minutes.** As you breathe, focus your mind on your breath and push all other distracting thoughts from your consciousness, suggests Rocco Lo Bosco, a massage therapist, yoga instructor, and author of *Buddha Wept*.

8 **Walk the stress off.** Stress hormones prepare your body for a physical response. A healthy way to respond to a rush of stress, then, is to get physical. Go for a brisk 15-minute walk and burn off your nervous energy. Use the time to think through the issue and return to a positive, peaceful frame of mind.

9 **When you get out of bed in the morning,** spend a few minutes consciously sensing your body from toes to head. Focus on the feet first. Notice how they feel from the inside out and mentally relax them. Then move upward to your ankles, then to your knees, on up your legs to your torso, chest, upper back, neck, head, and face. As you get used to the technique, you can bring your awareness inside your body and focus on relaxing each body part whenever you start to feel stressed, suggests Lo Bosco.

10 **Designate one person to whom you can vent your frustrations.** Complaining widely about your work or family frustrations is not a healthy hobby to have—not only does it keep you in a negative frame of mind, but it's not very good for your professional or personal relationships either. The solution: Designate one trustworthy friend or family member to be your confidant. Someone

who is discreet and knows just to listen and not to attempt to solve all your problems. Use that person to listen as you openly voice your stresses and how they are affecting you. Then, to the rest of the world, present yourself as positive and in control. Admit to stress, but don't detail it. You'll be amazed at how acting that way can make it a reality!

11 When you're ready to rip out your hair, phone a friend. People who have strong social ties live longer. A diversionary conversation with a close romantic partner, friend, or family member helps prevent stress hormones from triggering high blood pressure and other health complications.

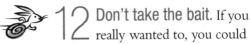 **12** Don't take the bait. If you really wanted to, you could spend your entire life angry at the world—at the rude salesclerks, the bad bosses, the crazy drivers, the lousy politicians, the unfair prices for a good piece of salmon. Happy, low-stress people choose not to get angry, even when the opportunity is dangled right in front of them. Practice this. The next time someone does something that could—maybe even *should*—anger you, smile instead and say to yourself, "I'm not going to take the bait."

13 Don't respond to anger with anger. Confrontations tend to escalate. Next time you suddenly find yourself on the receiving end of aggression,

 In**Perspective**

Learn to Breathe

You already know how to breathe, right? You do it every moment, every day, without even thinking about. Chances are, though, your breathing technique is not as healthy as you might think. Most of us breathe too shallowly, too quickly. Our lungs and heart would greatly prefer longer, slower, deeper breaths. This is true for general health, and it is also true for managing stress. Deep breathing helps dissipate the fight-or-flight reaction so many of us experience when we're stressed. It sends a signal to your brain to slow down, which results in hormonal and physiological changes that slow heart rate and lower blood pressure.

You might be surprised that there are lots of big books written on breathing method. That's because proper breathing technique is crucial for everyone from athletes to people with asthma to yoga experts. But for us regular folk, there are only a few things you need to keep in mind:

● In general, inhale slowly and deeply through the nose. A healthy inhale takes about five seconds.

● In general, exhale slowly through the mouth. Empty your lungs completely. Good breathers focus more on thorough exhalation than on inhalation.

● Engage your diaphragm for good breathing. The diaphragm is the sheet of muscle along the top of your abdomen that pulls your lungs down to draw in air, and then pushes your lungs up to expel carbon dioxide. With a good inhalation, your lungs puff up as your diaphragm drops. With a good exhale, your diaphragm rises. If you don't feel this muscle moving, deepen your breaths even more.

● Work toward breathing just six or eight deep breaths per minute. Most of us breathe more than 20 times a minute.

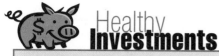

Healthy Investments

A Yoga, Pilates, or Stretching Book

For $20 or so, you can learn all types of moves that soothe your muscles, calm your spirit, and improve your health. Five to 10 minutes of stretching or yoga positions each day can go a long way toward defusing stress.

don't automatically respond with the same. Take a breath, pause, then respond calmly and honestly, without undue defensiveness. If the other person won't engage constructively or is being irrational, then smile and excuse yourself, with the message that you'll be happy to discuss the issue when the person regains his composure or reason.

14 **Carry around a lucky "rabbit's foot" that helps you feel calm.** Your "rabbit's foot" might come in the form of a photograph of your grandchildren, a favorite poem, or a Bible verse. Carry it around and focus on it whenever you need to relax, suggests Scott Sheperd, Ph.D., author of *Who's In Charge? Attacking the Stress Myth.*

15 **Every night before bed, take five minutes to look over your day.** Instead of asking yourself, "How did my day go?" ask "How did I handle my day, and how does that compare with six months ago?" Focusing on what you can control—your response to stress—will help you feel more in control.

16 **Decompress with a single alcoholic drink at the end of the day.** Not only will it help prevent heart disease—one of the side effects of

stress—but it will also disable your psychological inhibitions. "When we let our guard down a bit, we can ventilate some of our emotions and feelings that we would otherwise harbor within us," says James Campbell Quick, M.D., a distinguished professor at the University of Texas at Arlington. Just be sure to stop at one drink.

17 **Each Sunday, plan out your meals for one week.** Studies show that as late as 4 p.m., a majority of people don't know what they're going to have for dinner that night. Planning ahead prevents the end-of-workday stress of trying to figure out what to eat. "Knowing what's for dinner when you come in from work cuts down on stress and encourages better eating and family time," says Audrey Thomas, an organizational consultant and author of *The Road Called Chaos.*

18 **Decorate your office walls with your children's or grandchildren's pictures.** Studies find that viewing works of art—and yes, children's pictures are art—lowers stress hormones. If you don't want to hang up finger-painted stick figures, go to www.print-art.com to print out copies of works of art from the world's great masters.

19 **Relax with a cup of basil tea.** Thought to help induce a state of calm, this herb is easy to grow in a container garden and one of the easiest fresh herbs to find at your grocery store. Place three washed fresh basil leaves in a cup of hot water. Steep 10 minutes, then sip.

20 **If exercise isn't helping to lower your stress level,** switch from a repetitive type of exercise to a type that engages your mind. "Sometimes workouts are not effective at reducing stress because we use the time to think about all the stressful things we have going on," explains Larina Kase, Psy.D., president of Performance and Success Coaching and a psychologist at the Center for Treatment and Study of Anxiety at the University of Pennsylvania. Step aerobics, very active spinning classes (where you change positions a lot), and circuit training or interval training (where you alternate different activities) prevent your mind from drifting, providing the mental break you need. A good option at home is dancing. Play your favorite music, and really get into it. Involve your whole family to benefit one and all, and add a great "bonding" experience into the bargain.

21 **Go somewhere blue or green.** Cool colors, such as light blues and greens, help people to relax, feel calm, and relieve stress, says Dr. Kase. When you're at the end of your wits, sit in a room where you can surround yourself with cool colors or find a bench in a garden. Having lush green plants in your home or office can provide similar color-related benefits.

Two-Second**Quiz**

Get Mad or Get Even?

Answer: *Neither.*
Instead, get satisfaction by being a communicator. Let other people know when you're angry, and why. But be prepared to listen to their side, too, and try to find common ground. Common understanding is less dangerous than holding anger in or expressing it in aggression. And guys, if you feel challenged in this area, consider a brief course in conflict resolution.

22 **Take on just one new activity at a time.** When you try to master too many new activities at once, you can easily feel overwhelmed, explains Edward J. Cumella, Ph.D., a licensed psychologist and director of research and education at the Remuda Ranch Treatment Centers in Wickenburg, Arizona. "Both at work and at home, take on new commitments with care," he says. "When your job is pushing the envelope, don't do more at home. Don't buy a new house and simultaneously take on higher car payments. When your home life is stressful and changing, don't quit your job or change careers!"

23 **Schedule six to eight hours of free time each week.** Use the time to daydream, read a novel, take a nap, see a movie, or generally relax in whatever way feels best to you. This is your time. Guard it as closely as you do your PIN code for the ATM.

24 **Drop in on a yoga class.** Just one class is all you need to lower levels of the stress hormone cortisol, according to a study from Jefferson Medical College. Researchers took blood samples from 16 beginners taking their first week of yoga classes. Cortisol levels dropped after the first class.

25 **Several times during the day, immerse yourself fully in the task at hand.** Chew your food slowly and taste every bite. Notice the temperature and sensation of water as you wash the dishes. You can even just sit and breathe, noticing the temperature of the air as it travels in and out of your nostrils. This will help you let go of stressful thoughts and allow you to rest in the present moment. "When you are relaxed, you stop to smell

the roses, taste your meal, and enjoy your grandkids. Your life then seems more full of wonderful things, and that in turns makes you more optimistic, which makes you calmer and happier," says Rob Goldblatt, Psy.D., author of *The Boy Who Didn't Want to Be Sad*.

26 Count your blessings once a day.
Once every day, say to yourself (or to someone else): "I feel lucky to have _____ in my life" or "I feel privileged to have _____." Fill in the blanks with the names of family or friends, or with other positives, such as good health or a good career, suggests Dr. Winner.

27 Have a really good cry.
By crying tears you were holding in, you can eliminate depression, make it easier to think clearly, heal old pain and hurt, and achieve a sense of inner peace, says Southern California psychotherapist Tina Tessina, Ph.D., author of *It Ends With You: Grow Up and Out of Dysfunction*. Plus, she says, studies find that crying boosts the immune system and reduces levels of stress hormones.

28 When you're stressed or tired and someone wants more of you than you can give,
tell him you only have a few minutes to talk or that you are tired and not able to really listen right then. Believe it or not, he will trust you more because you are honest and you will not be taking on more issues than you can tackle, says Dr. Kase.

29 Practice some difficult assertiveness skills
such as declining a project, telling someone that you cannot talk now, expressing disagreement or disapproval or recommending an alternative. Increasing assertiveness skills can greatly reduce your feelings of stress at work and increase your sense of self-confidence, says Dr. Kase. Be assertive in a friendly but firm way.

30 Put Post-it notes on your bathroom mirror,
on your car dashboard, and on your office computer that say "Slow down" and "What's your rush?" "Your brain takes many cues from your body, and sometimes it misinterprets the cues, so use that to your advantage," says Patricia A. Farrell, Ph.D., a licensed psychologist and the author of *How to Be Your Own Therapist*. Slowing everything down—walking instead of running, listening to slow music, speaking more slowly than normal—will trick your brain into calming down your stress level too.

31 Think of your children or your pet.
Sometimes diverting your thoughts momentarily to those who love you, who matter more to you, and who bring you pleasure helps you instantly put things in perspective during very stressful moments. You don't have a pet? Get one. Studies find that pets, particularly dogs, are one of the best stress-relievers and health promoters around.

32 Carry a small notebook with you everywhere.
This is your "worry" journal. When you feel stressed, whip it out and scribble down everything on your mind *at that minute*. Close the journal. Close your eyes. Take 10 deep breaths. Now open the journal and read what you've written. You'll find your worries are not nearly as stressful as you thought now that you've gotten them out of your head and onto the page.

33 Spritz lavender scent into the air (don't forget to spray yourself). Studies find the scent is instantly relaxing.

34 Unclench your muscles. Until you do this exercise, you won't even know how tense you really are. It's called progressive relaxation and it works like this: Starting with your toes and working your way up, clench each muscle for 10 seconds, then thoroughly relax them. The whole exercise shouldn't take more than a couple of minutes, and you'll feel as if you've just undergone a massage.

35 Deprive your senses. You've heard of sensory deprivation, right? That's the theory behind those tanks in which people float in body-temperature water in a dark, enclosed capsule. Well, you don't always have access to one of those. Instead, find the darkest room in your house or office. Turn off all the lights, pull the shades, and close the door. Slip an eyeshade over your eyes and stuff earplugs into your ears. Then lie back on the couch or a few pillows, get comfortable, and let the relaxation take you away. (You might want to set an alarm clock just in case you fall asleep.)

36 Slip in a CD of solo piano music from Chopin. Or Enya, Ella Fitzgerald, Marvin Gaye, or Hawaiian guitar. Soothing music, researchers find, actually produces slower brain-wave patterns, like those observed when people are about to fall asleep or are taking certain medications.

37 Find your own credo, or words to live by. It could be something as simple as the Serenity Prayer, "God grant me the serenity to accept the things I cannot change ... " or as complex as the Rudyard Kipling poem "If," one of our favorites.

Defusing Anger

25 WAYS TO RELEASE YOUR EMOTIONAL STEAM

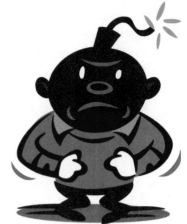

Furious. Burning. Annoyed. Enraged. Irate. Maddened. Outraged. Raging. Riled. Wrathful. All synonyms for one of the most common human emotions: anger. There's no way to get through life without getting angry. The key is to learn how to constructively defuse that anger so it doesn't wind up destroying your health.

Anger has an effect on health? Oh, yeah! In so many ways. Bottling up your anger can raise levels of homocysteine, a chemical linked to heart disease. It can raise your cholesterol levels and heart rate, suppress your immune system, lead to depression, and even give you a heart attack. On a heart-damaging scale of 1 to 10, 1 being a juicy apple and 10 being a double-cheese, triple-meat pizza, we'd put anger at about an 8.

But by defusing your anger in Stealth Healthy ways like the ones below, you can reduce your risk of these health conditions. Think of the effort involved in controlling anger in the same way you think of exercise—as something that isn't necessarily easy, but that is worthwhile, a productive challenge. Here's how to let the steam off safely and save your health:

1 **If you are angry with a politician, policy, or other public injustice, do something about it.** In one 2003 study, researchers from the University of Wisconsin tracked the brain-wave patterns in students who had just been told the university was considering big tuition increases. They all exhibited brain patterns signifying anger, but signing a petition to block the increases seemed to provide satisfaction. Put simply, working to right a wrong is life-affirming and positive. Stewing in a bad situation without taking action is the opposite.

2 **Forget about punching a pillow, a wall, or the object of your anger.** Contrary to popular belief, these common reactions don't decrease your anger. In fact, studies find, they only increase your hostility.

3 **Take three deep breaths.** When you're angry, your body becomes tense, says Robert Nicholson, Ph.D., assistant professor of community and family medicine at Saint Louis University. Breathing deeply helps lower your internal anger meter.

4 **Know why you feel angry.** Think like a detective and track down clues about the kinds of situations, people and events that trigger your anger, says Dr. Nicholson. Once you're aware of them, try to avoid them if possible. If you can't avoid them, at least you'll know to anticipate them, which will give you more time to prepare for them so they don't affect you so negatively.

5 **Keep in mind that whoever loses it, loses.** Losing your temper makes you look like the bad guy to everyone else, no matter who is really at fault, says Southern California psychotherapist Tina Tessina, Ph.D., author of *It Ends With You: Grow Up and Out of Dysfunction.* To get better at controlling your anger, visualize a scene in which you got angry and replay the tape several times, each time envisioning yourself responding a different way. You're actually rehearsing different reactions and giving yourself new options. The next time you're close to losing your temper, one of these options will pop into your mind, providing you with a better response.

6 **When you get really angry, walk away from the source.** Then take a five-minute walking break to get some fresh air, or do something else that provides calm and relief. If your anger stems from the traffic jam you're stuck in, turn up the radio and sing at the top of your lungs. The idea is to create a mental and/or physical escape from the situation.

7 **Picture a red stop sign in your mind or wear a rubber band on your wrist** and snap it whenever you find your anger beginning to boil. Then take a few minutes to put the issue into perspective and ask yourself if it's worth the humiliation that comes from becoming overtly angry.

 In**Perspective**

Type A vs. Hostility

Have you ever taken one of those personality tests? The ones where you fill out a bunch of questions, add up your score, and come up with a category into which your personality fits? Well, if you have what's known in the literature as a "hostile" personality, then you're more likely to have insulin resistance or pre-diabetes than someone with a different form of personality. Hostility is also thought to be the culprit behind the link between so-called type A personalities and heart disease.

Put simply, hostile people are impatient and aggressive. That differs from the type A personality, however, in that type A behavior itself—being driven, always in a hurry, a mega-multitasker—isn't detrimental. The hostile element, however—being quick to anger, aggressive, and easily irritated—seems to be the heart-damaging part of the equation. Hostile people are also more cynical, quicker to think the world is out to get them, and less likely to trust other people. They're also more likely to have heart disease.

In one study from Duke University, researchers found that physicians who scored in the top half on a hostility questionnaire administered at the age of 25 were four to five times more likely to have heart disease than low scorers by the time they reached age 50.

8 **Recognize your own personal signs of escalating anger.** Those might be clenched fists, trembling, flushing, sweating. Then use deep breathing to regain control of yourself before your anger erupts, suggests Catheleen Jordan, Ph.D., a professor of social work at the University of Texas at Arlington. If you're not sure about your own anger warning signs, ask a friend or family member. They'll know!

9 **Pinch yourself every time you hear yourself using the words "never," "always," etc.** Such thinking leads to a black-and-white, all-or-nothing mentality, and that, in turn, shortens your fuse. Instead, suggests Dr. Nicholson, look at things in shades of gray instead of black and white. Acknowledge that sometimes life is unfair and sometimes the person who is making you angry does the wrong thing. But don't fuel the fires with phrases like "always disappoints" or "never comes through."

10 **Take "self-control" time.** It works to get children to calm down, says Jon Oliver, author of *Lesson One: The ABCs of Life,* so it should work with angry grown-ups too. Here's how to do it:

▶ Sit up proud and relaxed wherever you may be (a couch, the floor, a chair, etc.).
▶ Place your feet flat on the floor in front of you.
▶ Extend your hands palm down and place them gently in your lap. Make sure your elbows are naturally back by your sides.
▶ Relax your shoulders so the muscles around them are neither tight nor tense.
▶ Breathe deeply in through your nose and exhale through your mouth to help your body relax into this position.

Two-Second Quiz

Hold In Anger or Express It?

Answer: *Express your anger.*
The real damage of a type A personality doesn't come from ambition, but from repressed anger. If you're angry, get it under control, then express it. But don't fixate on the anger; instead, concentrate on the underlying causes and issues. Try to be fair, but also be honest.

▶ Close your eyelids lightly and continue breathing deeply.
▶ When using self-control time as a regular part of the day, it should last approximately three minutes. When using it as a way to help regain self-control, it should last approximately one minute.

11 **When dealing with angry family members, find a way to make them laugh.** This is a trick family therapists often use, says Dr. Jordan. So, for instance, take a quick digital photo of yourself with a silly or contrite expression, print it out, and put it on a family member's pillow. Or do some silly dancing together, or hide a gift in the mashed potatoes served at dinner. The point is to do something together that is lighthearted and fun. Not only does this defuse the anger, but it reminds everyone that you are in this family together, forever, and that love and forgiveness remain in ample supply.

12 **Remember that anger is really a messenger.** So ask yourself exactly what is bothering you right now. Use the anger as a simple indication that something can and should be changed to improve things in the future.

13 Remember, too, that displays of anger don't accomplish anything except to anger or intimidate others. It is not a disciplinary tool, a communication method, or an emotional weapon. It is a damaging, personal, emotional state that is symptomatic of an underlying problem. So don't ever let yourself use anger as a threat—particularly with your children. Your anger should be your problem, not theirs.

14 When you're angry, look at your watch. Let the second hand sweep across the dial at least two minutes before you take any action, says Ron Potter-Efron, author of *Stop the Anger Now*. By then, you'll have had time to think and can act in a more appropriate way. Plus, it's kind of a Zen thing to watch time move.

15 Write a forgiveness letter or e-mail. You don't even have to send it. Just the act of writing it will lighten the load of anger you've been carrying. If you want to resume your relationship with the person or persons with whom you've been angry, however, then hit the send button. One major study from Hope College in Michigan found that when volunteers thought about a

person they were angry with, their blood pressure, heart rate, and muscle tension spiked. But when they imagined themselves forgiving the other person—just imagined it!—their blood pressure, etc., didn't rise nearly as much.

16 Embrace empathy. True empathy means getting into another person's head and heart to both understand and feel that individual's experience. You can do this in numerous ways: visualizing the situation through the other person's eyes; writing a story from the other person's perspective of the situation; telling the story to a friend taking the other person's perspective.

17 When you're angry with your parents, think about your kids. How do you want them to feel about you when they're your age? Wouldn't you want them to understand that you were only doing the best you could at the time? Suddenly that 20-year-old lingering hurt won't be as sharp.

 18 Acknowledge some core truths about people:

- Most people act out of the belief that they are doing the right thing.
- Most people are not malicious, mean-spirited, or backstabbing.
- Most people are more sensitive and insecure than they let on.
- Most people aren't very good judges of how their actions affect others.

In other words, we're neither villains nor saints. We're all just people—struggling to lead happy, healthy, meaningful lives in a complicated world. Even the people who anger you. Particularly them. With this in mind, forgiveness comes much easier.

Healthy Investments

An iPod (or Any Other Portable Music Player With Headphones)

Whenever you're in a situation in which you feel yourself beginning a slow burn, pull out the iPod (which you've stocked with your favorite songs), pop in the headphones, and mentally take yourself out of the situation.

---

19 Get angry with the person who can make a **difference,** not the poor soul who is simply caught in the crossfire. This advice is particularly important when you're dealing with people who work in the service industry. Is it the fault of the service technician that his company only allows him to book appointments in three-hour blocks? No, but his manager could probably fix things.

20 Write letters. Constantly. To the president of the company that just laid you off. To the friend who dissed you. To the politician who raised your taxes. Some you'll send, some you won't. But all will help you corral your anger and express it in a worthwhile, healthy way.

21 Understand that someone, somewhere, is gossiping about you, because that's what people do, but understand also that it has absolutely no impact on your life.

22 Take responsibility for your anger. Recognize that it's your choice whether or not you become angry.

23 Talk about your anger. This is different from expressing it; talking about it means unloading and decompressing with a friend, going over

Two-Second**Quiz**

Fly or Drive?

Answer: *Drive.*
It's hard not to get angry while traveling. But if your destination is less than 300 miles, lean toward driving. You have more control over the situation when you're in the driver's seat, the environment is your own, and fewer things can go wrong (e.g., weather, overbooked flights, missing crew). Plus, between airport parking, ticketing, check-in, security, and boarding, you often don't gain nearly as much time as you think by flying.

the situation with a neutral observer who can bring some perspective to the situation, or even talking out loud to yourself about it (preferably when no one else can hear you).

24 Get on your bike and go for a half-hour ride. Or jump up and down on a trampoline. Or go for a vigorous swim or attack the weeds in your garden. Any kind of vigorous, intense physical activity helps dissipate anger.

25 Get some perspective. Is this person or situation really worth spending your emotional energy on? Risking your health over? Putting your dignity and peace of mind at risk?

Dealing With Anxiety

17 WAYS TO STAY SETTLED

You know the feeling. You're doing fine, when all of a sudden your car dies, your daughter tells you she's dropping out of college, and you find out you need a new roof. Suddenly, you feel like you can't breathe. Your chest hurts and you're convinced you're having a heart attack. More likely, you're having an anxiety attack—an acute reaction to intense stress. Even if you don't wind up with the full-blown attack, anxiety can leave you feeling apprehensive, uncertain and fearful, paralyzing you into inaction or withdrawal.

An anxiety disorder isn't just a case of "nerves." According to the Anxiety Disorders Association of America, an estimated 19 million Americans ages 18-54 (more than 13 percent of the population) experience debilitating bouts of anxiety. It is the most common psychiatric condition in the United States. Primary symptoms include a rise in blood pressure, a fast heart rate, rapid breathing, an increase in muscle tension and a decrease in intestinal blood flow, potentially resulting in nausea or diarrhea.

Sometimes your anxiety disorder will be serious enough to require medication and therapy. But quite often, learning to better manage stress, as described two chapters ago, can make a big difference. We've also come up with 17 tips to help you cope when anxiety hits so it doesn't overwhelm you.

1 **Get out your bike, pull on your walking shoes, or grab your gym bag.** There's no better therapy for the "I can't breathe" feeling of an anxiety attack than to quickly escape the situation and get your blood moving and endorphins pumping through exercise.

2 **Cut out all caffeinated drinks, foods, and medications.** The caffeine only adds to that tense, jittery, anxious feeling, says Daphne Stevens, Ph.D., a clinical social worker and author of *Watercolor Bedroom: Creating a Soulful Midlife.* Sources of caffeine include chocolate, beverages like coffee, tea, soda, and some prescription and over-the-counter medications, like Excedrin.

3 **Avoid conversations likely to increase your anxiety when you're tired, overwhelmed, or stressed.** For instance, tell your kids that you're simply not available for problem solving after 8 p.m. Try to protect a "trouble free" time, especially before bed, when you don't address difficulties but focus instead on pure relaxation.

4 **Buy a white-noise machine and use it when you go to sleep.** The soothing sound will help you fall and stay asleep. A good night's sleep is critical when you're stressed, since sleep deprivation fuels anxiety even as anxiety leads to sleep deprivation. See "The Sleep Routine," (page 79) for 24 more tips on getting a good night's sleep.

5 **Choose one thing that is making you anxious.** Now sit down and write out all the fears you have about that one thing. If it's money, write down what would happen if you lose your job, if you can't pay your bills. What is the absolute worst thing that could happen? Now look at each item and mark it on a scale of 1 to 10, with 1 being highly unlikely it would ever happen, 10 being likely that it would happen. You'll be surprised at how few items rank above a 5. This understanding should help reduce your anxiety. If something does rank higher than 5, you may want to develop a contingency plan for it. Nothing works better to calm anxiety than turning from pure worry to an action plan.

6 **Rent a comedy and watch it.** Let yourself laugh out loud. The act of laughter stimulates endorphins that help blow stress hormones (which contribute to that feeling of anxiety) out of your system the way a good thunderstorm can blow away hot, humid weather.

 In**Perspective**

Coping With Disappointment

When you are middle-aged or younger, stress and anxiety are often born out of career issues, a too-busy schedule, and the struggle to achieve a balance between work, family, and self. But for those past their career peaks, past having young kids at home, past having to worry about how to get everything done in a day, stress often comes in different shapes and forms. And one of those forms is disappointment—in how life turned out, how children turned out, how the fanciful dreams of youth never quite came to reality.

Too often people want to skim over the discomfort associated with disappointment, says Leslie Levine, president of Life Integration Concepts and the author of *Wish It, Dream It, Do It: Turn the Life You're Living Into the Life You Want*, yet it's a normal and to-be-expected emotion. So don't ignore it. Understanding what you're disappointed about and why you're disappointed can be a wonderful learning experience. For instance, if you're disappointed in other people's behavior, perhaps you need to examine your expectations. Or if you're disappointed that you never became the doctor you always thought you'd be, maybe it's time to consider some kind of second career in health care.

What you don't want to do is become immobilized with disappointment, she says. So don't gloss over the emotion. Instead, sit with it and learn from it.

Ultimately, experts say, the trick is to forgive the past, have hope for the future, but to live in the present. Make today an outstanding day. Make tomorrow even better. Never give up on making new friends, learning something new, pursuing a dream, starting right now. With such an attitude, there's much less room in your life for disappointment and its negative health effects.

7 Follow the Relax, Detach, Focus steps. Created by Marcia Reynolds, M.Ed., author of *Outsmart Your Brain! Get Happy, Get Heard, and Get Your Way at Work,* the routine goes like this:

- Relax your body from the toes up.
- Detach from your thoughts.
- Center yourself in the moment (e.g., feel your head upon the pillow, or your feet on the ground, etc., depending on where you are).
- Focus on who you want to be and how you *want* to feel.

8 Turn on the news and watch the disasters unfurl. It will help you put your own problems into perspective and realize it's a large world, filled with both triumph and disaster. The challenges in your life that make you anxious may not seem as great when you put them in world context.

9 Don't borrow future problems. Many people get into a cycle of predicting and worrying about future concerns, says Larina Kase, Psy.D., a psychologist at the Center for Treatment and Study of Anxiety at the University of Pennsylvania and president of Performance and Success Coaching. Ask yourself, "Is this something I know can happen and is it something I can do something about right now?" If the answer to either of these questions is no, tell yourself you will revisit it later.

10 Simply experience your anxiety for 45 minutes. That's usually all it takes for you to become used to it and for the anxious feeling to dissipate, says Dr. Kase. The worst thing you can do is try to ignore it, she says, because anxiety tends to fight back if you push it down.

Breathe Away Anxiety

In "Defusing Stress," we discussed healthy breathing (see page 293). But proper breathing is particularly important during moments of great anxiety. At times like these, many people resort to chest breathing—the type of big, desperate inhales and exhales that make you rapidly puff up and deflate your chest, says Michael Crabtree, Ph.D., a professor of psychology at Washington & Jefferson College in Washington, Pennsylvania, and a licensed clinical psychologist.

To regain healthy breathing during periods of anxiety, he says, lie on the floor and place your hand on your chest. Using your hand as a gauge, try to reduce the amount of chest movement, while continuing to breathe normally. You don't want your chest to move; you want the other parts of your body to take over the breathing—using your diaphragm instead of the big chest inhales and exhales. Do this for five minutes.

Be aware that chest breathing still has a purpose, but only in times of extreme emotional arousal or physical challenge. "Most Americans use chest breathing because of developing instincts from fight-or-flight conditions," he says. It is in those types of physically dangerous situations that it is still necessary—not for everyday stress or anxiety.

11 Talk to yourself. Remind yourself of how you handled similar situations in the past, your strengths, and how long you will need to get through it. Show yourself that this anxiety is manageable and time-limited.

12 Go to the museum, see a movie, read a good book, or take up oil painting (or some other hobby). People who are bored tend to score higher on tests designed to measure levels of anxiety.

Two-Second **Quiz**

Laugh or Cry?

Answer: *Cry.*

When life is so challenging that you are having anxiety attacks, this is serious business. While laughing off the situation may seem like a mature, "I'm in control" response, it may be masking or denying some very unhealthy issues. Crying is a more honest, anxiety-releasing response, with positive physiological effects. It also signals to you and your loved ones that all is not well and that change may be in order.

13 Keep a journal of what makes you anxious. Then revisit these same items when you're feeling calm and develop plans to deal with them.

14 Name your fears. The most anxiety-producing thing of all is the unknown. So drag your worries out of the shadows. Worried about your son/daughter/spouse getting hurt or killed in a car crash? Discuss it—at least with yourself. Look up the statistics on driving and injury to relieve your mind. Do the same for whatever else makes you worry, whether that's West Nile virus, bioterrorism, cancer, or plane crashes. Once you name your fears and learn about them, you can take steps to minimize your risk. You'll also find the fears you name and tame are far less menacing than fears left to lurk in the shadows of your imagination.

15 Make sure you're getting several servings of whole grains, fruits, and vegetables every day, along with healthy protein sources such as fish, poultry, lentils, soy, or lean meats. The combination helps your brain make serotonin, a chemical that induces a state of calm relaxation.

16 Rent a meditation, t'ai chi, or yoga tape from the library. They are all effective, nonmedical ways of dealing with anxiety.

17 Share your anxieties with a confidant. You need to find someone who can help you understand why you worry too much. Try to play the same role for that person. We are usually better at placing someone else's worries in perspective than we are our own.

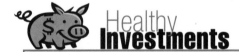 Healthy **Investments**

A Notebook to Keep by Your Bedside

Anxiety is often worst at night, and it can manifest as a litany of "coulda, shoulda, wouldas" at 3 a.m. When this hits, be ready with pad, pencil, and bedside light. Write down the ideas you get, the things you need to do, and so on. You will relieve your mind knowing you recorded your concerns as a to-do list for the next day.

Depression

17 WAYS TO
BANISH THE BLUES

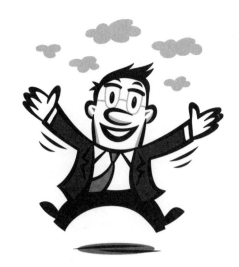

There comes a point in all of our lives when we come to a stark realization: Life sometimes isn't very fun. The realities of day-to-day existence are challenging, and setbacks common. Life may have been an eye-opening adventure in our youth, our teens, even our 20s, but as time passes, the glee of living gets harder to sustain.

Most of us cope just fine with this fact. With age, exuberance and excitement get replaced by a more subtle but deeper joy. We have families we love, jobs that are meaningful, friends that care, hobbies and vacations that provide real pleasure, accumulated wisdom that gives us a sense of value and uniqueness.

But rare is the person who doesn't encounter times of major loss or challenge along the way. And for millions of people, the path of life occasionally takes us through the dark regions of depression. Often it is a negative event, or a sequence of events, that triggers this condition. Sometimes it is a shift in our attitudes—from a life half-full to a life half-empty—that brings it on.

And sometimes it is body chemistry itself—an imbalance in the chemicals of the brain that deprives you of the feel-good hormones and casts a long shadow on your moods and emotions.

Depression is a serious condition, demanding a doctor's treatment. Here we aren't trying to give you a diagnosis or treatment—that's for professionals to do. But even if you are taking medication for depression, the following lifestyle tactics may increase the drug's effectiveness. If you're simply feeling low, they may give you the boost you need to pull out of it and help you avoid adding another expensive prescription to your list.

1 **Spend at least one hour each week with a close friend.** In a British study, when 86 depressed women were paired with a volunteer friend, 65 percent of the women felt better. In fact, regular social contact worked as effectively as antidepressant medication and psychotherapy. Regular social contact with a close friend may boost self-confidence and encourage you to make other positive changes that will help lift depression, such as starting an exercise program. Speaking of which—start an exercise program!

2 **Eat seafood twice a week or more.** A Dutch study found that people who consume diets rich in omega-3 fatty acids, a type of fat found in

cold-water fish such as salmon and mackerel, were less likely to suffer from depression than people whose diets were low in this important fat. Another study, this one conducted in England, found that pregnant women who didn't eat fish had twice the rate of depression as women who ate 10 ounces of fish a day. In fact, one reason researchers think the rate of depression has skyrocketed in this country is that we get so few omega-3 fatty acids in our diets. Another good idea for getting your omega-3s: Keep a container of ground flaxseed in the fridge. Use it to sprinkle on everything from ice cream to yogurt to cheese omelets. Mix it into muffin mix, shakes, and salad dressings. Flaxseed is an excellent source of omega-3 fatty acids.

3 Play with a dog a few minutes every day.
When non-pet owners played with a dog for just a few minutes a day as part of a University of Missouri study, blood levels of the brain chemicals serotonin and oxytocin—both mood elevators—rose. You don't need to own a dog to experience these feel-good effects (although dogs are great antidotes to the kind of chronic stress that can result in depression). Pet your neighbor's dog for a few minutes a day, volunteer at an animal shelter, or stop by your local pet store for some furry one-on-one therapy.

4 Take 600 milligrams of chromium picolinate a day if you have depression and insulin resistance.
This mineral may improve function of the hormone insulin, which, in turn, may help normalize levels of the mood-boosting brain chemical serotonin. In a study completed at Duke University, people with atypical depression—characterized by mood swings, carbohydrate cravings,

weight gain, and lethargy—boosted their mood and reduced their carbohydrate cravings and other symptoms when they began supplementing their diet with chromium. Consult your doctor first, though.

5 Eat a bowl of fortified breakfast cereal or take a multivitamin every day.
This will ensure you consume the recommended amount (400 micrograms) of folate, an important B vitamin that may help lift depression. Folate and other B vitamins help maintain nerve and blood cells, used in brain reactions and essential for the production and function of a number of mood-boosting brain chemicals. In a Finnish study published in the *Journal of Nutrition*, participants with the lowest folate consumption were at the highest risk for depression. Another study, published in the *Annals of Clinical Psychiatry*, found this vitamin helps enhance the effectiveness of antidepressant

Two-SecondQuiz

Exercise or Antidepressants?

Answer: *Exercise.*
A study of older adults found 10 weeks of regular exercise was 20 percent more effective at reducing depressive symptoms than medication. However, because depression may make you want to do anything *but* exercise, many physicians recommend combining the two treatments. With your physician's okay, start taking an antidepressant until you feel energetic enough to begin exercising. Then, once you get into a regular exercise routine, talk to your doctor about possibly reducing the dosage of your medication or weaning yourself off it altogether.

medication. Another good source? Avocados. They're one of the richest plant sources of B vitamins.

6 **Get a 12-minute massage three times a week.** It doesn't have to cost a lot. Whether you pay a professional or ask a spouse or friend to rub your back, the result is the same: a natural mood boost. In a study of depressed dialysis patients, participants who received a 12-minute massage three times a week were less depressed than those who didn't get the soothing rub. Another study of 84 depressed pregnant women found those who received two 20-minute massages a week from their partners reduced their incidence of depression 70 percent. Researchers suspect massage boosts serotonin levels (which jumped 17 percent in the women who received twice-weekly massages) and reduces levels of the stress hormone cortisol.

7 **Pull an all-nighter.** Staying up all night for one night—and therefore depriving yourself of sleep—has been shown to lift depression for as long as a month. Although researchers aren't sure why it works, they speculate that one night of sleep deprivation may reset the sleep clock, enabling people who *are* depressed to sleep better.

8 **Eat a whole wheat English muffin smothered with jam.** When you consume high-carbohydrate foods—such as the muffin with jam—you encourage the amino acid tryptophan to flood your brain, boosting serotonin levels. A slice of whole wheat bread slathered with honey or a snack of air-popped popcorn will also produce the same effect. Why the emphasis on whole grain? White flour

provides similar benefits, but the effects wear off quickly, taking you from peak to valley in an hour or so.

9 **Just bang on something.** Employees at a retirement community who took a drumming class felt more energetic and less depressed six weeks after the class than before they started it. Researchers

---

Diagnosing Depression

How do you know if you're just feeling blue or if you're truly depressed? "Everybody has a day or two when they feel some sadness," says Edward J. Cumella, Ph.D., a licensed psychologist and director of research and education for the Remuda Ranch Treatment Centers in Wickenburg, Arizona. "Maybe you're a little under the weather; maybe something unpleasant happened." This tends to pass, however, and is temporary.

Depression, on the other hand, drags on for weeks or months. It affects your mood, thoughts, and even physical body, including the way you eat and sleep. Studies find people with depression are also more likely to develop such serious diseases as heart disease and diabetes. Classic symptoms of depression include:

- Difficulty concentrating
- Short-term memory loss
- Pessimism
- Loss of enjoyment of activities you once found pleasurable
- Fatigue
- Irritability
- Changes in appetite
- Lack of sexual desire
- Difficulty sleeping

If your symptoms last for two weeks or more, you may need more than home remedies. Make an appointment to see your doctor.

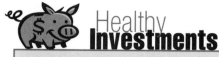

Healthy Investments

A Light Box

Bright light therapy has been shown to relieve depression during pregnancy as effectively as antidepressant medication. Additional research shows it also can ease seasonal affective disorder, a type of depression some people experience during the winter months when sunlight is in short supply. It may also ease other types of depression as well. The therapy involves sitting in front of a specially designed light box shortly after waking each morning for 20 minutes to an hour. You can purchase a light box for home use from a variety of companies, including SunBox, Northern Lights, and Apollo. They range in price from $200 to $400.

speculate that drumming helps to relax your body. Whacking a few notes out on your desk may help, but joining a weekly drumming circle may help more, particularly since it provides camaraderie with others, which, as noted earlier, also helps with depression.

10 Take a 10-minute walk three times a day during the winter. Many people feel depressed during the winter months, when they travel to and from work in darkness and don't get enough natural sunlight. Physical exercise, however, encourages the release of hormones and neurochemicals that boost mood, says Richard Brown, M.D., associate professor of clinical psychiatry at Columbia University and coauthor of *Stop Depression Now*. Walking outside during the day will give you a few short doses of sunlight, also shown to boost mood, particularly in the winter.

11 First thing in the morning, lie on your back with your head hanging over the edge of your bed. Grip a 5- or 10-pound dumbbell with both hands and extend it behind your head, letting your arms hang down toward the floor. Take 10 deep breaths, trying to expand your rib cage as much as possible. Bring the weight back and place it on the bed beside you. Scoot onto the bed so your head is supported, and take another 10 deep breaths. Repeat three times. The stretch will open your rib cage and chest, making it easier to take a deep breath. "The most common unrecognized source of mild depression is restricted trunk flexibility that interferes with full respiration," says Bob Prichard, a biomechanist and director of Somax Sports in Tiburon, California. "Most people with mild depression are shallow breathers because their chest and stomach are too tight to allow full, easy breathing," he says.

12 Drink one to two cups of coffee or tea each morning. Regular, modest caffeine intake decreases the risk of depression by more than 50 percent, says Edward J. Cumella, Ph.D., a licensed psychologist and director of research and education for the Remuda Ranch Treatment Centers in Wickenburg, Arizona.

13 Look in the mirror and force your lips into a smile. "Research shows that the physiology of smiling actually makes you feel happy," Dr. Cumella says. If you need a little extra help in the smile department, watch a funny movie, read the comics, buy a Peanuts or Calvin and Hobbes collection, or ask a friend to tell you one joke every day.

Two-Second**Quiz**

Work or Sex?

Answer: *Sex.*

A group of economists found that going from having sex once a month to having it at least weekly is roughly equivalent to the amount of happiness that an extra $50,000 of income would bring to the average American. The findings hold regardless of age or gender. The reason? Probably the fact that people with good relationships and healthy sex lives tend to be happier overall than those without.

14 Sleep in a different bedroom. Many people with depression also have insomnia. Switching your sleep location can help, says Dr. Cumella. You can also reduce insomnia by getting up at the same time every day, never napping for more than 20 minutes, shunning caffeine after 3 p.m., and relaxing for an hour before bed.

15 Go easy on yourself. When something goes wrong, resist the urge to mentally beat up on yourself. "Give yourself permission to be a human being and not a human doing," says Karl D. La Rowe, a licensed clinical social worker and mental health investigator in Oregon. When you catch yourself mentally berating yourself for some supposed failing, replace your negative thoughts with the phrase "I am doing the best I know how to do. When I know a better way and can do it, I will."

16 Break out of your routine today. Sometimes being stuck in a rut is just that. Get out of it and your mood may come along with you. Take a day off from work and go explore a town nearby. Go out to a restaurant for dinner—even though it's a Tuesday night. Take a different route as you drive to work, wear something that is totally "not you," or take your camera and go on a photography hike. For a major blue mood, consider that it might be time for you to take a vacation.

17 Get a day of vigorous outdoor recreation, like hiking, canoeing, or biking. Let the combination of nature and physical activity work their magic on your mood.

REMINDER

 Fast Results
These are bits of advice that deliver benefits particularly quickly—in some cases, immediately!

 Easy Gains
These are tips that give the biggest value for the least amount of effort.

 Super Effective
These are tips proven to be particularly effective through scientific research or widespread usage by experts.

Dealing With Guilt

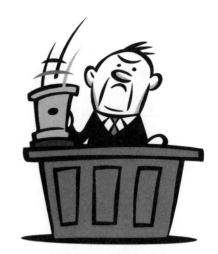

22 TIPS FOR A CLEANER CONSCIENCE

Ask anyone to define "guilt," and they hem and haw. It's a feeling that's kind of hard to describe. A feeling that I should have done something, should be doing something, should not have done something.

Actually, "guilt" comes from an Old English word that meant "delinquency." Today Merriam-Webster's Collegiate Dictionary defines it as "feelings of culpability, especially for imagined offenses or from a sense of inadequacy; self-reproach." It's a revealing definition—nowhere does it say that guilt is related to things you actually did wrong.

Sometimes you should feel guilty (if you've done something morally wrong, committed a crime, or intentionally hurt someone). But if you're like most of us, you walk around feeling guilty because of all the "shoulds" that come into your life—that is, the things you didn't do. That's not only bad for your mental and physical health, but completely unfair to you. Here's how to shed some of that guilt:

1 **Above all else, learn to forgive yourself.** If feelings of guilt haunt you, take some concrete steps to end this self-inflicted punishment. First, list the things you feel guilty about. It could be something stupid you said recently, an act of cruelty you did to a sibling in your childhood, or a detrimental personal habit that has hurt your relationship with a loved one. Then ask, How can I forgive myself and let it go? Perhaps it's prayer, writing a letter, having a talk, making a charitable donation, or committing to a personal change. Often it's merely having the courage to say, "I'm sorry." Then do what it takes so you can honestly, finally forgive yourself. You'll be amazed at the lightness and freedom doing this can bring.

2 **Set a no-guilt-allowed rule whenever you go on vacation or do something just for yourself.** Often women do not experience vacations, breaks, and other relaxing activities as stress-relieving because they feel guilty that they are not doing more productive things, says Larina Kase, Ph.D., a psychologist at the Center for Treatment and Study of Anxiety at the University of Pennsylvania. Tell yourself that you are taking a break and doing it for a reason (improved health, decreased stress, etc.) so there is no reason to feel guilty. As soon as you hear yourself say, "I should be..." remind yourself why you are choosing not to do that. Make sure anyone you're traveling with knows about the no-guilt rule too.

3 Take five minutes in the morning to feel guilty. Then either *do* what you're feeling guilty about (e.g., call your mother) or forgive yourself for what you did that you shouldn't have done, knowing that you've learned your lesson and won't do it again, says Rebecca Fuller Ward, a therapist in Little Rock, Arkansas, and the author of *How to Stay Married Without Going Crazy.*

4 Correct a mistake rather than feeling guilty about it. For instance, if you're feeling guilty because you went shopping on Saturday instead of visiting your mother in the nursing home, take time out of your schedule midweek for a visit. Many times, the things we feel guilty about are relatively easy to make right.

5 Ask yourself what your guilt is really about. If you're guilty about not serving on the church landscaping committee, is it because you really don't have the time, or because you don't like the other women? Maybe you want to do more for the church, but landscaping just isn't it. Take some time and really examine the motivation behind your guilt, rather than just wallowing in it.

Two-Second**Quiz**

Letter or Phone Call?

Answer: *Letter.*
When an apology is due, sit down and write a letter. Not only will it give you a better opportunity to think through your thoughts, but you always have the option of sending it or not sending it. Sometimes the simple act of writing is enough to give you peace of mind. If you do send it, the person to whom you're sending it has a lifetime reminder of your apology.

6 Recognize that a feeling of guilt doesn't always mean that what you did was wrong. For instance, if you're feeling guilty because you decided it was more important to relax with a book than to have coffee with your always-in-a-crisis friend, that means you're learning to set limits and take time for yourself. In cases like this, have the confidence to admit that you made the right choice.

7 Commit to saying no at least once a day—no guilt allowed.

8 Start a guilt journal. Every time you feel guilty about something, write it down in your journal. Write the time, the day, what you feel guilty about. Go back and reread this journal every couple of weeks to find the trends in your guilt. This will provide clues to the source of your guilt that will enable you to better deal with its underlying roots.

9 Stop asking, "What if?" Instead, start asking, "What now?" Put another way, stop thinking about things you've already done and can't change, and instead focus on the present—what you can do today to make your life and the world around you better.

10 Recall all the healthful benefits of some of the most guilt-inducing foods. For instance, dark chocolate is full of heart-healthy antioxidants. Red wine has fabulous benefits for your heart, cholesterol, and other health markers. A handful of mixed nuts imparts a healthy dose of monounsaturated fat and vitamin E. A box of popcorn gives you a good dose of fiber. Just remember: moderation in all things!

11 **Talk to a relative or friend who recalls the incident about which you're feeling guilty.** Often our own memories are not the most accurate; your feelings of guilt may be coming from something that really didn't happen the way you remember it.

12 **Don't get caught up in blaming.** For some reason, many people feel compelled to assign blame (often to themselves) for anything that goes wrong, big or small. But that's a bad approach to this complex world of ours. Instead, take a more forgiving approach to the world and recognize that sometimes things just happen on their own momentum, as a result of a cascade of events that cannot be blamed on any one person.

13 **List 10 things you like about yourself.** Most of us are highly critical of ourselves, without acknowledging the good, the funny, the right choices, the successes. Guilt becomes less of an issue when we are happy and secure in who we are. Keep this list in your purse, in your pocket, or on your computer at work. Look at it whenever you're feeling guilty about what you should or should not have done.

14 **Recognize that you can only do your best.** Nothing more. So maybe you weren't the kind of mother who got down on the floor to play with her kids, but you *were* the kind of mother who took her kids on outings to museums and parks. Maybe you aren't the kind of person to surprise your spouse with romantic gestures and gifts, but you do provide a perpetually open ear, helping hand, and unconditional support.

Blocking the Guilt

Has your mother, spouse, or priest given you one too many guilt trips lately? Desensitize yourself to guilt with the following exercise, courtesy of Dale V. Atkins, Ph.D., a psychologist and author of *I'm OK, You're My Parents: How to Overcome Guilt, Let Go of Anger, and Create a Relationship That Works*. The idea is to train yourself to react calmly when people try to make you feel guilty.

- Make a list of at least five typical guilt-inducing statements that people in your life use.
- Record each line into a tape recorder, using the exact inflection the person uses.
- Sit in the place and position you are usually in when you deal with this person's guilt offensives.
- Play back the tape.
- If possible, stay in the same room, but change your position to a restful one.
- Listen to the tape several times.
- Repeat the exercise whenever you anticipate conflict.

---

15 **Write a check to an aid agency.** That's doing something concrete with your guilt. If you're feeling guilty about eating that chocolate cake last night, go for a long walk today. If you feel guilty about the long hours you've been spending at work, call in sick tomorrow and spend the day with your kids and/or partner doing what *they* want.

16 **Make a sign that proclaims "I deserve this" and hang it above your desk.** The next time you feel guilty about your success, or begin to feel like you're a fake and don't deserve the success you've achieved, look at the sign and repeat the mantra 15 times.

Two-Second Quiz

Gift or No Gift?

Answer: *Gift.*

If you've had a fight with your partner, particularly a bad fight, a peace offering goes a long way toward restoring, well, the peace—as long as it is delivered with a sincere apology or message of reconciliation. But be careful never to try to win back favor with a gift alone—that's called a bribe. It's the apology that matters; the gift reinforces the message of love and commitment.

17 **Focus on the world around you.** There's no use feeling guilty for all the horrors of the world. You are just one person with a limited reach. Ask a clergy member or any anthropologist or social scientist and they'll all say our job as humans is to do our best, and nothing more.

18 **Determine your priorities, write them down**, and then post the list on your refrigerator and in your office. Next time you start feeling guilty about something you didn't do, check the list. If it's not in the top three priorities, you're off the hook.

19 **Accept some selfishness.** It really *is* okay to look out for yourself.

20 **Don't leave guilt unresolved**, particularly if it relates to an older relative such as a parent. Address the issues that matter to you so you're not left with regrets you can't address.

21 **Ask yourself, "Would I want someone *else* to feel guilty** about what's eating away at me?" "Would I forgive someone else for doing/not doing what I did/didn't do?" If the

answer to either of these is yes, then (to paraphrase the golden rule) do unto yourself as you would have yourself do unto others!

22 **Politely decline other people's guilt.** Mothers have an amazing capacity for making children feel guilty—even when their child is 60 years old. Some spouses, bosses, children, and religious leaders are also masters at making others feel bad about what they have (or haven't) done or said. Know what? They have no right to do that, and you have no obligation to listen. Only you are accountable for your actions. Assuming you haven't broken a law or a solemn promise, only you have the right to judge whether you did something wrong. A loved one can certainly tell you if you've done something to hurt him. But he doesn't have the right to tell you what your reaction ought to be.

Two-Second Quiz

Short or Long Apology?

Answer: *Short.*

The person you wronged doesn't want to hear about the kind of day you had, the jerk who cut you off on the interstate, the ketchup someone squirted on your tie. She just wants to know that you realize barking at her the minute you walked in the door was wrong. So say simply that you are sorry and that you know it was wrong. Then let her talk, rather than listening to you detailing all the reasons for your foul mood.

Dealing With the Uncontrollable

13 WAYS TO MAINTAIN A HEALTHY PERSPECTIVE

All you have to do these days is turn on CNN to realize how out of control the world is. First there are the big things—war, terrorism, famine, political gridlock. But then there are the smaller things that are out of your control, ranging from the weather to your job to your son or daughter. And if you're a controlling person—someone who has to have everything just so, in its right place in just the right way—then feeling out of control is one of the most stressful things that could ever happen to you.

We're here to tell you that the golden rule of life hasn't changed, and never will: Stuff happens. Much of it you can't control. What you *can* control is how you react to it and how much it affects you physically, financially, or otherwise. Here are 13 ways to gain back a bit of control when you feel like your world is spinning off its axis:

1 Above all else, distinguish what you can't control from what you can. Then direct your energies to influencing the latter, and accepting the former. This might sound simplistic, but you'd be amazed at how many people still think they can control traffic, or the weather, or their boss's mood, or the stock market. Make a list of all the things in your life that you *can't* control, no matter how hard you try, and post it on your refrigerator and your computer. Then accept it. Of course you can care about these things, and try to influence their outcome. But it's essential that you untie your emotional well-being from those things you cannot alter.

2 When things feel out of control, clean a closet or drawer. It worked for therapist Rebecca Fuller Ward, author of *How to Stay Married Without Going Crazy*. The night her mother had a heart attack, she cleaned out her pantry. "*That* I could control," she says.

3 Take up a new hobby. Mastering a new skill, whether it's paddling a kayak or learning to knit, will return a sense of control to your life.

4 When bad things happen, sit down and write out what you might have done differently. This self-assessment is not to blame and beat up on yourself; it's a chance to say, I may not control everything,

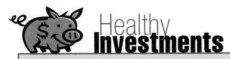

A Mudroom

The idea here is that there is one place in your house in which chaos can be contained, and you don't care how messy it gets. If your house is old and there just isn't space for a back-of-house mudroom for all those coats, shoes, and backpacks, designate another room as the official house "chaos" room. It can be the basement, garage, coat closet, even a kid's room (just close the door). At the same time, create a "sanctuary" room in your house that is kept orderly at all times. Use it to regain peace those times that the chaos of life overspills its boundaries.

but I do control me! What can I do with *me* that will make this situation work better and turn out more to my liking? So, if you get a bad evaluation at work, don't respond to it by blaming your boss or blaming your bad luck. Instead, says Patricia Farrell, Ph.D., author of *How to Be Your Own Therapist,* be honest with yourself about what you could have done differently that year— come into work on time, met all your deadlines, etc.—to garner a better result. Understanding your role in the situation will help you realize that the world actually is a fairly controllable place.

5 **When things feel out of control, pick one thing in your life to work on that you can make a difference in.** For instance, start an exercise program, write in your journal one day a week, balance your checkbook, or take your car in for an oil change.

6 **Build in contingencies.** For instance, say you have an outdoor party planned for 20 people but a tropical storm hits the day of the party. Well, while you

can't control the weather, you *can* control where you hold it (move it inside), *when* you hold it (postpone it), and *how* it's held (if you were planning a cookout, whip up a couple of big lasagnas).

7 **Make a list.** Nothing puts more control back into your hands than taking all the "to dos" swirling through your head and writing them down. Now make a plan for how you will accomplish each one. For instance, if one of the things on your list is Christmas shopping, set a date, a time, and a time limit to go shopping. If one of the things on your list is to clean the house, break it into manageable parts. So on Monday you clean the kitchen, on Tuesday the bathrooms, and so on.

8 **Build up tolerance to chaos by giving yourself small out-of-control experiences.** For instance, if you typically are the lead driver of the family car, have your spouse take the wheel next time you all go out together, suggests Larina Kase, Ph.D., a psychologist at the Center for Treatment and Study of Anxiety at the University of Pennsylvania. Ask someone to interrupt you periodically, have your partner make the weekend plans without

Two-Second**Quiz**

Messy or Neat Desk?

Answer: *Neat.*
We've all heard someone say he knows just where everything is from behind a desk that looks like a Superfund site. Guess what? He's lying! Take the time to clean up your work space and consider it a good investment. Clutter around you tends to add to the clutter in your mind, making everything feel just the slightest bit out of control.

your input, turn over the bill paying to your partner. These will help you learn to accept being out of control.

9 Practice positive self-talk. It would be great if someone else did this for you, but often you have to do it for yourself, says Dr. Farrell. Self-talk means saying things like, "I'm going to be okay," "I'll get through this," or "Right now, I have to give myself a few minutes and then I can begin coming up with a plan to handle this."

10 Take time to de-stress before addressing the maelstrom. Put your feet up, do some relaxation breathing, have a cup of tea. Calming yourself down is one area in which you do have control, notes Dr. Farrell.

11 Create a perception that you have control. There is a good deal of research showing that the perception of control is more important than actual control, says Dr. Kase. For instance, people are able to tolerate a hot room if they know they have the option of turning down the heat. Come up with some little things that you can do to make out-of-control situations more manageable.

12 Iron something. Ironing is a relatively mindless activity that still provides very visible results. The sense of control you gain as you turn a crumpled ball of fabric into a crisp garment will carry over into other areas of your life, promise!

13 Focus on what you're doing, not the outcome. You can often control the specific task or motion, but you can't always control the outcome. Just

---

Coping With Grief

There's nothing more uncontrollable than the death of someone you love. But there are ways to cope, says Tina Tessina, Ph.D., psychotherapist and author of *It Ends With You: Grow Up and Out of Dysfunction*. She offers the following tips to help you move through what may seem like endless grief. Note the pattern in her suggestions—maintaining your love for the person and honoring his or her memory, while still moving on with life:

● Think of your grief as a certain number of tears you must shed before the intensity of the sadness, anger, and guilt subsides. The more opportunities you take to grieve and feel all the related feelings, the sooner you will reach your magic number of tears.

● Create a special place in your house, with a picture, a candle, and perhaps some small mementos of your loved one. When you feel sad, spend some time there, and "talk" to the person you lost about how you're feeling.

● Get a scrapbook and make a memory album of the good times you had together. Put in photos, greeting cards, menus, or postcards. You can also write in it. Refer back to it in times of sadness.

● On your loved one's birthday or anniversaries, buy a card or write a letter and burn it to send it.

consider baseball slugger Mark McGwire, says Michael Crabtree, Ph.D., a professor of psychology at Washington & Jefferson College in Washington, Pennsylvania. "He was just a .200 hitter with the Oakland A's because he was focused on his low batting average and hitting home runs—not on just swinging the bat. When he started focusing on that, it changed his whole approach and he became a much better hitter," Dr. Crabtree says.

Enhancing Your Sense of Humor

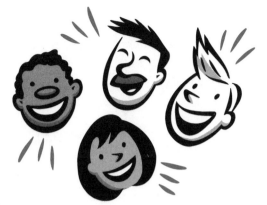

19 WAYS TO BRING OUT THE LAUGHTER INSIDE YOU

What is the greatest reward of being alive? Is it chocolate, sex, ice cream, tropical vacations, hugs from children, a perfect night's sleep, or the satisfaction of a job well done? A thousand people, a thousand different answers. But one supreme pleasure that spans all people is laughter. Little can compare to the feeling of a deep, complete, heartfelt laughing spell. No matter your age, wealth, race, or living situation, life is good when laughter is frequent.

Life is also healthier. Research finds that humor can help you cope better with pain, enhance your immune system, reduce stress, even help you live longer. Laughter, doctors and psychologists agree, is an essential component of a healthy, happy life.

As Mark Twain once said, "Studying humor is like dissecting a frog—you may know a lot but you end up with a dead frog." Nonetheless, we're giving it a try. Here are our 19 Stealth Healthy tips for getting—or growing—your sense of humor, based partly on the idea that you can't *be* funny if you don't understand what funny *is*.

1 First, regain your smile. A smile and a laugh aren't the same thing, but they do live in the same neighborhood. Be sure to smile at simple pleasures—the sight of kids playing, a loved one or friend approaching, the successful completion of a task, the witnessing of something amazing or humorous. Smiles indicate that stress and the weight of the world haven't overcome you. If your day isn't marked by at least a few dozen, then you need to explore whether you are depressed or overly stressed.

2 Treat yourself to a comedy festival. Rent movies like *Meet the Parents; Young Frankenstein; Pee-Wee's Big Adventure; Monty Python and the Holy Grail; This Is Spinal Tap; Animal House; Blazing Saddles; Trading Places; Finding Nemo.* Reward yourself frequently with the gift of laughter, Hollywood style.

3 Recall several of the most embarrassing moments in your life. Then find the humor in them. Now practice telling stories describing them in a humorous way. It might take a little exaggeration or dramatization, but that's what good storytelling is all about. By revealing your vulnerable moments and being self-deprecating, you open yourself up much more to the humorous aspects of life.

4 **Anytime something annoying and frustrating occurs, turn it on its head and find the humor.** Sure, you can be angry at getting splashed with mud, stepping in dog poop, or inadvertently throwing a red towel in with the white laundry. In fact, that is probably the most normal response. But it doesn't accomplish anything other than to put you in a sour mood. Better to find a way to laugh at life's little annoyances. One way to do that: Think about it as if it happened to someone else, someone you like—or maybe someone you don't. In fact, keep running through the Rolodex in your head until you find the best person you can think of to put in your current predicament. Laugh at him, then laugh at yourself!

Two-Second**Quiz**

To Tease or Not to Tease?

Answer: *Tease.*
But there are rules. One, do it with love, not hostility. Two, both teaser and teasee must be in on the fun. Third, you must be willing and able to reverse roles. Teasing is a way of highlighting the humor in our idiosyncrasies. Get used to being teased as a way of seeing the humor in yourself. But if someone's feelings get hurt, it's time to revisit the ground rules.

5 **Read the comics every day and cut out the ones that remind you of your life.** Post them on a bulletin board or the refrigerator or anywhere else you can see them frequently.

6 **Sort through family photographs and write funny captions** or one-liners to go with your favorites. When you need a pick-me-up, pull out the album.

7 **Every night at dinner, make family members share** one funny or even embarrassing moment of their day.

8 **When a person offends you or makes you angry, respond with humor rather than hostility.** For instance, if someone is always late, say, "Well, I'm glad you're not running an airline." Life is too short to turn every personal affront into a battle. However, if you are constantly offended by someone in particular, yes, take it seriously and take appropriate action. But for occasional troubles, or if nothing you do can change the person or situation, take the humor response.

9 **Sign up to receive the Top 10 list** from David Letterman every day via e-mail. You can find it at www.cbs.com/latenight/lateshow.

10 **Spend 15 minutes a day having a giggling session.** Here's how you do it: You and another person (partner, kid, friend, etc.) lie on the floor with your head on her stomach, and her head on another person's stomach and so on (the more people the better). The first person says, "Ha." The next person says, "Ha-ha." The third person says, "Ha-ha-ha." And so on. We guarantee you'll be laughing in no time.

11 Read the activity listings page in the newspaper and choose some laugh-inducing events to attend. It could be the circus, a movie, a stand-up comic, or a funny play. Sometimes it takes a professional to get you to regain your sense of humor.

12 Add an item to your daily to-do list: Find something humorous. Don't mark it off until you do it, suggests Jeanne Robertson, a humor expert and author of several books on the topic.

13 When you run into friends or coworkers, ask them to tell you one funny thing that has happened to them in the past couple of weeks. Become known as a person who wants to hear humorous true stories as opposed to an individual who prefers to hear gossip, suggests Robertson.

14 Find a humor buddy. This is someone you can call just to tell him something funny; someone who will also call you with funny stories of things he's seen or experienced, says Robertson.

15 Exaggerate and overstate problems. Making the situation bigger than life can help us to regain a humorous perspective, says Patty Wooten, R.N., an award-winning humorist and author of *Compassionate Laughter: Jest for the Health of It*. Cartoon caricatures, slapstick comedy, and clowning articles are all based on exaggeration, she notes.

16 Develop a silly routine to break a dark mood. It could be something as silly as speaking with a Swedish accent (unless you are Swedish, of course).

Do You Even *Have* a Sense of Humor?

To evaluate your own sense of humor, Patty Wooten, R.N., an award-winning humorist and author of *Compassionate Laughter: Jest for the Health of It,* provides these questions to evaluate your own sense of humor (or lack thereof):

- Do I see the existence or possibility of amusing stories in the absurd moments in my life?
- Do I spontaneously laugh out loud when I notice something funny?
- Am I able to share my amusing insights with others?

If all you're doing is answering no, then you need to spend some extra time with this chapter.

---

17 Create a humor environment. Have a ha-ha bulletin board where you only post funny sayings or signs, suggests Allen Klein, an award-winning professional speaker and author of *The Healing Power of Humor.* His favorite funny sign: "Never wrestle with a pig. You both get dirty, and the pig likes it."

18 Experiment with jokes. Learn one simple joke each week and spread it around. One of Klein's favorites relates to his baldness: "What do you call a line of rabbits walking backward? A receding hare line."

19 Focus humor on yourself. "Because of my lack of hair," Klein says, "I tell people that I'm a former expert on how to cure baldness."

Improving Memory

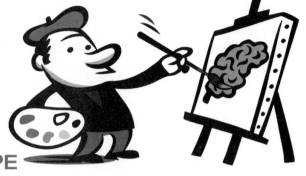

27 TRICKS TO KEEP YOUR BRAIN IN SHAPE

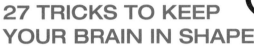

Five things you need to buy at the grocery store—forgotten! The name of your neighbor's son—lost! The reason you needed to go to Wal-Mart—gone! The magazine you wanted to show a coworker—left at home!

Relax. These little memory meltdowns are an inevitable part of life. In most cases, they have nothing to do with Alzheimer's, nothing to do with disease or injury, and everything to do with stress, too much work, and our daily craziness.

The good news is that the imminent aging of the baby boomers has spurred massive research into the origins and maintenance of memory. If you think you have a serious memory decline, seek medical attention, of course. It is possible it could be related to heart disease or the onset of Alzheimer's. But if you are just trying to have fewer "senior moments" than your bridge opponents, we're here to help with the following 27 tips. And remember: Aging alone doesn't cause a decline in brain function—live well, and you can keep learning and thinking clearly until your ripest old age.

1 **Use it or lose it: The golden rule of brainpower.** The brain functions like a muscle in that the more you use it, the stronger it gets. Watching lots of unstimulating TV; having a job routine; cooking, cleaning, and shopping the same way over and over—all contribute to a brainpower loss. Learning new things, varying your routines, having provocative discussions, going on adventurous vacations, and playing a musical instrument all cause your brain to make new connections and function better.

2 **Take a B-complex vitamin pill.** As you age, your body becomes less efficient at absorbing certain B vitamins from food. Yet the B's are critical for maintaining a sharp memory. A study of 260 healthy men and women over age 60 found that those with low blood levels of vitamins C or B_{12} scored the worst on memory and cognitive functioning tests. Those with low levels of the B vitamins riboflavin or folic acid scored worst on a test of abstract thinking. Another study found that giving women a B-complex supplement improved their performance on memory tests. B vitamins also help lower levels of artery-clogging homocysteine, linked to memory loss. Two other supplements to take along with your B's are vitamins E and C. Studies find taking the two together can protect against Alzheimer's. But taking the supplements

separately (for example, one in the morning and one at night) had no effect.

3 Add whole grain bread back into your diet. If you've been following a high-protein, low-carb diet and simultaneously finding your memory going, it's probably not a coincidence. More than any other organ, the brain relies on glucose for fuel. And glucose comes from carbs. One study of 22 older people from the University of Toronto found that those whose diets contained the greatest percentage of calories as carbohydrates performed best on memory and task tests. Make sure you're getting your carbs from fruits, vegetables, and whole grains, not ice cream, candy, and cake.

4 Make up a batch of tuna salad on Sunday nights and make sure it's gone by Friday. Tuna, even the canned kind, is high in omega-3 fatty acids, important for maintaining memory. Try it stuffed into a tomato, added to a regular green salad, or on toast for breakfast.

5 Eat a vegetarian dinner at least once a week. Low in saturated fat and high in fiber, it will boost your efforts to maintain healthy cholesterol levels. That's important when we're talking about memory, because high cholesterol levels eventually damage

blood vessels, affecting long-term memory and speeding the progression of Parkinson's and Alzheimer's diseases.

6 Eat cereal mixed with one cup of blueberries for breakfast several days a week. Not only do studies find that eating cereal in the morning can help your performance on certain cognitive tests, but a study in rats who got blueberries every day for two months found the fruit boosted levels of enzymes that help brain cells communicate with each other. Although the study was done in rats, the lead researcher says the results were so compelling that he now eats a cup or two of blueberries every day—just in case.

7 Skip dessert tonight. And tomorrow night as well. It might just help you drop a few pounds—a good thing when it comes to memory. That's because Swedish researchers found that older women diagnosed with memory problems tended to be an average of 11-17 pounds overweight compared to women who had fewer memory lapses. Other studies find overweight women and men have a higher risk of developing Alzheimer's disease.

8 Get a book on tape (or CD) and listen to it while you walk briskly, three times a week. A University of Illinois study found that older adults who walked that often had higher scores on memory tests than adults who just did stretching and toning exercises. Listening to the book *while* you're walking also exercises your brain while you're exercising your body.

9 Go to bed early the night after learning something important. So if you're learning a new computer program at work, make sure you get a good night's

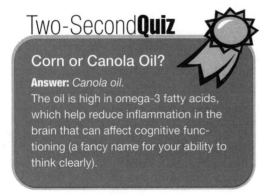

Two-Second**Quiz**

Corn or Canola Oil?

Answer: *Canola oil.*
The oil is high in omega-3 fatty acids, which help reduce inflammation in the brain that can affect cognitive functioning (a fancy name for your ability to think clearly).

sleep after your training. A Harvard study found that a good night's sleep improves your ability to remember something you learned during the day.

10 Stuff a chicken with sage and lemons and roast in a 350°F oven until done (about 2 hours). A couple of small studies suggest that the anti-inflammatory effects of sage may boost memory for several hours after eating the herb. Plus, lemons are chock-full of antioxidants important for maintaining healthy cell function. Other sage options: Try a tea made with a teaspoon of the dried herb, use in salad dressing and rice dishes, or add to flavor pork or fish. Try growing some in your garden. Sage is a perennial that overwinters well in most climates.

11 Switch the television station to PBS. The higher-level programming on public television will do more to engage your brain than any reality show or sitcom ever could. As we said, the more engaged your brain, the healthier your brain functions, including memory.

12 Snack on grapes instead of cookies. Researchers find that people with a high intake of trans fats—found in baked goods like cookies—are more than twice as likely to develop Alzheimer's disease as those who eat the least. Grapes, on the other hand, have phytochemicals and antioxidants that help lead to improved blood flow and overall health.

13 Have a glass of wine with dinner. A study of 746 men and women found that those who drank one to six alcoholic beverages (beer, wine, or liquor) a week were 54 percent less likely than abstainers to develop dementia

Healthy Investments

A Book of *New York Times* Crossword Puzzles

Doing crossword puzzles is to the brain what a treadmill is to your heart and legs. Puzzles activate nearly every important area of the brain, from visual to language centers to memory systems.

(including Alzheimer's disease and vascular dementia) over six years. Stop with one, though; the same study found that 14 or more drinks weekly increased the risk of dementia by 22 percent.

14 Whip up a batch of curried chicken tonight. An Italian study found that this common spice blend appears to enhance an enzyme that protects the brain against oxidative conditions that could lead to memory loss and Alzheimer's.

15 Cut some tofu cubes into your soup. Soy products like tofu have isoflavones that also appear to help preserve memory and hinder protein changes that contribute to Alzheimer's.

16 Read for an hour every day. But forget Jackie Collins novels. Pick a topic about which you know very little and read five books on that topic. Then move on to the next topic. Your brain will soak up the knowledge like a parched rosebush, sending out blooms in the form of neurons that help maintain a healthy memory.

17 Take up oil painting. Or fishing, or needlepoint, or ballroom dancing, or piano. The idea here is to continue stretching your mind around new things and new experiences, which studies find can help stave off dementia and improve memory.

18 Memorize a poem every day. Sure, it reminds you of your days in elementary school ("I think that I shall never see / A poem lovely as a tree ... "), but it's also a great exercise for those memory muscles, a.k.a. the brain. Not into poetry? How about memorizing the phone numbers of all your friends, or the addresses of all your family members?

19 Do one thing every day that will force you out of your comfort zone. It might be taking a different route to work, writing or using the mouse with your nondominant hand, or approaching a total stranger and striking up a conversation (in a safe place, mind you). This kind of challenge is the perfect "weightlifting" exercise for those brain cells.

20 Listen to music while you are exercising. A study of 33 adults undergoing cardiac rehabilitation found that those who listened to music while they worked out improved their scores on a verbal fluency test—a test that measures overall brainpower.

21 Spend a day exploring in an unfamiliar town. The challenge that comes from following a map, coupled with the novelty that new sights, sounds, and smells bring, serves as a healthy wake-up call for your brain.

22 Get a course book from your local college and pick one class to take next semester. A study from Chicago's Rush Alzheimer's Disease Center found that people who had higher levels of education exhibited fewer signs of Alzheimer's disease even when autopsies revealed they *had* the disease.

23 Do one thing at a time. If you're trying to have a phone conversation while checking e-mail, chances are good you won't remember a word you talked about. A growing body of research finds our increasing tendency to multitask actually harms our brains.

24 Have a bag of toasted pumpkin seeds for a brain-boosting snack. They're high in iron, shown to improve test scores in college students.

25 Pay better attention next time someone tells you his name, or when you throw your keys into the basket on the counter, or when you park your car. Often the reason we can't remember things is that we're on autopilot when we do them (or hear them). But if you stop for a second when someone introduces himself and repeat the name out loud, or stop when you get out of your car at the mall and look—really look—at the spot in which you're parked, you'll remember those things better.

26 Study, read, and work in a quiet room. Studies find that noise exposure can slow your ability to rehearse things in your mind, a way of building memory links.

27 Talk with your hands. No, we're not talking about sign language, but about using your hands to emphasize what you're saying. Turns out it's easier for us to speak when we're gesturing, leaving more mental resources available for transferring information into memory.

PART SEVEN

Stealth Habit
CONTROL

It's not the occasional splurge that hurts your health—it's the unhealthy habits we partake in every day. Here's compassionate advice for kicking the habits that bind you.

Cigarettes
25 Ways to Put the
Butts Behind You

Overeating
27 Ways to Stop
Compulsive Consumption

TV Addiction
17 Ways to
Escape the Tube

Alcohol
18 Ways to Cut Back
on Your Drinking

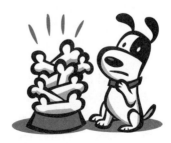

Cigarettes

25 WAYS TO PUT THE BUTTS BEHIND YOU

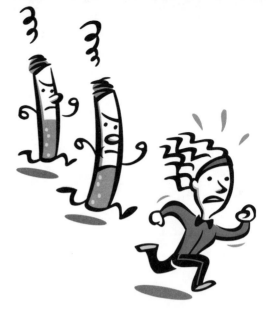

For all the intense efforts to reduce smoking in America over the past two decades, the progress has not been stellar. Today one in four men and one in five women still smoke. For those who never smoked, this is a befuddling fact. Don't smokers understand that cigarettes are the number one killer in America, that they dramatically increase risk for heart disease, stroke, cancer, high blood pressure, and almost every other health concern, small or large? How could any habit be worth this?

Truth is, most smokers do understand. They also understand the huge financial toll of smoking, with a pack of 20 cigarettes costing $7 in some areas (imagine: $2,500 spent a year on cigarettes by pack-a-day smokers—often people of only modest resources).

Then why do millions still smoke? In good part, because the nicotine in cigarettes is highly addictive. In good part, because smoking provides psychological comfort to some people. Perhaps most of all, because quitting is so hard.

Researchers and businesses have responded strongly to the last point. Never have there been so many tools, systems, and programs available for quitting smoking. And with every month that passes, there is more research showing the benefits of quitting, and the drawbacks of not quitting.

So if you smoke, consider again whether it is time, finally, to quit. If yes, you'll need to think through the best approach, perhaps working with your doctor or an expert. But the following 25 tips will help you succeed.

1 **Make an honest list of all the things you like about smoking.** Draw a line down the center of a piece of paper and write them on one side; on the other side make a list of all the things you dislike, such as how it can interfere with your health, work, family, etc., suggests Daniel Z. Lieberman, M.D., director of the Clinical Psychiatric Research Center at George Washington University Medical Center in Washington, D.C. Think about the list over time, and make changes. If you are brave enough, get feedback from family and friends about things they don't like about your use of cigarettes. When the negative side outweighs the positive side, you are ready to quit.

2 **Then make another list of why quitting won't be easy.** Be thorough, even if the list gets long and discouraging. Here's the important part:

Next to each entry, list one or more options for overcoming that challenge. For instance, one item might be: "Nicotine is an addictive drug." Your option might be: "Try a nicotine replacement alternative." Another reason might be: "Smoking helps me deal with stress." Your option might be: "Take five-minute walks instead." The more you anticipate the challenges to quitting, and their solutions, the better your chance of success.

3 Set a quit date and write a "quit date contract" that includes your signature and that of a supportive witness.

4 Write all your reasons for quitting on an index card and keep it near you at all times. Here are some to get you started: "My daughter, my granddaughter, my husband, my wife..." You get the idea.

5 As you're getting ready to quit, stop buying cartons of cigarettes. Instead, only buy a pack at a time, and only carry two or three with you at a time (try putting them in an Altoids tin). Eventually you'll find that when you want a smoke, you won't have any immediately available. That will slowly wean you down to fewer cigarettes.

Two-Second**Quiz**

Tobacco Treatment Program or Quit on Your Own?

Answer: *The program.*
People who take part in these programs double their chances of quitting for life, studies find. Visit www.quitnet.com to find a program near you.

6 Keep a list of when you smoke, what you're doing at the time, and how bad the craving is for a week before quitting to see if specific times of the day or activities increase your cravings, suggests Gaylene Mooney, chair of the American Association for Respiratory Care's Subcommittee on Smoking and Tobacco-Related Issues. Then arrange fun, unique things to do during those times, like some of the ones we recommend here.

7 Prepare a list of things to do when a craving hits. Suggestions include: take a walk, drink a glass of water, kiss your partner or child, throw the ball for the dog, wash the car, clean out a cupboard or closet, have sex, chew a piece of gum, wash your face, brush your teeth, take a nap, get a cup of coffee or tea, practice your deep breathing, light a candle. Make copies of the list and keep one with you at all times so when the craving hits, you can whip out the list and quickly do something from it.

8 When your quit date arrives, throw out anything that reminds you of smoking. That includes all smoking paraphernalia—leftover cigarettes, matches, lighters, ashtrays, cigarette holders, even the lighter in your car.

9 Instead of a cigarette break at work, play a game of solitaire on your computer. It takes about the same time and is much more fun (although, like cigarettes, it can get addictive). If your company prohibits games like that, find another five-minute diversion: a phone call, a stroll, or eating a piece of fruit outdoors (but not where smokers congregate).

10 Switch to a cup of herbal tea whenever you usually have a cigarette. That might be at breakfast, midmorning, or after meals. The act of brewing the tea and slowly sipping it as it cools will provide the same stress relief as a hit of nicotine.

11 Switch your cigarette habit for a nut habit—four nuts in their shell for every cigarette you want to smoke. This way, you're using your hands and your mouth, getting the same physical and oral sensations you get from smoking.

12 Carry some cinnamon-flavored toothpicks with you. Suck on one whenever a cig craving hits.

13 Make an appointment with an acupuncturist. There's some evidence that auricular acupuncture (i.e., needles in the ears) curbs cigarette cravings quite successfully, says Ather Ali, N.D., a naturopathic physician completing a National Institutes of Health-sponsored postdoctoral research fellowship at the Yale-Griffin Prevention Research Center in Derby, Connecticut. You can even do it yourself by taping "seeds" (small beads)

onto the acupuncture points and squeezing them whenever cravings arise.

14 Swing by the health food store for some *Avena sativa* (oat) extract. One study found that, taken at 1 milliliters four times daily, it helped habitual tobacco smokers significantly decrease the number of cigarettes they smoked.

15 Think of difficult things you have done in the past. Ask people who know you well to remind you of challenges you have successfully overcome, says Dr. Lieberman. This will give you the necessary self-confidence to stick with your pledge not to smoke.

16 To minimize cravings, change your routine. Sit in a different chair at breakfast or take a different route to work. If you usually have a drink and cigarette after work, change that to a walk. If you're used to a smoke with your morning coffee, switch to tea, or stop at Starbucks for a cup of java—the chain is smoke-free.

17 Tell your friends, coworkers, boss, partner, kids, etc., how you feel about situations instead of bottling up your emotions. If something makes you angry, express it instead of smothering it with cigarette smoke. If you're bored, admit to yourself that you're bored and find something energetic to do instead of lighting up.

18 If you relapse, just start again. You haven't failed. Some people have to quit as many as eight times before they are successful.

19 Put all the money you're saving on cigarettes in a large glass jar. You want to physically see how much you've been spending. Earmark that money for something you've always dreamed of doing, but never thought you could afford, be it a cruise to Alaska or a first-class ticket to visit an old college friend.

20 Switch to decaf until you've been cigarette-free for two months. Too much caffeine while quitting can cause the jitters.

21 Create a smoke-free zone. Don't allow anyone to use tobacco in your home, car, or even while sitting next to you in a restaurant. Make actual "No Smoking" signs and hang them around your house and in your car.

22 Find a healthy snack food you can keep with you and use in place of cigarettes to quench that urge for oral gratification. For instance, try pistachio nuts, sunflower seeds, sugarless lollipops or gum, carrot or celery sticks. The last ones are best if you are concerned about weight gain.

23 Picture yourself playing tennis. Or go play tennis. British researchers found volunteers trying to quit smoking were better able to ignore their urges to smoke when they were told to visualize a tennis match.

24 Quit when you're in a good mood. Studies find that you're less likely to be a successful quitter if you quit when you're depressed or under a great deal of stress.

Two-Second Quiz

Cigars or Cigarettes?

Answer: *Sugarless gum.*
Even though most cigar smokers dismiss their habit by saying they never inhale, Greek researchers found that smoking one cigar (Cuban, by the way) raised the heart rate, blood pressure, and pulse pressure in the healthy men who puffed away, as well as increased the stiffness of their aortas and other large arteries. The effects lasted about two hours. Turns out that even if you're not inhaling, you're absorbing more nicotine from a cigar via your mouth and nose cells than from a cigarette. For the record: One 7-inch cigar can hold as much tobacco as an entire pack of cigarettes.

25 Post this list in a visible location in your house. Whenever you're tempted to light up, take a look at all the ways smoking can damage your health:

▶ Increases risk of lung, bladder, pancreatic, mouth, esophageal, and other cancers, including leukemia
▶ Reduces fertility
▶ Contributes to thin bones
▶ Affects mental capacity and memory
▶ Reduces levels of folate, low levels of which can increase the risk of heart disease, depression, and Alzheimer's disease
▶ Increases likelihood of impotence
▶ Affects ability to smell and taste
▶ Results in low-birth-weight, premature babies
▶ Increases risk of depression in adolescents
▶ Increases risk of heart disease, stroke, high blood pressure
▶ Increases risk of diabetes
▶ Increases your child's risk of obesity and diabetes later in life if you smoked while pregnant

Alcohol

18 WAYS TO CUT BACK ON YOUR DRINKING

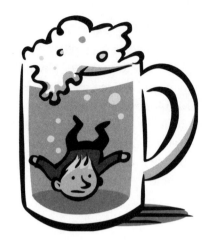

You'd think that it would be obvious to someone if he or she had a drinking problem. But that's not the case. Unlike other health-destroying habits like smoking or illegal drugs, drinking is something that most adults do, and that is quite healthy in moderation. Moreover, bars, cocktails, wine, and beer are woven into our cultural fabric, as so many liquor ads and commercials attest.

So how do you know when your drinking has become a problem? Look to the small signs. Maybe you've been waking up in the middle of the night with a raging thirst, drenched in sweat, needing to go to the bathroom. Maybe getting out of bed in the morning is a bit harder these days, and you seem to have an awful lot of headaches. Been taking the recycling to the center instead of leaving it out for the trash people to collect because you're too embarrassed about the large number of wine and beer bottles? Or putting on a few pounds, even though you're not eating any differently?

Maybe it's time to speak honestly to yourself and cut back on your drinking. This chapter will help you do it.

One caveat, though: Alcoholism is a serious disease. If you think you might be, or know you are, an alcoholic, you're going to need more than just the tips in this chapter to help you quit. Instead, the tips here are designed more for the social drinker who wants to cut back but who doesn't need to stop drinking altogether for health reasons. If you need more help, please see your doctor.

1 Other than on special occasions, limit your drinking to the level associated with optimal health: up to two drinks per day for men, one for women. And no stockpiling: Going without alcohol today doesn't increase the amount you can have tomorrow. In particular, you can't save up for a weekend binge.

2 Meet friends, dates, or business associates at a coffee bar, not a tavern. If the point of the get-together is fun, casual conversation in a friendly,

loose environment, there are many ways to do that without the alcohol. Coffee shops like Starbucks are good places to meet. Other possibilities include bistro-style restaurants, bowling alleys, and even sushi bars.

3 Watch sporting events with friends at your home or theirs. A night at a sports bar almost guarantees a morning with a headache. Guys, how can you resist the temptation to guzzle beer in a room filled with beer guzzlers?

4 Never, ever drink alone. Make it a rule. Not because it is so evil—indeed, there are plenty of times when a glass of wine by yourself is appropriate. Rather, do it for the discipline. If you learn to drink alone, it makes it too easy to begin drinking in excessive amounts.

5 Never, ever drink for courage. Throughout time, people have turned to drink to overcome social inhibitions. In fact, there's an old expression for alcohol: "liquid courage." And it's true—a few drinks can take the fright out of a party, business gathering, or speech. Trouble is when you rely on alcohol for bravery. No one should need alcohol to function socially. So find other ways to bolster your confidence. It's harder, but healthier and more honest—and you're less prone to making alcohol-induced gaffes.

6 Never, ever drink for solace. It's the old stereotype: down-trodden businessman, sitting at the bar, necktie yanked down, clothes disheveled, muttering, "Pour me another one, bartender." Sad, isn't it? Numbing yourself from the challenges of the world through alcohol. Again, we say, Drink for joy, not for pain. Drink to feel alive, not to feel dead.

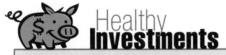

Healthy Investments

Properly Sized Glasses

A serving of wine is 5 ounces, a serving of beer 12 ounces, a serving of liquor 1.5 ounces. Yet some wineglasses are large enough to contain nearly a full bottle of wine! Buy a set of glasses for your drinking, regardless of what you drink, and use a permanent marker to mark the spot at which you should stop pouring.

Two-Second Quiz

Wine or Gin and Tonic?

Answer: *Wine.*
Not only does a glass of wine provide more volume for the alcohol (meaning it lasts longer so you'll drink less), but the health benefits of wine are legendary. Choose red wine over white for maximum health benefits.

7 Never, ever drink out of habit. You know what we mean: "Seven o'clock, time for my martini." "Done with cutting the lawn, time for my beer." "Friday night, time to hit the bar with the gang and have my weekly margaritas." Think through your week to see if you have a specific drinking routine or habit. If yes, commit to finding a substitute for it.

8 In particular, choose a pleasant substitution for your after-work drink. It could be a nonalcoholic drink, like a spiced ice tea or a fruit smoothie. Or it could be a walk, or a hot bath, or a sliced peach. Do this for two weeks until it becomes your new habit.

9 Switch to mixed drinks with a lower-proof alcohol. There are lots of alternatives to the standard, high-power alcohols of gin, vodka, or whisky. For example, a flavored cognac with seltzer has half the alcohol content of a gin drink, and probably twice the flavor.

10 Always drink double-fisted: your drink, and a large glass of water. Don't use alcohol to quench your thirst. That's what water is for. Sip on alcohol for the flavor and the pleasure.

11 **Keep the wine bottle off the dinner table.** Instead, keep a pitcher of water on the table. It makes it too easy to keep pouring until it's empty. Instead, pour one glass, then cork the bottle and put it away.

12 **Discover the glories of seltzer water.** It mixes with wine, whisky, vodka, cognac, indeed almost any alcohol other than beer. Making your drinks with seltzer cuts down on alcohol consumption, in part because the bubbles in the seltzer help fill you up.

 13 **When you're at a party, drink a full glass of water** or other nonalcoholic beverage before and after every alcoholic drink. We guarantee that the amount of alcohol you drink will drop substantially.

14 **Create a list of rules for drinking.** For instance, no more than one drink a day. Only drink on weekends. Only drink wine spritzers. Only drink when you're dressed up in your best clothes, etc. Post the list near the liquor cabinet/wine cellar.

15 **Keep a drinking diary.** You can find a sample from the National Institute on Alcohol Abuse and Alcoholism (www.niaaa.nih.gov). Tracking how much you drink will provide you with some surprising information that will encourage you to cut down or quit.

16 **Make a list of reasons why you want to cut back on drinking.** This could be: lose weight, sleep better, fewer headaches, get more done, improve blood sugar control, better sex, perform better at work. Post the list in a prominent place and read through it every time you think about having a drink.

17 **Track how much money you're spending on alcohol every week.** Now commit to spending half that amount. Put the savings into a special account (or even a jelly jar) and use it for something special for you (*not* a bottle of 2000 Bordeaux).

18 **Tell everyone you know that you're cutting back on your drinking.** Hopefully, this will prevent people from urging you to have "just one" or "just one more."

In**Perspective**

Do I Have a Problem?

If you're wondering if your drinking—or a loved one's—has crossed the line, answer the following questions:

1. Have you ever felt you should cut down on your drinking?

2. Have people annoyed you by criticizing your drinking?

3. Have you ever felt bad or guilty about your drinking?

4. Have you ever had a drink first thing in the morning to steady your nerves or to get rid of a hangover?

One yes answer suggests a possible alcohol problem. More than one yes answer means it is highly likely that a problem exists.

Overeating

27 WAYS TO STOP COMPULSIVE CONSUMPTION

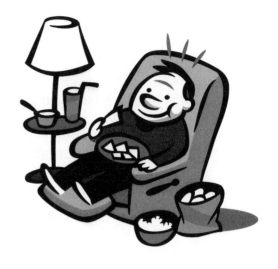

What is it about food? Serve us a plate with normal-sized portions and no other food on the table, and we'll eat it and likely be quite satisfied. But put us before an all-you-can-eat buffet, and suddenly our hunger sensor goes on the blink and we eat until we have to loosen our belts and unbutton our pants. Whether you need to lose weight or you're just tired of leaving the table feeling like you swallowed a beach ball, the following Stealth Health tips will help you curb your appetite and eat just enough—and no more.

1 Purge your home of low-nutrition snack food. That means ice cream, candy, potato chips, packaged cookies, doughnuts, cake, and any other salty or sugary snacks that you munch on between meals. Learn to live without this stuff. Period. These are the foods that we eat compulsively and that make us overweight. From now on, only eat these foods when offered them at a social event, or when you and the family deserve a special treat. Then go to the ice-cream parlor and get a single scoop of your favorite.

2 In its place, stock your home with mounds of fresh fruit, dried fruit, carrots, celery, tomatoes, granola bars, and high-fiber breakfast cereal. Here's your new snack food. For more healthy snack ideas, go to Part 2, "Stealth Healthy Cooking." Delicious, healthy ideas are spread throughout!

3 Never, ever buy a snack at gas stations, drugstores, or discount chains. Yes, they want to tempt you with doughnuts, potato chips, candy bars, or hot dogs—that's why they put the stuff all around the cash register. It makes them a lot of money. It makes *you* poorer, heavier, and less healthy.

4 Never, ever stop at a food store just to buy a snack. No drive-through windows for the 99-cent special at Burger King. No stopping at the doughnut shop for a quick glazed. No quick pizza slice at Mario's. This type of compulsive, unhealthy eating is causing our nation's weight problems.

5 Make this simple salad for a big, healthy splurge. Feel desperate for a big bowl of crunchy food? Throw into a bowl half a head of iceberg lettuce, ripped up; a fistful of bite-size carrots; half a tomato, sliced up; and half a cucumber, sliced. Drizzle on olive oil, shake on a little balsamic vinegar, sprinkle on some oregano, salt, and pepper, and mix. This is a huge bowl of flavorful food at relatively few calories.

6 Another splurge food: watermelon. It's more than 90 percent water, and the other 10 percent has plenty of healthy nutrients and reasonable calorie levels. If you want to indulge in a hearty helping of food, dig deeply into a hearty portion of watermelon.

7 Yet another splurge food: vegetable soup. Need comfort food? Heat up a large bowl of soup made with lots of vegetables and beans. It's flavorful, hearty, and generally high in nutrition and low in fat.

8 One more great snack option: nuts in their shell. The truth is, compulsive eating is often about boredom, stress, and other non-food issues. The great thing about nuts is that the effort to crack the shells and extract the nut meat without breaking it is highly therapeutic and distracting. In addition, nuts are very healthy to eat (in moderation). Choose walnuts, almonds, pecans, Brazil nuts, or hazelnuts. It's too easy to open and overindulge in peanuts and pistachios. The only drawback to this snack is the mess the shells make. Be sure to have a bowl to put shells in as you go.

9 If you need to retrain your appetite, start out by eating out. Restaurants have a reputation for rich food and large portions, but if you've been eating with wild abandon, you can go to a restaurant, ask the waiter to bring you half the normal

portion, eat it, feel satisfied, and leave. Then there are no kids' plates to clean off or leftover mashed potatoes singing to you from the fridge, notes Victoria Moran, author of *Younger by the Day: 365 Ways to Rejuvenate Your Body and Revitalize Your Spirit.* After a few days of this, you'll be in the swing of eating regular meals and you can eat at home without overdoing it. Just avoid restaurants that offer all-you-can-eat buffets, the option of "supersizing," or those known for huge portions. Otherwise, the whole point of this exercise is moot!

10 Get picky. Moms complain about children who are finicky eaters, but you're not a child, and you owe it to yourself to be a bit persnickety when it comes to what goes into your mouth. As a rule of thumb: If it doesn't look good, don't eat it. Watch naturally thin people: You won't see them scarfing down wilted lettuce, or what's left in the bowl when the soup's gotten cold. Follow their example.

11 Get into the habit of ordering the small size. There's no need to feel deprived. Today's small was the medium or large just a few decades back. Eat (or sip) slowly. Savor the flavors. Before long, small will feel just right. Besides, remember that ordering the small size leads to wearing the small size.

12 **Always choose the best from what's available.** Sometimes you'll have lots of great choices—at a farmers' market, let's say, or a restaurant that caters to people interested in their health. Other times you'll be on an interstate and have to choose from three fast-food places. Either way, if you pick the best in your current situation—a combination of what's most nutritious, most attractive, the right price, and simply what you have a hankering for right now—you'll find yourself lean and healthy in the long run.

 13 **Always allow a half-hour between your last bite of dinner and dessert.** This gives your brain time to get the fullness signal and, most likely, will make it easier to skip the sweet

stuff, notes Susie Galvez, author of *Weight Loss Wisdom: 365 Successful Dieting Tips.*

14 **Only eat portions the size of the palm of your hand.** Any more will be considered overeating.

15 **Always put what you're eating on a plate or in a bowl.** Never eat out of a bag, carton, or box.

16 **Eat a healthy snack before going out to eat.** It will help you avoid the tempting bread basket.

17 **As soon as you feel the first stirrings of fullness,** remove your plate from the table or, if you're dining out, cover your plate with a napkin. This tells your brain that food time is over, says Galvez.

18 **Dine to soothing music, not the television.** This signals that mealtime is to be enjoyed and savored. You'll be

In**Perspective**

Binge-Eating Disorder

How do you know if you're simply eating too much or whether you have an actual eating disorder called binge-eating disorder? Well, *how* do you eat?

If your overeating generally occurs when you eat out, encounter a buffet, or are served your all-time favorite food, you probably have nothing to worry about. But if you find you have episodes in which you eat faster than normal, eat until you're uncomfortably full, eat large

amounts of food when you're not even hungry, eat alone because you're embarrassed by how much you're eating, feel disgusted with yourself, depressed or very guilty after overeating, then you might have a problem.

An estimated 2-5 percent of Americans experience binge-eating disorder in a six-month period, surveys find. Key symptoms are recurrent episodes of binge eating characterized by eating an excessive amount

of food within a short period of time and by a sense of lack of control over eating during the episode. To be diagnosed with the disorder, however, you must have had these symptoms at least two days a week for six months.

If you think you might have binge-eating disorder—or if you make yourself vomit after bingeing, a condition called bulimia—see your doctor immediately. Therapy and medications can help you bring it under control.

more aware of what you're eating, will eat slower, and will get the "full" signal sooner, thus eating less.

19 **Buy (or package) snacks and other foods into single-serving containers.** For instance, don't leave a half-gallon of ice cream in your freezer; it's too easy to add that second or third scoop when you're dishing it out. Instead, when you get home from the grocery store, scoop the appropriate serving size into individual containers and freeze. Do this after you've eaten, so you're not tempted to increase the size or sneak a bite.

20 **Don't talk while you're still chewing.** Instead, put your fork down, chew, and swallow your food before you begin talking. Again, this will force you to slow down while eating, and you'll be full before you know it (yet you *will* know it!)

21 **Scrape all leftovers into the trash.** Make it a habit. You don't need to clean off everyone's plates yourself.

22 **Write down every morsel you eat in a food diary.** It's likely you've been overlooking some calories,

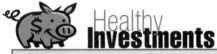

Healthy Investments

A Dinner Belt

The idea is to have one belt that you wear while eating, to gauge your level of fullness. Wear it cinched firmly around your waist when you are about to eat dinner, using the same hole each evening. As soon as you feel the least amount of strain against the belt, put your fork down and cover your plate with your napkin. You're done.

and it's time to start looking them over! Seeing all you ate in black and white will help keep you from overeating.

23 **Nix the restrictive or fad diets.** They will only make you crave certain foods, leading to binge eating.

24 **Limit the amount of artificial sweeteners and artificially sweetened foods you eat.** A Purdue University study published in July 2004 found that consuming artificially sweetened foods and beverages may throw off your natural ability to monitor calories and increase your likelihood of overeating.

25 **Practice the 20-minute distraction strategy.** When you find yourself looking for food, even though you are not hungry, do something else for 20 minutes, suggests Jill Fleming, R.D., author of *Thin People Don't Clean Their Plates.* The activity needs to involve your brain as well as your hands, such as playing the piano or cleaning a closet.

26 **Set your kitchen timer for 20 minutes** every time you think you want something to eat. If you still want to eat when it rings, fine. If not, you weren't really hungry to begin with and the urge will have passed, says Fleming. Conversely, when you sit down to eat, set your time for 10 minutes. After 10 minutes, stop eating, put down your fork, walk around the house. After 10 minutes of this, you can go back to eating.

27 **Have a nutritious snack** like a handful of peanuts, a piece of fruit and cheese, or a yogurt about an hour or so before dinner. Keeping your appetite in check is one of the best ways to avoid binges.

TV Addiction

17 WAYS TO ESCAPE THE TUBE

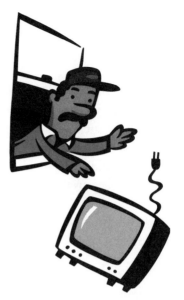

This country boasts a population of 275 million people—and 248 million televisions, according to the 2000 Census. Nearly every household (98.2 percent) has at least one TV and most have more, with an average of 2.4 sets per home. We spent an average of $255.18 per person for cable and satellite TV in 2004 and watch the equivalent of about 70 days of television a year (more if you're over 65), a truly scary thought when you consider the quality of most programming these days. Plus, there's the fact that TV watching has been linked to higher rates of obesity and diabetes.

Tired of wasting the equivalent of two months of your life every year glued to the tube? Spending more than an hour sitting in front of the television each evening? Like kicking any habit, half the battle of TV addiction is acknowledging the problem and making the commitment to change. Assuming you have the commitment, here are specific tips on getting the job done:

1 Give your extra TVs to charity. Allow your home one TV in a room dedicated to nothing but reading or TV watching. Donate the rest to a school or charitable organization in your community. You'll not only get the tax deduction and a feeling that you did good, but it will be that much harder to veg out in front of the tube!

2 Only turn on the TV to watch a particular show. In other words, don't just turn it on and go surfing for something worthwhile. Hours are quickly wasted, switching from one show to the next, watching all and none at the same time.

3 Then, when you sit down to watch a particular show, set a timer or an alarm clock in another room for the length of the show. When it beeps, you'll have to get out of your chair to turn it off, a signal to also turn off the tube.

4 Throw out the remote control. It's amazing how much less television you'll watch if you have to get up every time you want to change channels or adjust the volume. Plus, it eliminates all those hours you spend channel surfing.

5 Rearrange the furniture. Design your family room so that the television becomes not the focal point of the room, but an afterthought that requires twisting around or rearranging the furniture to view.

6 Hide the television. Put it behind an armoire, hang a blanket over it, or stick it inside a cabinet. Do whatever you can to ensure it fades into the background and can't be seen for what it is—a dangerous time sucker.

7 Eat meals, especially dinner, with the television OFF.

8 Set a rule that you can't watch TV if the sun is shining. Instead, you have to go for a walk, ride a bike, or get some other kind of healthy physical activity for at least an hour before you can turn on the tube. This rule also works great for your kids or grandkids.

9 Make a TV-watching plan each week. Sit down with the viewing guide and pick out the shows you want to watch that week. Watch only those shows, and when they're over, turn the TV off.

10 Set a rule that you must read 30 pages of a book or magazine before you can turn on the TV. Depending on how fast you read, you may never watch TV again!

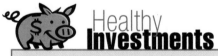

Healthy Investments

TiVo

This cool toy enables you to watch the TV programs you're interested in when you want to watch them, regardless of when they're on. You'll spend much less time channel surfing.

11 Create a list of one-hour evening projects. List everything you can possibly dream of: cleaning a particularly messy cupboard, organizing recipes, touching up the paint on your bedroom walls, sharpening kitchen knives, sorting through your sewing materials. Then create an old-fashioned job jar, and try to do one each evening.

12 Switch to games. With your spouse and/or children, relearn the fun of Scrabble, backgammon, or even chess. Get out the playing cards and have a hearts or gin rummy battle. Play Ping-Pong, pool, or darts in the basement. Go outside and practice your golf swing with practice balls. All of these are more fun, healthy, and life-affirming than sitting in front of the television.

13 Develop a fast-moving news routine. Most news shows are scheduled down to the minute. So investigate the handful of shows you watch and figure out when they run the features you are most interested in. For example, the local weather is on the Weather Network at eight after the hour; the recap of the day's headlines on CNN at fifteen after; the sports scores on ESPN SportsCenter shortly after. Add it all together, and you have a total national news briefing in about 15 minutes. Sounds like the perfect evening television routine. Watch it when you get home, and then turn off the television for the rest of the night.

14 Say no to *Jaws* for the 15th time. Often we can be strangely drawn into watching things we've seen many times before. There's something comforting in the repetition. Well, resist it.

Watching the same James Bond movie or *Trading Spaces* episode again and again is unhealthy for your body and your brain.

15 **Get outdoors every night.** Make it a point to leave your home or apartment at least once after dinner, if only for a short walk around the block. Too many people consider their day pretty much done once they've eaten dinner, when in fact, evening can be a wonderful time for getting things done and having fun.

16 **Change your TV-viewing chairs.** Make them somewhat hard and upright—chairs you don't want to lounge in for hours. Move your most comfy chairs to the living room, and use them for listening to music and reading.

17 **Say no to pundits and celebrity talkfests.** One way to cut down on television is to rule out certain types of shows. We suggest, start with any show in which you are watching a person talk. It is rare that a television interview or conversation is deeply insightful. Other categories to consider boycotting:

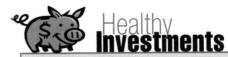

Healthy Investments

Knitting Needles and a Ball of Yarn

Learn to knit while you watch television; it will keep you from eating your way through the evening, and you'll accomplish something productive.

- *Entire ball games.* Why spend three hours watching a baseball or football game when the critical action can be captured in five minutes?
- *Any show with a laugh track.* How good can it be if it requires canned laughter to tell you a scene is funny?
- *Shows filled with guns and violence.* Who needs the mental baggage of all that killing and mayhem?
- *Reality shows built on a cruel premise.* If it torments the participants, or causes them ridicule, or extols values contrary to yours (like all the shows glorifying plastic surgery), then don't watch.

What does that leave you with? Quality news coverage; good movies; shows you can learn from; shows that celebrate people and the good in life.

REMINDER

 Fast Results
These are bits of advice that deliver benefits particularly quickly—in some cases, immediately!

 Easy Gains
These are tips that give the biggest value for the least amount of effort.

 Super Effective
These are tips proven to be particularly effective through scientific research or widespread usage by experts.

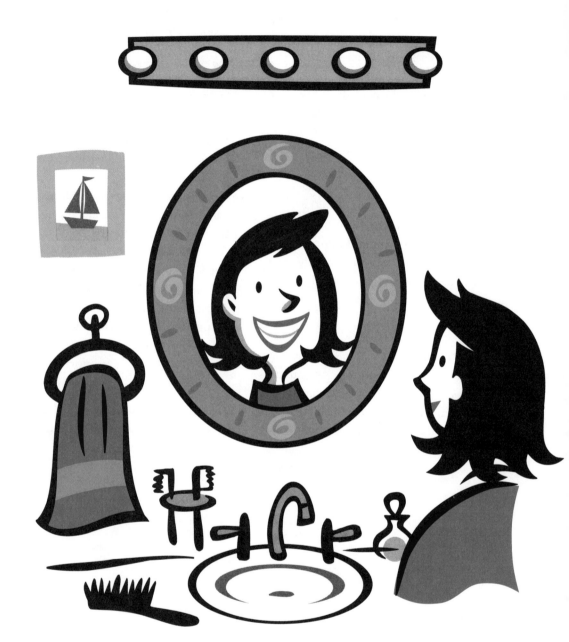

PART EIGHT

Stealth Healthy

LOOKS

Let's be honest. Looking good feels good. But a nice appearance isn't just vanity; healthy skin and teeth contribute to overall health. Here are easy, fast ways to look your best.

Healthy Skin
39 Fast Tricks to
Enhance Your Glow

Maintaining a Healthy Smile
22 Ways to Keep Your
Gums and Teeth Clean

Healthier, More Attractive Hair
32 Ways to Add Body,
Personality, and Longevity

Healthy Nails
14 Ways to Keep 'Em Strong

Grooming
32 Ways to Look
(and Smell) Your Best

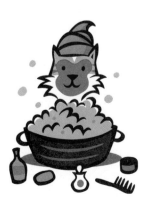

Healthy Skin

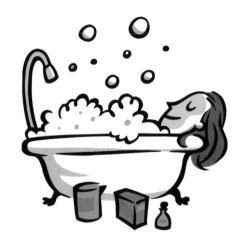

39 FAST TRICKS TO ENHANCE YOUR GLOW

Beauty, the saying goes, is only skin-deep. But the importance of skin goes a lot deeper. Most of us think of skin as just our body's visible outer layer, but doctors consider skin an organ, meaning that it is very much alive and charged with many important duties. In particular, the skin is the first layer of your immune system, serving as a shield between you and legions of germs such as viruses and bacteria. It also protects your insides from sun, cold, scrapes, cuts, and moisture. And, of course, your sense of touch is crucial for everyday function.

Like any part of your internal body, your skin can be healthy or ill. It can be well nourished or malnourished. It can be exercised, and it can wear down with age or abuse. In particular, as we age, our skin becomes thinner and drier. Plus, other, more unpleasant things happen to our skin. Things like wrinkles, age spots, dark circles, and large pores, which tend to turn up like uninvited guests at a wedding.

While you can't control your age, you can control numerous other factors that accelerate this aging process, including excessive exposure to sunlight, loss of estrogen during menopause, poor dietary habits, stress, and cigarette smoking.

Unlike the other organs of your body, you can apply medicines, moisturizers, and other healthy potions directly to the skin. For that reason alone, there is absolutely no reason you can't have healthy, attractive skin throughout your life. To keep your skin and face young and healthy, and to maintain its natural, protective moisture, follow these Stealth Healthy tips.

1 **Skip the long, steamy showers and opt for shorter, cooler sprays.** Long, hot showers strip skin of its moisture and wash away protective oils, says Andrea Lynn Cambio, M.D., a New York City dermatologist. So limit showers to 10 minutes and keep the water cool.

2 **Check the dryness of your skin by scratching a small area on your arm or leg with your fingernail.** If it leaves a white mark, your skin is indeed dry and needs both moisture and exfoliation (that is, removal of the outermost layer of dead skin cells).

3 **Treat your neck and chest like an extension of your face.** Your neck and upper chest area is covered by very sensitive skin, making it a prime spot for telltale signs of aging such as dryness, sun spots, and wrinkles, says Susie Galvez, owner of Face Works Day Spa in Richmond, Virginia, and author of *Hello*

Beautiful: 365 Ways to Be Even More Beautiful. To keep this area youthful, use facial cleansing creams that hydrate and cleanse gently rather than deodorant soaps, which can be drying. Top it all off with a good facial moisturizing cream. If this area is extra dry, use a facial moisturizing mask twice a month.

4 Run a humidifier every night in the winter to moisturize the air in your bedroom. Not only will it ease itchy, dry skin, you'll be able to breathe the moist air more easily.

5 Take 160 milligrams of soy isoflavones per day or pour soy milk over your cereal. Soy consumption may support skin health by supplying high-quality protein needed for building and maintaining collagen, the material essential to connective tissues, says Aaron Tabor, M.D., CEO and medical research director at Revival Soy in Kernersville, North Carolina. Soy isoflavones may also act as antioxidants to protect collagen from damage caused by free radicals, highly reactive molecules that can weaken or destroy cell membranes. Free radicals can also damage DNA, create age spots and wrinkles, and depress the immune system, increasing the risk of skin cancer. Good sources of soy isoflavones include soy milk (20-35 mg soy isoflavones per serving) and tofu (20-30 mg soy isoflavones per serving).

6 Switch from a deodorant soap to one with added fat, like Dove, Oilatum, or Neutrogena. Deodorant soaps can be drying, whereas added-fat soaps leave an oily, yet beneficial, film on your skin.

7 Keep your beauty products clean and simple, particularly if you have sensitive skin. Stay away from products with color, fragrance, or those that produce bubbles or have "antibacterial" on the label, says Dr. Cambio. These can all irritate skin.

8 Smooth a couple of drops of olive oil over your face, elbows, knees, and the backs of your arms every evening. The oil contains monounsaturated fat, which refreshes and hydrates skin without leaving a greasy residue.

9 For soft, young-looking hands and feet, slather on moisturizing cream and then slip on thin-fabric socks and gloves while you sleep.

10 Tone your skin with a sage, peppermint, and witch hazel combination. Sage helps to control oil, peppermint creates a cool tingle, and witch hazel helps restore the skin's protective layer. Combine 4 ounces of witch hazel with 1 teaspoon each of sage and peppermint leaves and steep for one to three days before applying to your skin.

Healthy Investments

Prescription Peeling Agents Like Retin-A and Tazorac

These topical medications help smooth out wrinkles and skin blotchiness, says Vicki Rapaport, M.D., a Beverly Hills dermatologist. Retin-A is a vitamin A derivative approved for long-term correction of fine wrinkles. It works by producing a thicker, healthier epidermis (the top layer of the skin).

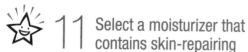

11 Select a moisturizer that contains skin-repairing humectants. Is that a new word for you? Humectants attract water when applied to your skin and improve its hydration. Good ones include glycerin, propylene glycol, and urea. Also look for skin products that contain alpha-hydroxy acids (AHAs), compounds that help reduce wrinkles and improve dry skin, acne, and age spots. AHAs, which naturally occur in grapes, apples, citrus, and sour milk (think buttermilk or yogurt), work by speeding up the turnover of old skin cells, making skin look younger.

12 Use a loofah daily to keep ingrown hairs and scaly skin under control. While in the shower, gently scrub bumpy or scaly skin with a circular motion to remove dead cells. For extra-smooth skin, sprinkle a few drops of an alpha-hydroxy product on the loofah before scrubbing.

13 Take rose hips every morning to help build collagen. Rich in vitamin C, rose hips (available at drugstores) can help keep skin smooth and youthful. Follow label directions.

14 Pop a high-potency multivitamin every day. Many nutrients are vital to healthy skin, including vitamins C, A, and B. The most reliable way to get them all every day is to eat well, as well as take a daily supplement.

15 Use unscented baby powder to keep areas where skin meets skin—like the inner thighs, underarms, beneath large breasts—clean and dry. This is important to prevent a common skin condition called intertrigo, which occurs when such areas remain moist, fostering the growth of bacteria or fungi.

16 If you're gearing up for a day in the sun, steer clear of scented lotions and perfumes. Scented products can lead to blotchy skin when exposed to the sun, says Galvez.

DoThreeThings

If you do only three things to improve the look and feel of your skin, make them these three, agree several of our experts:

1. **Drink at least eight 8-ounce glasses of** water a day to stay hydrated. This helps flush toxins through your kidneys instead of your skin.

2. **Follow a healthy diet rich in fruits, vegetables, and fish.** When researchers from Monash University in Australia studied the diets of 453 people ages 70 and older from Australia, Greece, and Sweden to see if there was any correlation between what they ate and the number of wrinkles in their skin, they found those who ate the most fruits, vegetables, and fish had the fewest wrinkles. Conversely, the researchers found, foods high in saturated fat, including meat, butter, and full-fat dairy, as well as soft drinks, cakes, pastries, and potatoes, increased the likelihood of skin wrinkling.

3. **Protect your skin from the sun all year round with a sunblock with an SPF of 30 or greater.** Just because there's snow on the ground doesn't mean your skin can't be damaged by the sun, says Andrea Lynn Cambio, M.D., a New York City dermatologist. Time outdoors is time well spent, but be sure to keep your skin either well covered or well protected with sunblock. In particular, the sun is at its most damaging between 11 a.m. and 3 p.m.

17 To treat dry, rough, itchy skin, try these bath add-ins:

▸ **Half a pound of sea salt and one pound baking soda.** Soak until the water is cool to detoxify your skin and soothe the itch.

▸ **Two cups Epsom salt.** In addition to soaking in it, while your skin is still wet, rub handfuls of Epsom salt on the rough areas to exfoliate skin.

▸ **A few bags of your favorite tea.** The tea provides antioxidants as well as a delicious scent.

▸ **One cup uncooked oatmeal tied into an old stocking or muslin bag.** Oats are not only wonderful for your inner health, says Galvez, but provide a healthy glow on the outside as well, leaving a film on your skin that seals in water.

▸ **Equal parts of apple cider vinegar, wheat germ, and sesame oil.** Apple cider vinegar is both antibacterial and alkalinizing (meaning it helps maintain the proper acid balance), while sesame oil and wheat germ add moisture.

▸ **One cup powdered milk with one tablespoon grapeseed oil.** The lactic acid in the milk will exfoliate your skin, and the grapeseed oil will give your skin a powerful dose of antioxidants.

18 Apply ice wrapped in a towel to dry, itchy skin. A few minutes on, a few minutes off. Allow the moist cold to relieve your skin and draw warming blood to it, but don't let your skin get so cold as to sting or hurt.

19 Smooth aloe vera gel over extra-dry skin. The acids in aloe eat away dead skin cells and speed up the healing process. Cut off an end of an aloe leaf, split open, and spread the gel on the dry area.

---

10 Foods to Eat for Your Face

The following foods are all rich in antioxidants and other nutrients shown in laboratory studies to benefit skin health:

1. Salmon
2. Green tea
3. Olive oil and olives
4. Sardines
5. Brazil nuts
6. Blueberries
7. Flaxseeds
8. Nonfat dairy products
9. Canola oil
10. Avocados

---

20 Plunk your rough, dry elbows into grapefruit halves. First exfoliate your elbows in your bath or shower, then cut a grapefruit in half and rest one elbow on each half, letting them soak for 15 minutes, recommends Galvez. The acid in the grapefruit provides extra smoothing power.

21 Hang room-darkening shades in your bedroom. They help avoid sleep disturbances or insomnia caused by ambient light. Sleep is critical to your skin's health because most cell repair and regeneration occurs while you're getting your z's; if you're not getting enough rest, your skin cannot renew itself.

22 Cook with garlic every day. A 1996 Danish study found that skin cells grown in a culture dish and treated with garlic had seven times the life span of cells grown in a standard culture. They also tended to look healthier and more youthful than untreated cells. Plus, garlic extract dramatically inhibited the growth of cancerous skin cells.

How to Choose Makeup

Check any woman's bathroom, and chances are you'll find a plethora of makeup, much of it old and barely used. But choosing a makeup should be as simple as choosing an ice-cream flavor—once you know what's best for you. Along those lines, follow this advice:

▼ FOUNDATION

✔ If you're blessed with great skin, **use as little foundation as possible,** suggests Dianne M. Daniels, image consultant and color analyst at Image & Color Services in Norwich, Connecticut. If you do use foundation, choose a sheer liquid foundation instead of a corrective foundation and top it off with a dusting of loose powder.

✔ For a bit more coverage, **go for a crème-to-powder** foundation.

✔ Mature skin usually requires a heavier crème foundation—**a powder finish may actually accentuate lines** in your face.

✔ Make sure you apply the right amount of foundation to your face. Too much is like pointing a neon sign at your wrinkles, says Daniels. Instead, **dip a fine brush or makeup sponge in a lightweight foundation and dab it on** skin blotches and brown spots to even them out. Then take a damp sponge and apply foundation to your entire face, making sure to match the color of your neck and blend in well so there's no obvious line at your chin.

✔ For instant radiance, **mix liquid bronzer with your foundation or moisturizer** before applying it to your face.

✔ **Use a makeup sponge instead of your finger to apply foundation.** Dipping your finger into your foundation spreads bacteria, which can cause breakouts. And use a fresh, disposable makeup sponge every day.

▼ CONCEALER

✔ **Hide pimples with red neutralizer** (available at your local beauty supply store). Just dab it on the pimple before putting on foundation.

✔ **Buy a good concealer.** It can hide a multitude of flaws, such as pimples, dark circles, or patchy lip tone. Look for a creamy, yellow-based concealer that's one shade lighter than your skin tone.

✔ Don't use concealer all over your face. **Just dab a bit on where needed,** but don't try to substitute it for a good foundation.

✔ **Cover lids, brow bone, and eye corner** with concealer. It evens out skin tone and provides a base for eye makeup so the color stays in place longer.

✔ **Skip under-eye concealer** if you have under-eye lines. The skin under your eyes is too thin to hold the heavy concealer, says Andrea Lynn Cambio, M.D., a New York City dermatologist. Instead, dab on foundation.

▼ CHEEKS

✔ Match the shade of your lips without lipstick to your blush color to get the most natural color. Or you can **match your cheek color after you've exercised or gotten overheated.**

✔ Smile broadly, then **brush blush on the puffy tops of your cheekbones.** Brush upward and outward to your hairline.

▼ LIPS

✔ **Match your lip liner to the shade of your lipstick.** Lip liner shouldn't look like it's outlining your mouth. Instead, apply a sheer, frosty lip gloss over your regular lipstick for a more subtle, elegant look.

✔ **Choose the right color lipstick.** That would be pink shades for light complexions, and dark, earthy tones for dark skin.

✔ **Put a little concealer on your upper and lower lip** to prevent lipstick from bleeding past your lips. Follow up with a little translucent powder.

✔ **Exfoliate your lips** once or twice a week to keep them soft and kissable. Once they're exfoliated, douse your lips with a lip balm enriched with vitamins E and C.

▼ EYES

✔ Zigzag your mascara wand while applying mascara for **clump-free eyelashes**, suggests Susie Galvez, owner of Face Works Day Spa in Richmond, Virginia, and author of *Hello Beautiful: 365 Ways to Be Even More Beautiful*.

✔ Apply eyeliner with a brush. It provides a smoky look while gently blurring the color. It also **gives your eyeliner more staying power.** For best results, look for a thick angled sable or synthetic-fiber brush.

✔ Remove waterproof, smudgeproof mascara with makeup remover before going to bed. Nothing makes you look more worn-out than residual mascara under your eyes in the morning.

✔ Draw attention to your eyes and make them look bigger with **a dab of gold or silver** eye shadow applied to the center of your eyelid just above the lash. When you blink, **people will be attracted to the light** and therefore, to your eyes.

✔ **Brush Japanese rice powder onto lashes** before applying mascara to enhance thin or short eyelashes, recommends Janet M. Niegel, M.D., an ophthalmologist in West Orange, New Jersey.

✔ Accentuate the outer corner of your eyes with a gray-brown powder and extend it toward the edge of the eye to **make close-set eyes look farther apart,** says Gina Michele Bisignano, model and beauty expert in Los Angeles.

✔ Use a **white eyeliner on the inside rim** of your eyes to make your eyes look more open and brighter, thus making them look bigger.

▼ BASICS

✔ Use a **moisturizing makeup remover** that leaves your face feeling clean and soft.

✔ **Throw foundation away after three months.** After a few months, the oils in foundation can go bad and smell rancid, says Gabriela Hernandez, makeup artist in Los Angeles. Powder makeups like blushes and eye shadows last a little longer, but make sure to throw them out after a year.

✔ Keep your makeup style fresh and current. **A subtle change now and then will keep your look fashionable.** If you'd rather not change your colors completely, change the texture. For example, if you love a particular shade of eye shadow, choose the same shade in a sparkly version. The small change will get noticed, but it won't be too dramatic.

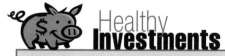

A Wide-Brimmed Hat

It provides an extra layer of protection from skin-damaging UVB and UVA rays. It also shields your eyes from direct sunlight. And it keeps the sun off your hair, which is a good thing too.

23 Go for a run, ride your bike, work out in the garden on a hot day—anything that gets you sweating. Sweating is nature's way of eliminating toxic chemicals that can build up under skin. Plus, regular exercise maintains healthy circulation and blood flow throughout your body, including your skin. If you're exercising outdoors, though, remember to wear a sunscreen on your face that protects against UVA and UVB rays, or a moisturizer with sunscreen protection.

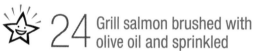

24 Grill salmon brushed with olive oil and sprinkled with toasted, crushed walnuts. There, you've just gotten a skin-healthy dose of poly- and monounsaturated fats, particularly omega-3 fatty acids, which studies suggest may affect the amount of sun and aging damage your skin experiences. By extension, make sure olive oil is the primary source of fat in your cooking each and every day, and try to have salmon twice a week or more.

25 Brew a pot of tea, chill, then store in the fridge and drink throughout the day. Tea, as you probably know, is a great source of antioxidants, molecules that fight the free-radical damage caused by sun exposure and cigarette smoking. One Arizona study, for instance, found that the more tea people drank (particularly tea with lemon) the less likely they were to develop squamous cell skin cancer.

26 Switch moisturizers every time the seasons change. Your skin needs more moisture in the winter than in the summer. So the same day you bring those sweaters down from the attic for the winter, buy a heavier moisturizer. When you trade in the sweaters for shorts, switch to a lighter one.

27 Here's one for men: Recognize that skin-preserving products like cleansers and moisturizers aren't just for women. Men need skin care just as much as their wives and sisters. To prevent wrinkles and skin cancer, use a moisturizer containing a sunscreen with an SPF of at least 15 daily. Also use a gentle exfoliant weekly and a nighttime moisturizer that contains alpha-hydroxy acids to encourage skin regeneration.

28 Prepare a homemade oat scrub and use on your face every other day. Oats moisturize and exfoliate your skin at the same time. Grind enough rolled oats in a food processor or coffee grinder to fill ½ cup. Combine with ⅓ cup ground sunflower seeds, ½ teaspoon peppermint leaves, and 4 tablespoons almond meal. Mix 2 teaspoons with a small amount of heavy cream. Scrub your face and neck with the mixture, then rinse thoroughly with cool water.

29 Add a teaspoon of grapeseed oil to your toner. The oil acts as an anti-aging serum by helping your skin cells repair and rejuvenate themselves, suggests Gina Michele Bisignano, a model and beauty expert in Los Angeles.

30 **Avoid these three skin destroyers:** Smoking, tanning salons, and sunbathing. All three will age your skin prematurely, many doctors agree.

31 **For double protection, apply a cream containing vitamin C to your face over your sunblock.** The cream helps prevent facial skin damage, dehydration, and wrinkles, says Galvez. Also try creams containing vitamin E or beta-carotene.

32 **Use a spritzer with rose, sandalwood, or bergamot essential oils mixed with water.** These oils are great for hydrating the skin, says Melinda Minton, spa consultant and health and beauty expert in Fort Collins, Colorado. To create an herbal spritzer, mix a few drops of essential oil with water in a small spray bottle and spritz on your face whenever your skin needs a little boost. Your skin is more pliable when it's hydrated, so a spray helps stave off frown lines and general movement wrinkles. The hydrator also keeps pollutants out and keeps your skin's natural lubricants in. An added bonus: Your makeup will stay on longer and look more natural.

33 **Make your own cleansing, moisturizing masks.**

▸ **Mix 1 tablespoon plain yogurt with a few dashes of sesame oil.** Leave on for 15 minutes, then rinse.
▸ **Mash a banana well and mix with a little honey for an instant dry-skin fix.** Leave on for 15 minutes, then rinse.
▸ **Mix ¼ cup whipping cream, ½ teaspoon olive oil, 2 tablespoons ripe mashed avocado, and 1 teaspoon calendula petals.** Leave on for 5 minutes,

then rinse. A study completed at the Department of Food Engineering and Biotechnology, Technion-Israel Institute of Technology, found avocado oil significantly increased the collagen content in skin, maintaining its youthful look. Not only does the oil in avocado act like an emollient, but the fruit also contains moisturizing vitamin E. Another good avocado mix is 1 tablespoon mashed avocado, 2 egg whites. and 2 tablespoons honey blended until smooth. Leave on for 15 minutes, then rinse.

A Skin-Care Glossary

Confused about skin-care terminology? Here's what several common terms mean:

- **Collagen.** A protein that contributes to the elasticity of skin tissue.

- **Emollient.** A lotion or cream that helps make skin smoother and softer.

- **Exfoliant.** Any product that helps to remove dead cells from the skin's surface.

- **Humectant.** A product that promotes the retention of moisture in the skin.

- **Hydration.** The process of bringing more water into skin tissues.

- **SPF.** Stands for sun protection factor, a numeric scale used to establish the effectiveness of a product at blocking the harmful rays of sunlight from reaching the skin. The higher the number, the greater the protection.

- **AHA.** Stands for alpha-hydroxy acid. A natural acid, often derived from fruit, that helps slough off dead skin and speed up cell renewal. AHAs have emerged as one of the most important ingredients in skin care.

- **Lightly scramble an egg and apply to your face while still warm, leaving it on until it hardens**. To remove the egg, place a warm, wet washcloth on your face and allow the moisture to soften it. Eggs are great for tightening wrinkles and smoothing skin. If you have oily skin, apply an egg white only; if you have normal skin, use the whole egg.
- **Simmer an apple covered in water just until soft. Remove from the water, mash, then add to the apple 1 teaspoon lemon juice and 1 teaspoon crushed peppermint leaves**. Apply the mixture to your face, leave for five minutes, then rinse. This works great on oily skin.
- **Mash peeled mango flesh until it turns soft and pulpy.** Then massage into skin, leave on for a few minutes, and rinse. This helps clean and tighten pores.
- **Add 1 tablespoon of peppermint, yarrow, sage, or hyssop to 1 cup boiling water.** Steep for 30 minutes, then strain and cool before dabbing it on your face. This makes a great skin toner for oily skin.

34 Clean your face and neck with a natural cold cream and follow with a rosewater and glycerin rinse twice a day to remove skin-damaging pollutants.

35 Keep your hands off your face! Because your hands touch so many surfaces, they are a magnet for dirt and germs. Rub your eyes, stroke your chin, cup your cheek, and you've transferred everything on your hands to your face. As an extension of this, use headphones or a headset when talking on the phone. This, too, keeps hands and germs away from your face.

36 Stop with one glass of wine or one alcoholic drink. Overdoing it enlarges the blood vessels near the surface of your facial skin.

37 De-shine your face throughout the day by periodically dabbing on loose powder to blot excess oil. Don't use pressed powder, which actually contains oil as an ingredient.

38 Never, ever rub your eyes— apply compresses instead. The skin on your face is extremely delicate, especially under your eyes. So use a very light touch on your face at all times, says Dianne M. Daniels, image consultant and color analyst at Image & Color Services in Norwich, Connecticut. If your eyes itch, apply a cold compress or washcloth to the area, or try a cotton pad moistened with toner or witch hazel.

39 Use a single family of skin-care products. If you buy and use lots of different skin-care products, there's a good chance some contain the same ingredients, thus making them redundant, says Cara DeCenso, an aesthetician at Ajune in Manhattan. And some brands just aren't very compatible with others, though you'd have no way of knowing that until you already paid for and opened them. You'll get much better results if you use products that are designed and formulated to work together, such as Clinique, Mary Kay, Albolene, or Neutrogena. You may have to shell out a little more cash, but experts agree you'll get better results.

Maintaining a Healthy Smile

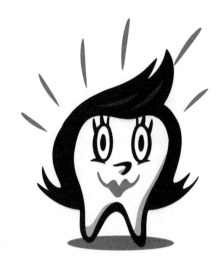

22 WAYS TO KEEP YOUR GUMS AND TEETH CLEAN

From the time your first tooth poked its way through your tender gums, those pearly whites have played an enormous role in your life. Not only do the 32 nuggets in your mouth help you talk and chew, they can make or break your appearance. Although aesthetics are important, however, even more important is tooth and gum health. In the last few years, researchers have uncovered a link between periodontal (gum) disease and increased risk of heart disease. One study found that men with periodontitis had a whopping 72 percent greater risk of developing coronary disease than those with healthy gums.

To keep your choppers in tip-top shape (heck, just to keep them in the first place), we've come up with the following 22 tips that go far beyond just brushing and flossing.

1 **Go on a white-teeth diet.** What goes in, shows up on your teeth. So if you're quaffing red wine and black tea, or smoking cigarettes or cigars, expect the results to show up as not-so-pearly whites. Other culprits to blame for dingy teeth include colas, gravies, and dark juices. Bottom line: If it's dark before you put it in your mouth, it will probably stain your teeth. So step one: Brush your teeth immediately after eating or drinking foods that stain teeth. Step two: Regularly use a good bleaching agent, either over-the-counter or in the dentist's office. Step three: Be conscious of the foods and drink in your diet that can stain your teeth, and eat only when a toothbrush is around. If there isn't one, eat an apple for dessert—it will provide some teeth-cleaning action.

2 **Hum while you brush.** The ideal amount of time to brush in order to get all the bacteria-packed plaque out is at least two minutes, British researchers found. Today you can actually purchase a song called "The Brush Along Song," which runs exactly 2½ minutes, to accompany your brushing. (www.alianda.com/brushalong/brush2.html) It's targeted toward kids, but so what? Isn't there a kid within all of us? Otherwise, keep a timer in the bathroom and set it for two minutes.

3 Grip your toothbrush like a pencil. Does your toothbrush look like it just cleaned an SUV? If so, you're probably brushing too hard. Contrary to what some scrub-happy people think, brushing with force is not the best way to remove plaque. According to Beverly Hills dentist Harold Katz, D.D.S., the best way to brush is by placing your toothbrush at a 45-degree angle against your gums and gently moving it in a circular motion, rather than a back-and-forth motion. Grip the toothbrush like a pencil so you won't scrub too hard.

4 Drink a cup of tea every day. Flavonoids and other tea ingredients seem to prevent harmful bacteria from sticking to teeth, and also block production of a type of sugar that contributes to cavities. Tea also contains high amounts of fluoride.

5 Chuck your toothbrush or change the head of your electric toothbrush at least every two to three months. Otherwise, you're just transferring bacteria to your mouth.

6 Use alcohol-free mouthwash to rinse away bacteria. Most over-the-counter mouthwashes have too much alcohol, which can dry out the tissues in your mouth, making them more susceptible to bacteria. Some studies even suggest

a link between mouthwashes containing alcohol and an increased risk of oral cancer. To be safe, be a teetotaler when it comes to choosing a mouthwash.

7 Clean your tongue with a tongue scraper every morning to remove tongue plaque and freshen your breath. One major cause of bad breath is the buildup of bacteria on the tongue, which a daily tongue scraping will help banish. Plus, using a tongue scraper is more effective than brushing your tongue with a toothbrush, says Dr. Katz.

8 Even if you're a grown-up, avoid sugary foods. Sugar plus bacteria equals oral plaque. Plaque, then, leads to bleeding gums, tooth decay, and cavities. Plus, the acid in refined sugars and carbonated beverages dissolves tooth enamel.

9 Instead, eat "detergent" foods. Foods that are firm or crisp help clean teeth as they're eaten. We already mentioned apples (otherwise known as nature's toothbrush); other choices include raw carrots, celery, and popcorn. For best results, make "detergent" foods the final food you eat in your meal if you know you won't be able to brush your teeth right after eating.

10 Gargle with apple cider vinegar in the morning and then brush as usual. The vinegar helps help remove stains, whiten teeth, and kill bacteria in your mouth and gums.

11 Brush your teeth with baking soda once a week to remove stains and whiten your teeth. Use it just as you would toothpaste. You can also use salt as an alternative

Healthy Investments

A Dental Water Jet

Dental water jets clean your teeth three times deeper than brushing and flossing alone. Fill the machine with mouthwash, water, or an antibacterial rinse and let the jet's pulsation go to work on your teeth once a day.

toothpaste. Just be sure to spit it out so it doesn't count as sodium intake! Also, if your gums start to feel raw, switch to brushing with salt every other day.

12 **Practice flossing with your eyes shut.** If you can floss without having to guide your work with a mirror, you can floss in your car, at your desk, while in bed, and before important meetings. In which case, buy several packages of floss and scatter them in your car, your desk, your purse, your briefcase, your nightstand.

13 **Keep rubber bottle openers and a small pair of scissors in your purse or desk drawer.** That way, you won't have to use your teeth as tools, which can damage them. In fact, never, ever use your teeth as tools for anything except eating.

14 **Drink one 8-ounce glass of water for every hour that you're at work.** That way, when you get home, you'll have finished your recommended daily eight glasses. If you work at home or part-time, make sure that you drink at least one eight-ounce glass every hour for eight hours. Not only does water help keep your digestive system healthy, control weight, and hydrate your skin, but it also helps keep your teeth even more pearly white. The more water you drink, the more bacteria you flush off your teeth and out of your mouth, which means less risk of gum disease, fewer cavities, and fresher breath.

15 **To check the freshness of your breath,** lick your palm and smell it while it's still wet. If you smell something, it's time for a sugar-free breath mint.

Two-Second Quiz

Manual or Electric Toothbrush?

Answer: *Electric.*
A major review of studies on the subject conducted over the past 37 years found that rotational oscillation toothbrushes (i.e., electric toothbrushes) were more effective than manual toothbrushes in reducing plaque and gingivitis.

16 **Suck—don't chew—extremely hard foodstuffs such as peanut brittle, hard candy or ice.** Chewing these hard foods creates tiny fractures in the enamel of your teeth that, over the years, combine to result in major cracks.

17 **Ladies: Choose a medium coral or light red lipstick.** These colors make your teeth look whiter, whereas lighter-colored lipsticks tend to bring out the yellow in teeth.

18 **Chew Big Red gum once a day.** Researchers at the University of Illinois at Chicago have found that the cinnamon-flavored chewing gum reduced bacteria in the mouth that cause bad breath. The reason? The gum contains cinnamic aldehyde, a plant essential oil used for flavoring that inhibits the growth of bacteria responsible for cavities and periodontal infections. Actually, any kind of sugar-free gum chewed after meals will help remove food particles and wash away bacteria (from the extra saliva chewing gum generates).

19 **Eat a container of nonfat yogurt every day.** Think of your teeth as external bones; just like your bones, they

need adequate calcium to remain healthy and strong.

20 Keep an extra toothbrush by your nightstand or under your pillow as a regular reminder to brush your teeth when you first get out of bed and before you get back in at night. They're the two most crucial times, says Kathleen W. Wilson, M.D., an internist at the Ochsner Health Center in New Orleans and author of *When You Think You Are Falling Apart*. That's because saliva (which keeps cavity-causing plaque off teeth) dries up at night, so it's best to have all plaque cleaned off the teeth before sleep. It's also important to brush first thing in the morning to brush off plaque and bacteria (morning breath!) that may have built up as you slept.

21 Pour liquids into a cup instead of drinking out of a glass bottle. You could inadvertently bang the bottle against your tooth, chipping it.

22 Carry your own (plastic) bottle of water with you so you can avoid water fountains. Someone could bump you from behind and you could chip or break a tooth on the fountain, says Jeff Golub-Evans, D.D.S., a New York City cosmetic dentist.

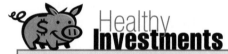

Healthy Investments

A Sports Mouth Guard

This small investment will protect your teeth and gums if you participate in any kind of contact or physical sport, including skiing, skating, basketball, or boxing.

Healthier, More Attractive Hair

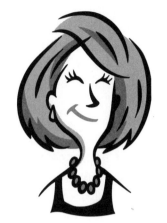

32 WAYS TO ADD BODY, PERSONALITY, AND LONGEVITY

Considering it is technically dead tissue, we spend an awful lot of time, money, and energy on our hair. And well we should. In addition to being fun to style and color, hair serves a valuable biological purpose: It keeps your head warm and helps regulate body temperature.

Hair, like nails, is an extension of your epidermis, the outer layer of your skin. It is composed mainly of protein. The typical hair cell stays with you for three to five years until it falls or grows out. Most of the time, it gets replaced. Because you spend so much time with your hair, particularly if you're a woman, it deserves good care. So here are some Stealth Health tips to help you keep your hair shiny, healthy, and beautiful:

1 Take one to three 250-milligram capsules of borage oil, evening primrose oil, or flaxseed oil one to three times a day. All are rich in omega-3 fatty acids like gamma-linolenic acid, great for keeping hair (and nails) moisturized, says Kathleen W. Wilson, M.D., an internist at the Ochsner Health Center in New Orleans and author of *When You Think You Are Falling Apart.*

2 For soft, natural highlights, squeeze some lemon juice on your hair before heading into the sun. Or use shampoos and styling products that contain citrus fruits, suggests celebrity hairstylist Federico of Beverly Hills. Citrus adds subtle streaks to your hair without adding damage.

3 Check the drain after each shower for the amount of hair. The typical person loses from 50 to 200 hairs a day (out of 80,000 to 120,000 hairs on the head). So it's normal to have a very small clump of hair left on the drain after washing. But if that amount starts increasing, see your doctor. It could mean your scalp has an infection, or that baldness is beginning to set in, or in rarer circumstances, that you have a nutritional deficiency.

4 **Mash a ripe avocado (pit removed) with one egg, then apply to wet hair.** Avocados are rich in vitamins, essential fatty acids and minerals that will help restore luster to your hair, says Stephen Sanna, expert colorist at the Pierre Michel Salon in New York City. Leave on for at least 20 minutes, then rinse several times. Repeat once a week for damaged hair and once a month for healthy hair.

5 **Mix a few drops of your favorite fragrance into your hair gel before applying.** You'll wind up with hair that not only looks, but smells, great, says Susie Galvez, author of *Hello Beautiful: 365 Ways to Be Even More Beautiful*.

6 **Transform ordinary shampoo into an herbal experience by mixing in a few drops of essential oils.** Dilute an eight-ounce bottle of shampoo by half with water and add about 20 drops of essential oil of lavender.

Two-SecondQuiz

Brunette or Blonde?

Answer: *Brunette.*
The "blondes have more fun" message comes directly from the marketing of hair-coloring products (arguably among the most successful ad campaigns ever). The large majority of people on this planet have black or dark hair. From a health standpoint, people with naturally blond hair are more susceptible to sunburn and skin cancer. And truth is, there are plenty of negative stereotypes about blondes. If becoming a blonde will really change your self-esteem for the better, pursue it. Otherwise, brunette is just fine.

7 **Use one part apple cider vinegar** and two parts very warm water to help balance the pH level of your scalp and bring out natural red highlights. It may be smelly, but it works, says Federico. Simply pour the vinegar mixture onto your hair, massage it into your scalp, and let it dry for a few minutes. Then wash hair as usual.

8 **Mix one egg with a small amount of shampoo,** apply to your hair for five minutes, and rinse well. This "shampoo omelet" helps to feed the protein in your hair.

9 **Men: If you're going bald, go short.** One of the worst mistakes balding men make is the comb-over. A sexier, more modern style is the closely trimmed, Bruce Willis look. An added bonus: Your hair will be easy to maintain.

10 **Bathe your hair in botanical oils.** Available at health food stores, olive, jojoba, and sweet almond oils are all wonderful elixirs for hair. If your hair is thick and heavy, coconut oil works wonders. Dampen your hair and apply small amounts of the botanical oil until your hair is thoroughly covered. Cover with a shower cap and warm towel for a half-hour, then rinse and shampoo as usual.

11 **Only spritz three times with hair spray.** In addition to making you look like you just stepped out of 1962, too much hair spray can weigh down your hair, leaving it flat. Instead, try a bionutrient styling spray containing the B vitamin panthenol. It will condition your hair and help protect it from environmental and styling damage.

12 To get beautiful streaks at home, mix honey and alum, an aluminum compound sold in most drugstores. Combine the two ingredients into a thick paste and paint the mixture on with your fingertips. Sit in the sun for 45 minutes, then shampoo and rinse your hair. You should have highlights three shades lighter than your natural hair color.

13 Wrap wet hair gently in a towel and let the cotton absorb the moisture for a few minutes instead of rubbing. This helps protect against split ends.

14 Get dressed and put your makeup on before styling your hair. This way, your hair will be almost dry. Hair is most susceptible to damage when wet.

15 Shampoo gray hair every day with a blue-colored shampoo. By nature of its light color, gray hair gets duller, dirtier, and drier than darker shades, which is why it's so important to shampoo and condition it daily. The bluish shampoo helps hide any yellowish (read: aging) tinge.

16 If you want to hide roots and try a new do at the same time, zigzag your part line.

17 Allow at least four weeks between single-process color treatments and at least eight weeks between high- or low-light treatments, Stephen Sanna recommends.

18 Mix a few drops of sandalwood oil with a few drops of olive or jojoba oil, rub the mixture between your

Correct Shampoo Technique

Few people realize there's a correct way to shampoo your hair, says George Caroll, a stylist, hair product designer, and consultant to the entertainment and beauty industry in Hollywood. He says proper shampooing not only improves the look of hair but also helps slow hair loss and promote healthier hair growth. He recommends the following:

- Before you even step into the shower, brush your hair from front to back with a stiff boar-bristle brush. This will stimulate circulation and prevent the buildup of styling products.

- Wet hair with warm water. (Hot water can strip your hair of protective oils.) Apply shampoo at the nape of the neck and shampoo the hairline first, followed by the top of your head.

- Massage your entire scalp at least three times to push nutrients into the hair bulb and free your hair follicles of clogging deposits.

- After rinsing your hair thoroughly, apply your conditioner. If you are doing all this outside the shower, wrap a "steam towel" (a wet towel that's been microwaved for two minutes) around your head and leave it on for 30-60 seconds. The steam will make moisturizing conditioners work more effectively by allowing the conditioner to be evenly absorbed into each hair strand.

- Finish with a cool-water rinse, which is not only stimulating but also helps tighten scalp pores, firm hair fibers, reduce hair limpness, and increase sheen and body.

palms, then smooth it through the ends of your hair for instant sleekness and a way to instantly curb and condition brittle, flyaway hair. Or you can squirt a few drops of hand lotion in your palm and smooth it through your hair.

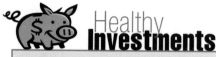

Healthy Investments

A Satin Pillowcase

Cotton or flannel can cause damaged ends. With a satiny smooth pillowcase, your hair slides over the fabric instead of sticking to it.

19 **Create instant highlights** by applying champagne- or gold-hued eye shadow to your hair with an ordinary makeup sponge.

20 **Use a humidifier at night in your bedroom, especially in cold weather.** Your home heating probably keeps the air very dry, which can dry out your hair.

21 **To keep your hair bouncy and healthy,** occasionally shampoo your roots only and then apply conditioner to just your ends. Then rinse.

22 **To reduce damage to your tresses** and add pouf to your do, dry your hair until 90 percent of the moisture is removed, then stop. Most people falsely believe they must use a hair dryer until their hair is bone-dry. Not true. The style should fall into place if your hair is healthy and well cut.

23 **If you usually wear your hair in a ponytail,** take it out for a few hours a day to give your hair a break. Also, try not to pull hair back too tightly. And never sleep with any sort of accessories in your hair.

24 **For an amazing haircut,** ask your stylist to cut the ends of your hair so they're slightly jagged instead of blunt. This provides extra body and texture.

25 **Make your own conditioner.** Here are some simple ways to condition your hair using some everyday household ingredients:

- Rub enough mayonnaise into your hair to coat it, wait up to an hour, and wash it out. You'll be amazed at how soft and shiny your hair is, thanks to this great protein source.
- Substitute condensed milk for your regular conditioner. The protein provides an extra-special shine.
- Mix 2 ounces olive oil and 2 ounces aloe vera gel with 6 drops each of rosemary and sandalwood essential oils. Olive oil is an emollient, aloe hydrates, and rosemary adds body and softness.

26 **Comb conditioner through your hair before hitting the pool to protect it from the harsh chemicals.** When you finish with your swim, rinse with ¼ cup apple cider mixed with ¾ cup water to help cleanse hair, recommends Susie Galvez, author of *Hello Beautiful: 365 Ways to Be Even More Beautiful*, then follow with more conditioner. Do the same before hitting the beach.

27 **Use moisturizing conditioner two to three times a week to combat fine, thin hair.** Many people think conditioners will flatten thin hair, but actually, using a moisturizing conditioner a few times a week will help your hair block out humidity, which can make hair flat.

28 **Match your hair color to be just a few shades lighter than your complexion,** which tends to lighten as you age. Highlight or bleach gray hair to give your hair a more uniform look and brighten your skin tone at the same time.

Dye or Natural?

Answer: *Stay natural.*
Although the evidence is mixed, several studies in recent years suggest an increased risk of non-Hodgkin's lymphoma, adult acute leukemia, and multiple myeloma in women who used permanent hair dye for 15 years or more. Even if the risks of hair dye are slight, they certainly exceed the risks of *not* dyeing your hair! So that's the way to go. Another option? Use temporary dye that washes out after a few shampoos. Studies find no increased risk of cancer in women using that form of hair color.

29 Use a gentle shampoo for oily hair. Ironically, harsh shampoos can actually lead to more oil because your scalp tries to compensate. Use a shampoo that's gentle enough for everyday use.

30 If you're trying to grow out your bangs, ask your hairdresser to add a few long layers around your face to help the bangs fade in as they grow.

31 Flip your head over, spray the underneath layers with hair spray, and shake out to instantly style your hair without rewashing and blow-drying.

32 Use styling gel correctly. Here's how to get the hold you want without looking like you stepped out of a grease pit. Place a dime-size dollop of product in the palm of one hand, then dab a tiny amount onto the fingertips of your other hand, leaving most of the gel in your palm. Starting at the back of your head near your scalp line, work the gel from your fingertips into the root area of your hair and continue until the dollop disappears.

REMINDER

 Fast Results
These are bits of advice that deliver benefits particularly quickly—in some cases, immediately!

 Easy Gains
These are tips that give the biggest value for the least amount of effort.

 Super Effective
These are tips proven to be particularly effective through scientific research or widespread usage by experts.

Healthy Nails

14 WAYS TO KEEP 'EM STRONG

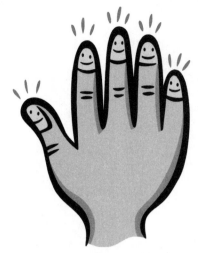

The longest fingernails ever recorded measured a total of 226 inches for five fingers—more than four feet for each nail—and took 43 years to grow. One can only imagine the difficulties that person had driving a car, typing, or gardening.

No one really knows just *why* we have nails, but the thinking is that they developed as an evolutionary outgrowth of hooves and claws. Whatever the reason, nails make it easier to pick up small things, clean a frying pan, and scratch an itch. They also provide an external sign of your health, with weak, brittle nails often signaling some nutritional deficiency. Ignore your nails and you could wind up with painful ingrown nails or annoying fungal infections.

Follow these 14 Stealth Healthy tips for not only well-groomed, but healthy nails on all 20 fingers and toes.

1 To keep your nails hydrated, rub a small amount of petroleum jelly into your cuticle and the skin surrounding your nails every evening before you go to bed or whenever your nails feel dry. Keep a jar in your purse, desk drawer, car—anywhere you might need it. Not a fan of petroleum jelly? Substitute castor oil. It's thick and contains vitamin E, which is great for your cuticles. Or head to your kitchen cupboard and grab the olive oil—it also works to moisturize your nails.

2 Wear rubber gloves whenever you do housework or wash dishes. Most household chores, from gardening to scrubbing the bathroom to washing dishes, are murderous on your nails. To protect your digits from dirt and harsh cleaners, cover them with vinyl gloves whenever it's chore time. And for extra hand softness, apply hand cream before you put on the rubber gloves.

3 When pushing back your cuticles (it is not necessary to cut them), come in at a 45-degree angle and be very gentle. Otherwise the cuticle will become damaged, weakening the entire nail, says Mariana Diaconescu, manicurist at the Pierre Michel Salon in New York City.

4 Trim your toenails straight across to avoid ingrown toenails. This is particularly important if you have diabetes.

5 Dry your hands for at least two minutes after doing the dishes, taking a bath/shower, etc. Also dry your toes thoroughly after swimming or show-

ering. Leaving them damp increases your risk of fungal infection.

6 Air out your work boots and athletic shoes. Better yet, keep two pairs and switch between them so you're never putting your feet into damp, sweaty shoes, which could lead to fungal infections.

7 Wear 100 percent cotton socks. They're best for absorbing dampness, thus preventing fungal infections.

8 Stretch out the beauty of a manicure by applying a fresh top coat every day, says Susie Galvez, owner of Face Works Day Spa in Richmond, Virginia, and author of *Hello Beautiful: 365 Ways to Be Even More Beautiful.*

9 To make your nails as strong and resilient as a horse's hooves, take 300 micrograms of the B vitamin biotin four to six times a day. Long ago, veterinarians discovered that biotin strengthened horses' hooves, which are made from keratin, the same substance in human nails. Swiss researchers found that people who took 2.5 milligrams of biotin a day for 5.5 months had firmer, harder nails. In a U.S. study, 63 percent of people taking biotin for brittle nails experienced an improvement.

10 Add a glass of milk and a hard-boiled egg to your daily diet. Rich in zinc, they'll do wonders for your nails, especially if your nails are spotted with white, a sign of low zinc intake.

11 File your nails correctly. To keep your nails at their strongest, avoid filing in a back-and-forth motion—only go in one direction. And never file just

after you've gotten out of a shower or bath—wet nails break more easily.

12 Massage your nails to keep them extra strong and shiny. Nail buffing increases blood supply to the nail, which stimulates the matrix of the nail to grow, says Galvez.

13 Polish your nails, even if it's just with a clear coat. It protects your nails, says manicurist Diaconescu. If you prefer color, use a base coat, two thin coats of color, and a top coat. Color should last at least seven days but should be removed after 10 days.

14 Avoid polish removers with acetone or formaldehyde. They're terribly drying to nails, says Andrea Lynn Cambio, M.D., a New York City dermatologist. Use acetate-based removers instead.

Two-Second**Quiz**

Quick-Drying or Regular Nail Polish?

Answer: *Regular.*
Quick-drying nail polishes may save time, but at the expense of your nails. Most of these formulas contain more formaldehyde and alcohol than regular polishes, both of which are drying and make nails prone to splitting. To fast-dry nails naturally, chill them. Dump a tray of ice cubes in your bathroom sink and fill it with cold water. After each coat of nail polish, dip your wet nails into the cold water for a minute or two. Miraculously, they'll be dry when you take them out.

Grooming

32 WAYS TO LOOK (AND SMELL) YOUR BEST

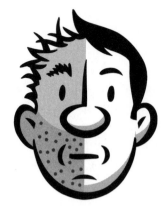

When it comes to grooming, little things can make a big difference. A cleanly plucked brow, clipped nose hairs, neatly filed fingernails and toenails, or a close shave can mean the difference between looking good and looking great.

No one wants to spend hours in front of the mirror primping or spend hundreds of dollars at a salon. So here are some Stealth Health grooming tips that will help you look polished, refined, and youthful—without investing a lot of money or time. Some are for men only, some for women only, and some for both.

Unisex Grooming

1 Track the amount of time you're spending on "grooming," and stop at 45 minutes. That's the most it should ever take to shower, take care of your skin, apply makeup, and style your hair. Any longer, and you need to get an easier haircut, use less makeup, and cut down to one skin-care product.

2 If you're prone to ingrown hairs, lather with shaving cream or gel for five minutes to soften hairs. Then shave in the direction of the hair growth with a new blade, says Andrea Lynn Cambio, M.D., a New York City dermatologist. Follow with a gentle moisturizer.

3 Shave slowly, with short strokes, and rinse the blade often in hot water. Your skin is not flat, so long strokes increase your chances of cuts or scrapes. Try not to press down with the blade, especially around sensitive areas.

4 Apply your shaving cream with a shaving brush for an extra-lustrous shaving session (whether for your legs or your face). It will create tons of lather, which will make the hairs softer and easier to remove.

5 If you have no time for a shower but need to be at your freshest, fill your sink with water and add 4 tablespoons baking soda. Then dip a sponge or washcloth in the sink and rub yourself down, recommends Susie Galvez, owner of Face Works Day Spa in Richmond, Virginia, and author of *Hello Beautiful: 365 Ways to Be Even More Beautiful.*

6 Ward off smelly feet with odor-absorbing insoles. Foot odor is a very common problem. Keep your feet smelling fresh by scrubbing them daily and drying them completely when you get out of the shower. Then insert odor-absorbing insoles, such as Odor-Eaters, into your shoes.

7 Schedule a weekly manicure and a monthly pedicure. This works for men *and* women. You can do it yourself, but a pro will always do a better job. The simple detail of well-filed nails, clean cuticles, and smooth toenails (if you're wearing open-toed shoes) goes a long way toward telling bosses, coworkers, and clients that you're a person who cares about the little as well as the big things.

8 Wear loose-fitting clothes to allow air to circulate around your body and perspiration to evaporate. Tight-fitting clothes cause sweat to be trapped in a film on your skin, which can result in body odor or noticeable embarrassing perspiration stains.

9 Buy clothes made from natural fibers like cotton. They allow skin to breathe, reducing body odor, says David Bank, M.D., dermatologist and director of the Center for Dermatology, Cosmetic, and Laser Surgery in Mount Kisco, New York. Avoid synthetic, man-made fibers, such as nylon or spandex, which tend to limit ventilation.

10 Apply antiperspirant when your underarms are a little moist and wet, like right after a warm shower or bath. It enables active ingredients to enter the sweat glands more readily.

11 Avoid sitting in direct sunlight. It heats your body and causes perspiration, especially in warmer weather.

12 Apply a cornstarch-based body powder in the morning to help skin stay drier throughout the day and reduce odor.

13 Take a yoga class. The education you get in stress management will help you better control perspiration and body odor. After heat, stress is probably the top cause of sweating.

14 Wipe a cotton ball soaked in rubbing alcohol, vinegar or hydrogen peroxide onto your underarms during the day to cut down on odor-causing bacteria. Or try witch hazel or tea tree oil, both of which help keep you dry, kill bacteria, and deodorize.

15 Fix some greens for dinner each night. Dark green leafy vegetables like spinach, chard, parsley, and kale are rich in chlorophyll, which has a powerful deodorizing effect on your body.

16 Roll antiperspirant across your feet before putting on your socks to control foot odor.

Two-SecondQuiz

Antiperspirant or Deodorant?

Answer: *Antiperspirant.*

If you want maximum protection, choose an antiperspirant, says David Bank, M.D., dermatologist and director of the Center for Dermatology, Cosmetic, and Laser Surgery in Mount Kisco, New York. Bacteria that feed on chemical components in underarm sweat cause odor. A deodorant works by controlling the bacteria, but does nothing to control wetness. An antiperspirant controls both.

For Women Only

17 **Tweeze your brows right after you step out of the shower.** Your pores are open, enabling the hairs to slide out when you pluck. Avoid brow shaping when your skin is most sensitive: first thing in the morning, after you've been outside in extremely hot or cold weather, or during your period, when your nerve endings are at their most sensitive, says Galvez.

18 **Carry a makeup touch-up kit with you wherever you go.** Look for double-duty products, like a lip/cheek/eye cream or a two-ended product with mascara on one end and eyeliner on the other. Other good kit items include cotton balls soaked in makeup remover and then stored in a film canister, pressed powder, nail file, and lip gloss.

19 **Check out your face in a small hand mirror in front of a window at least once a day.** You'll catch a glimpse of any sun spots or wrinkles you need to cover up or facial hairs you need to pluck, makeup that's uneven, even long nose hairs, says Galvez. The natural sunlight makes the inspection more revealing.

20 **Apply makeup in natural light.** Even if this means bringing your makeup and a mirror into the living room. The light from a bulb is often a different shade from that of natural light, and rarely does a bulb-lit room have evenly distributed light. If you must do your work in a bulb-lit room, make sure you are using the correct wattage—at least 60 watts for overhead lights and 25 watts for makeup mirrors.

Healthy Investments

A Magnifying Makeup Mirror

Even if you're not planning to use makeup, it gives you an up-close-and-personal look at any nose, ear, or chin hairs that need to be plucked, wax buildup in ears, large pores, blackheads, or other stuff only you want to know about.

21 **Rub some olive oil on your bikini line to keep it soft** and free of those unsightly red bumps. For best results, apply the olive oil to the area immediately after shaving.

22 **For instantly fresh feet, spray your soles with chilled cologne** or chilled peppermint or rose geranium herbal water. You can make your own by adding a couple of drops of the essential oils to a spray bottle of water and storing in the refrigerator.

23 **To make eyes appear closer together, tweeze your brows** on the outer edges and let them grow in closer toward the nose. To make your eyes appear farther apart, tweeze your brows to expand the open space above the nose, advises Gina Michele Bisignano, a model and beauty consultant in Los Angeles. "In other words," she says, "make the brows shorter."

24 **Wait a few minutes after applying your daily moisturizer before starting on your makeup.** If your moisturizer doesn't have time to penetrate your skin, your makeup may smear or go on unevenly.

For Men Only

25 If you have a unibrow, consider laser hair removal to tidy up the area. This procedure can also be used to remove stray nose and ear hairs. Excessive or unruly facial hair is generally considered unattractive.

26 Shave *after* your shower. Steam and hot water soften the bristles of your beard and open up the pores of your skin, making shaving easier and less painful.

27 Or, shave *in* the shower. Most men can get a terrific shave without any lather or cream whatsoever by shaving as the last part of a shower. Five minutes of hot, steamy water provides all the moisture and hair softening your beard needs, and the rinse-off and cleanup take just seconds.

28 Change the blade in your razor every three or four days. You could be shaving with the most expensive razor on the market, but if the blade is dull, it will leave you with a red, blotchy face and neck.

29 Shave some or all of your facial hair off for a more youthful look. If you have a full beard, try a goatee. If you have a goatee, go for the clean-faced look.

Two-Second Quiz

Electric or Straight Razor?

Answer: *Straight.*
It may be faster and simpler to shave with an electric razor, but it's harsher on your skin and can strip away natural oils. It also doesn't shave quite as effectively as a straight razor.

30 Trim the other hair on your body. Many men losing the hair on their heads start to gain it other places, like on their ears, nose, or back. To look clean and contemporary, trim, wax, or pluck unwanted hair.

31 When the weather gets warmer, trim your armpit hair. There will be less hair to trap bacteria and hence, less odor.

32 Extend the life of your razors by soaking them in mineral oil. Fill a shallow dish with mineral oil and soak them for a few minutes—the oil will stop the oxidation process that can dull edges. Then use a little rubbing alcohol to clean off the oil.

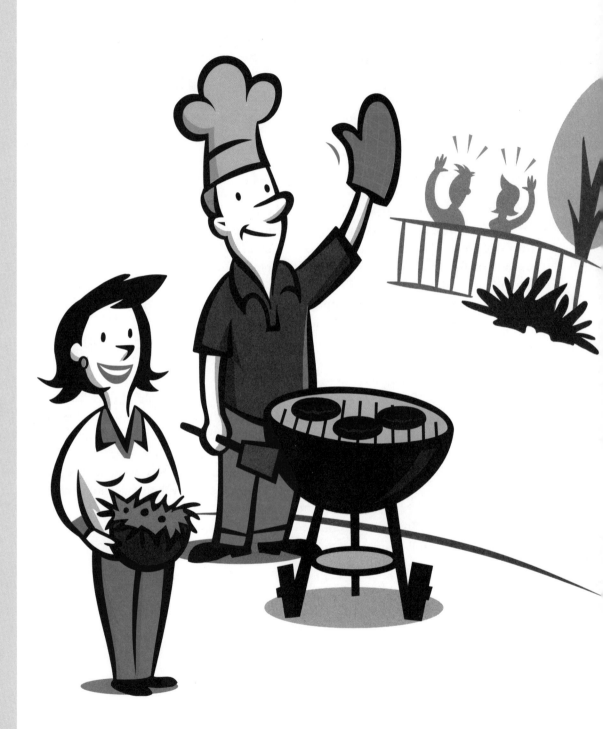

PART NINE

People

AND PLACES

Your relationships have a very real effect on your physical health. Here's how to make sure the people around you are helping—not hurting—your well-being.

A Better, Healthier Marriage
33 Ways to Grow Closer

Your Children
17 Ways to Sustain the Love and Respect

Your Parents
14 Ways to Maintain a Healthy Peace

Neighbors and Friends
11 Ways to Maintain a Healthy Circle Around You

Coworkers
16 Ways to Maintain Peace and Fun at Work

On an Airplane
18 Stealthy Strategies for a Healthy Flight

In a Hotel
20 Ways to Stay Healthier and Safer

In the Garden
15 Secrets for Healthier Digging

In a Crowd
12 Ways to Stay Safe and Healthy

Out in the Snow
12 Ways to Keep Safe and Warm

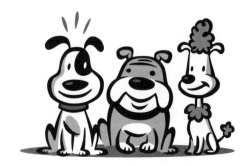

A Better, Healthier Marriage

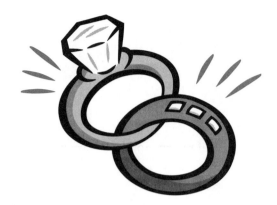

33 WAYS TO GROW CLOSER

All couples get married expecting that their relationship will remain as warm, loving, and intimate as it was on their wedding day. And for many couples, it does. There's no secret and no luck involved: These couples have simply learned to devote time and attention to their marriage. Not just sometimes, but every day.

You see, it's not diamonds and flowers that make a marriage, but the little things. Each morning, he makes you coffee, while you make sure the freezer is always stocked with his favorite ice cream. You're still spontaneous, taking a Friday afternoon off to explore the countryside and stop at an out-of-the-way roadhouse for lunch. You're each other's best friend, there when things go right—or wrong—but still appreciate your time apart. Above all, you learn through the years to accept each other's shortcomings and to forgive each other for transgressions both large and small.

The fact is, like a garden, you must attend to love. While the sun and rain will do their part to make a garden bloom, you still have to pull the weeds, fertilize, and provide tender loving care.

The good news is that in any relationship, particularly an intimate one, taking small, simple steps can bring big results. So check out the tips below. Most fall in the category of what we like to call "random acts of romance." You're sure to find more than a few ways to keep your love alive, vital, and evergreen, no matter how long you've been brushing your teeth side by side.

1 **Say thank you at least once a day.** You thank others for the little courtesies they do you. But do you thank your partner for his or hers? If she makes you breakfast every morning, thank her—and mean it. (How many wives make such a loving gesture?) If he took out the trash without your asking, thank him—even if it's his job. Saying, "Thanks!" once a day can help you avoid taking each other for granted.

2 **Praise your partner for the little things.** If there's something you appreciate about your partner, from the way she makes scrambled eggs to how hard he's working on the kitchen-remodeling project, speak up! Praising your partner

reminds him (or her) that you love him (or her), and knowing you are loved makes you more willing to iron out differences.

3 Do small kindnesses for your partner.
The good we do tends to come back to us. When you're thoughtful to your partner, she's more inclined to be thoughtful in return. So pick up each other's favorite dessert, clip or e-mail articles you think your spouse might like, make a favorite dinner, take on the other's chores, give your spouse a day off with no chores or expectations.

4 Deliver on your promises.
Failing to keep your word can destroy the unity and trust in a relationship. It's better to say, "Let me think about it" than say you will do something but drop the ball.

5 Play a game of show and tell.
Though it sounds X-rated, what we're suggesting is that you and your partner take turns choosing an arts or cultural event to attend together each month. The point is to show your partner what you love, so that he/she can experience it as you do (or close enough). To make this work, both of you have to be flexible: You may have to attend the Saturday-night race at the local dirt track, and he may have to go to the community theater with you. But the reward lies in experiencing each other's delight and sharing something of yourselves with each other. And who knows—you may have a lot more fun than you ever imagined.

6 Kiss under a full moon.
On a gorgeous evening, spread a blanket under the night sky and drink in the beauty and quiet of your surroundings together. You can talk if you wish, or simply savor the silence and being together, side by side, under the stars.

7 Make a fun, flirty change to your appearance.
Want to make him sit up and take notice? Color your hair, wear lipstick if you normally don't, or wear a pretty nightie to bed instead of your flannel pajamas. Want her to suddenly get the urge to run her fingers over your chest? Try a sexy black shirt or unusually tight trousers. The simplest change in your appearance can show your partner you care enough to catch his/her eyes, helping rekindle the chemistry that brought you together in the first place.

Do **Three** Things

If you do only three things to strengthen your relationship with your partner, make it these three, say relationship experts:

1. **Be kind to him or her.** Every day there are opportunities for simple gestures that show you care. A compliment, a hug, a note, or a favor takes only a moment, and yet they can brighten your spouse's day and your marriage.

2. **Give a full pardon.** When your partner has hurt you, extending forgiveness frees you from the bitterness and hurt that can eat away at your relationship. But don't think you have to forgive him or her instantly. Forgiveness is a process, rather than an event, so be as kind as you can be to your partner while you heal.

3. **Say, "I'm sorry."** If you hurt your partner, swallow your pride and offer a simple but sincere apology. Let your partner know that you didn't mean to cause hurt. At the same time, show that you take your mistake seriously by asking, "What can I do to make it up to you?"

8 **Play the newlywed game.** Do something for your partner that you did when you were newlyweds. Bake him a batch of homemade brownies. Send her flowers after a night of lovemaking. Tuck little notes into his briefcase or leave sexy messages on her voice mail.

 9 **Have a conversation about the big things in life.** When you were courting, did you talk for hours about current events or the meaning of life? If all you seem to talk about now is the grocery list or how much to spend on a new sofa, reintroduce meaningful conversation into your relationship. Asking her about her day isn't enough. Try this: One night while you're in front of the TV or in the car, make a provocative (but not hurtful) remark about something your partner deeply cares about—the guy in the White House, a favorite sports team—something that will get his/her dander up. He'll disagree, of course, which will get the ball rolling. Keep it rolling!

10 **Develop a common interest.** The couple that play together, stay together. To keep your relationship fresh and vibrant, think of an activity that both you *and* your partner enjoy, and do it together. The possibilities are endless: gardening, sports, attending classes or cultural events together, walking, hiking, working on home projects. How to get your partner to join you? Be sneaky. Say you need his/her help in the garden, want to do minor remodeling to the bathroom, that a friend just happened to give you two tickets to whatever. Chances are, he/she will have a wonderful time and want to do it again. In time, it may become a regular part of your life together.

11 **Do service projects together.** Giving to others moves you out of yourself and your own problems and supports a broader, more spiritual view of life. Again, try to pick a service or organization that appeals to you both, whether it's a mentoring program for disadvantaged

In**Perspective**

A Happy Marriage Is Good for Your Health

Happily married? Chances are, you're also healthier than someone in an unhappy marriage or someone who's single, according to a study of 493 midlife women.

Researchers at San Diego State University and the University of Pittsburgh examined the health of women who were happily married, unhappily married, and single. They studied factors such as blood pressure, cholesterol, glucose levels, and weight, as well as lifestyle choices like diet, exercise, and smoking.

The results? Women who reported that their marriages were highly satisfying tended to have lower blood pressure, cholesterol levels, and body fat—all factors in a healthy heart—as well as lower levels of depression, anxiety, and anger, which affect heart health. Other studies find similar results for men.

How might a happy marriage influence health? According to the researchers, it may be that the support of a happily married spouse protects one against the health risks associated with social isolation, which has been linked to heart disease. Also, a partner's influence may encourage you to swap unhealthy lifestyle behaviors, like smoking, in favor of healthy ones.

youth or working weekends in the local soup kitchen.

12 Rekindle your spirituality. If you're both interested in spiritual or religious activities, try some religious study together. If you both pray, praying together can be extremely intimate. Same goes for meditation or other spiritual or religious rituals.

13 Get active together. Are you both a few pounds heavier than when you first met? Engaging in a physical activity that you both enjoy can be as good for your marriage as it is for your body, and can reinforce the fact that you're a team of two. You needn't run a marathon together (although training for one could provide a lot of couple time). How about tennis? Golf? Swimming? Even gardening can be a workout, if you're landscaping the yard or tending a large flower or vegetable garden.

14 Set movie night once a month. All right, so he loves sci-fi and action, while you prefer romantic comedies. She is strictly chick-flick and you're super hero. Doesn't matter. To find common ground, select movies for the characters, not the genre. For example, in *The English Patient*, one gets espionage and adventure; the other gets a love story. In *Jerry Maguire*, there's football for one, Tom Cruise for the other. And if he wants to have a John Wayne film festival, gently direct him toward shoot-'em-ups that appeal to women, such as *The Last of the Mohicans*, starring Daniel Day-Lewis.

15 Each morning, ask, "What's on your agenda today?" Does he have a big meeting? Is she dreading a phone call to an important client? Is she having lunch with an old friend? Talking about the daily details of your lives is just as important as sharing hopes, dreams, and fears, so asking about those details is a great way to build understanding and rapport. And don't forget to ask how that meeting, phone call, or lunch turned out. Your thoughtfulness will make your partner feel loved and cared for.

16 Treat your spouse with respect and admiration in public. Whether you're at a party, a business meeting, or just strolling down the street, give him or her subtle signals of your connection. Hold his hand. Smile at her. Put your arm around her. And never, ever, make fun of your partner in public.

17 Walk out your disagreements. When you and your partner are at odds, ask him if he'd like to go for a walk to hash things out. Being outdoors and walking at a steady pace can melt away the tension so it's easier to talk honestly, form compromises, or apologize.

18 Learn—and use—the Serenity Prayer. When you see his towel on the floor instead of in the hamper, resist the urge to complain. While it's understandably irritating, it will undoubtedly happen again...and again...and again. When you start to sweat the small stuff, recite the Serenity Prayer: "God grant me the serenity to accept the things I cannot change, the courage to change the things I can, and the wisdom to know the difference." You'll be amazed at how quickly your resentment melts away.

19 Give your demands a makeover. You want him to hang a shelf? Mow the lawn? Asking her to throw in a load of laundry? Make sure you ask, rather than demand. We all tend to respond better to requests than orders. For example, instead of saying, "You should...," say, "Could you...?" And instead of saying, "Why didn't you...?" say, "Next time it would help me if you could try to..."

20 Try to air grievances at the same time each week. We know what you're thinking—who would do this? But consider this: If you and your partner discuss what's bothering you in a structured, formal way, these issues won't come up so often at other times, and if they do, you'll be able to discuss them more calmly. One more thing: Make the meeting formal. Sit down, turn off the television, and let the answering machine pick up calls.

21 Cuddle in the morning. You may associate snuggling with bedtime, and it is a lovely way to end the day. But cuddling in the morning will keep you feeling close to each other all day. So set the alarm clock five minutes early and snuggle. You can talk, or not. What's important is that you both start the day connecting physically and feeling secure and loved.

22 Schedule time for lovemaking. Yes, you're both busy. But don't let your schedules stand in the way of an activity that's so crucial to a loving, intimate relationship. The lovemaking may not be as spontaneous as you'd prefer, but there's something nice about looking forward to a night (or morning, or afternoon) of sex.

23 Always turn in together. This may take some compromise on both your parts. If your partner is dead tired, give up your nightly ritual (television,

surfing the Internet, whatever) and follow him to bed at least a few nights a week. Talk about the day, or simply snuggle while each of you reads. And if you're the morning person, maybe you can stay up to watch the eleven o'clock news. The point is, you're together when the house is quiet and the demands of the day are done. Make the most of it!

24 Make sure your bedroom is a sanctuary. Your bed is not the place to argue, or bring up complicated subjects, or discuss difficult parenting issues. Your bed is a place for good things only—sleep, companionship, romance. If it becomes a place for hard talks and critiques, one of you will eventually feel your bedroom is emotionally unsafe, and you'll start to avoid each other. If this is already going on, you need to stop it—declare the bedroom a safe zone, and that all serious discussions are to take place earlier and elsewhere.

25 Pursue your own interests. Go ahead, take that writing class—or pursue any other interest you might have outside of those you share with your partner. It makes you more interesting to your partner and everyone else. Moreover, a little "me time" allows both you and your partner to grow as individuals and reduces the pressure on each of you to fill the other's every need.

26 Have a regular girls' (or boys') night out. Every woman needs time with other women, just as every man needs a night out with the guys. If it's been a while since you've connected with friends or relatives, get on the phone and start arranging a day—or night—spent in their company.

27 Take a weekend getaway. If you present the idea to your partner as an adventure, he'll be more inclined to get into the act. Once you've gotten him excited, the fun begins: deciding where you'll go, what you'll do, and how you'll get there. And to make sure he's invested in the idea, let him in on the planning. Pore over maps and the travel section of the newspaper together. Discuss whether you should splurge on a room with a hot tub or a fireplace.

28 Renew your vows. Renewing your vows renews your commitment not only to your partner but also to keeping passion and intimacy in your relationship. You can do it once a year by taking a romantic getaway on your anniversary or make it a once-in-lifetime event.

29 Write him a love letter or send her a love e-mail. Don't worry that you're "not a writer"—be simple and sincere, rather than trying too hard to be romantic. On simple but good-quality stationery, describe to your partner how he/she makes you feel. Mention specific qualities he/she possesses that you appreciate, or little quirks you find endearing. Recall your past times together and describe your hopes for the future. Slip the letter into an envelope and tuck it in a briefcase or purse. (Just be careful your partner doesn't pull it out at an important business meeting.) If your partner is the type to snort at a love letter, send an e-mail at work.

30 Read the comics out loud to each other and share funny stories from your day. A 2004 study found that sharing humorous experiences significantly reduced the amount of conflict couples felt.

31 Go shopping (or watch a ball game) with a close friend. One study found that couples who have individual friendships outside their marriage were more satisfied with their marital relationships than those who didn't.

32 Demonstrate your love by working to improve something about yourself that bugs your partner. For instance, if she prefers you thin, join the gym or take up a nightly walk (preferably with her). If he's a neat freak, stop throwing your dirty socks on the floor and leaving your dishes in the sink. Saying "I love you" is always nice, but showing it is really fundamental.

33 Always put your marriage first, even if you have a houseful of kids. This is a golden rule: Of all your relationships, your spouse always comes first. After all, the kids are going to leave someday soon; hopefully, your partner isn't. Plus, giving up your life as a couple to indulge your children simply sets an uninspiring example: Grow up, become an adult, then you, too, can subjugate your existence to that of your children. Putting your marriage first means things like deliberately setting aside time for the two of you, whether it's a weekly date, a nightly bath together, or dinner alone a few nights a week (feed the kids early).

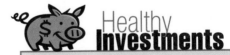

Healthy Investments

A CD You Both Love

One study found that when couples listened to music they both liked, they felt more caring toward their spouse. It's just something else they can share.

Your Children

17 WAYS TO SUSTAIN THE LOVE AND RESPECT

You remember them in diapers. You recall their first words. You cherish the days when they were innocent, loving, and eager for your hugs. Maybe that's why it's so hard to remember that your children are now teenagers or—where did the time go?—actual adults.

Once a parent, always a parent. And yet, as your children grow and evolve, so must your relationship with them. You need to be supportive but not intrusive; offer emotional support without being overly involved in their lives; and hope they make wise choices, while understanding that those choices are theirs to make.

Offering your love and support while respecting your children's choices can help you build a more enduring relationship with them. The tips below can help you bond with your kids even though they're no longer kids. And remember: This, too, is a matter of health for you. For nothing can break your heart as much as a strained or ruined relationship with your grown child. And nothing can make your heart soar as much as watching their lives prosper—and them wanting you to be an integral part of it.

1 **Set a standing dinner date.** There's something comforting and secure about the family gathered around the dinner table, perhaps because that tradition is rapidly disappearing. Yet the evening meal is often the one time of day when the family can gather in one place and reinforce their unity. So make dinner a family affair, even if you're sharing takeout at the dinner table. You can use the opportunity to share the news of the day, make weekend plans, and enjoy one another's company. As a bonus, research shows that adolescents who have dinner with their families at least several times a week are less likely to smoke and use drugs and tend to make higher grades.

2 **Back off, but stay close.** "It's normal for teens to want to spend more time with friends than parents," says Debbie Glasser, Ph.D., a licensed clinical psychologist, past chair of the National Parenting Education Network, and founder of NewsForParents.org, a nationally recognized news provider for parents. But don't take this as your cue that your job as a parent is diminished. Find ways to remain involved in your child's life. For example, while your years of volunteering

in his classroom may be over, you can still remain involved in his school by joining the PTA or organizing a school fundraiser. While play dates are a thing of the past, you can still get to know his friends by inviting them to the house after school. "Staying involved during these years may be more challenging now, but it's an important way to enhance your relationship with your child," says Dr. Glasser.

3 **Share your own feelings with your teen.** Of course, spare the intimate details of very personal subjects, but confiding that you, too, occasionally feel angry, insecure, or awkward shows your teenager that you're not just a parent—you're human. Not only will your child feel closer to you, but he or she may feel safe enough to disclose uncomfortable issues or feelings when they arise.

4 **Respect your teen's privacy.** Don't read her diary, eavesdrop on his phone conversations, or badger her with questions. If their behavior is troubling you, address it directly, using five little words: "Can we talk about it?" Some examples: "I've smelled smoke when you walk into the room several times now. Have you been smoking? Can we talk about it?" Or, "You seem very quiet lately, and I'm worried about you. Can we talk about it?"

5 **Seek their opinions.** Teenagers have opinions about, well, everything, and they aren't shy about sharing them, says Dr. Glasser. So allow them to make more independent decisions. For instance, let them decide when and where to study, what to wear, what after-school activity to pursue, what sports team to join. However, keep in mind that some decisions are nonnegotiable. "Parents

need to set limits that protect their child's health, safety, and well-being—at every age," says Dr. Glasser. These might include curfews, decisions about drinking and sexual activity, issues around grades and college. Still, find opportunities to solicit your teen's two cents when you can. Promise not to make decisions without hearing, and considering, their perspective and preferences.

6 **Trust your children to make smart choices.** Of course, they'll make the wrong ones occasionally. But especially if they're over 18, give them the chance to figure out solutions to problems on their own, without interference. After all, didn't you want the same from your parents when you were their age?

7 **Call before you drop by.** If you have an adult child, always call before you go to his home, unless it's absolutely necessary. (Do you like it when guests show up on your doorstep uninvited?) If you're the parent of a teen, knock before you enter her room.

8 **Accept their holiday absences with grace.** Yes, you may be disappointed that your children—and their children—spend Thanksgiving or Christmas without

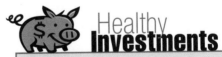

Healthy Investments

Space

If you can afford the costs involved in making sure your home gives everyone the option to have his own space, it is very much worth it. You can be together without crowding one another, get privacy when you need it, share what you want, but not what you don't.

you. But don't nag or complain about it. You may win a battle over which in-law's house they visit for Christmas, but lose your child's respect—and a strong, enduring relationship.

9 **When you catch yourself about to say,** "If I were you … " change the subject or leave the room for a moment to collect yourself. Your reward: a closer relationship with a child who appreciates that you respect his autonomy.

10 **Think about the things you value in your other relationships.** It's a good bet that trust, respect, and attention top the list, along with shared good times and unconditional acceptance. There you have it: the recipe for the perfect parent–child relationship.

11 **State your views, then invite reaction.** "Does that seem fair to you? Can you think of a better way to deal with this? What would you do in my position?" It's easy for a teen to be unreasonable if you take on the burden of reasonableness all by yourself. Share it and they'll find it harder to dismiss your position. Plus, you're more likely to land on middle ground you can both accept.

12 **Be there when they want you or need you, rather than when you want to be.** A lifetime of love, trust, and respect will ensue if you are reliably around whenever a reasonable and acceptable request is made of you.

13 **Be honest.** Many parents offer praise when they shouldn't, as well as when they should. That just undermines trust. We've all heard, "When you haven't got anything nice to say … " But in fact, if

In**Perspective**

For a Better Relationship, Lay Down the Law(s)

If you're the parent of a teen, be a parent rather than a pal. Chances are, your teen will welcome your rules and expectations—even if he grumbles about them under his breath.

Teens whose parents establish house rules have better relationships with their parents—and a lower risk of smoking, drinking, and using drugs—than the typical teen, according to a study conducted by the National Center on Addiction and Substance Abuse. The find-

ings were part of the center's annual national teen substance abuse survey.

The study, which analyzed a hands-on versus a hands-off approach to parenting, found that teens living in hands-on environments have parents who monitor their children's TV and Internet use, know and restrict the CDs they buy, know where their teens are after school and on weekends, impose a curfew, eat dinner with their teens six or seven nights a week, and

assign them chores, among other actions.

What's more, the survey found that 57 percent of teens with hands-on parents reported having an excellent relationship with their mothers and 47 percent reported an excellent relationship with their fathers. Only 24 percent of teens with hands-off parents reported an excellent relationship with their mothers and only 13 percent said they had an excellent relationship with their fathers.

both your praise and criticism are heartfelt and valid, your child will learn to trust you.

14 Cultivate love, but demand respect. This may sound a bit Machiavellian, but Machiavelli may well have been a good dad! Don't try so hard to be your child's friend that you fail to set limits, protect your own integrity, and earn respect. You can be friends long after your child is grown as long as you are the parent first.

15 Live your priorities. Kids should be among them, but not replace them. If you lose yourself in the process of indulging your kids, they will likely grow bigger egos than is healthy for them or you and belittle the value of your life.

16 Acknowledge that things have changed since you were their age. And they have. Music, clothes, technology, language, style, educational methods, the job market, even sexual mores and attitudes have evolved significantly in recent years. And the speed of change is only accelerating. You cannot

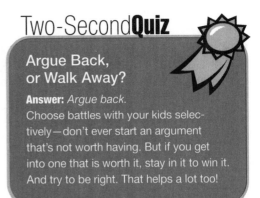

Two-Second Quiz

Argue Back, or Walk Away?

Answer: *Argue back.*
Choose battles with your kids selectively—don't ever start an argument that's not worth having. But if you get into one that is worth it, stay in it to win it. And try to be right. That helps a lot too!

keep up with it all, nor should you. But you do need to strike a balance: Don't live in the past, but don't try to bluff that you know exactly what's going on among teens today either. The middle ground is to live in the present, but your grown-up present. That includes being conversant about the Internet, HDTV, cell phones, the state of the economy, the world marketplace. Your kids will respect you if you are contemporary in a mature way, and don't base your observations of their lives on a past irrelevant to them.

17 Decode your child's "love language." While you may love your children dearly, they may not understand the ways you show your love—and you may not understand the ways they're best able to receive it. Some children need lots of hugs and cuddles; others may not be as touchy-feely. Some children want you to spend time with them, while others need lots of independence. The next time you spend time with your child, pay attention to the cues he or she sends so you can better interpret the way your child needs to be loved.

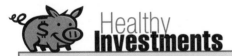

Healthy Investments

A Top-Notch TV, Computer, and/or Stereo

Let's face it, this stuff matters to young people. If you are the family with the plasma TV or the fastest Internet access, the kids will congregate at your house rather than elsewhere. And that has lots of benefits. Just be sure that you aren't stretching your budget beyond reason to do this—that just teaches your children to be overly materialistic. Also, don't buy it just for your kids; make this stuff for the whole family, including you.

Your Parents

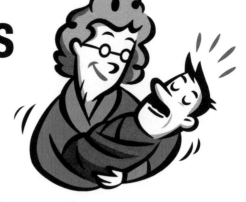

14 WAYS TO MAINTAIN A HEALTHY PEACE

Of course you love your parents—that's a given. But at times, maintaining the bond between parent and adult child can be as challenging as that between parent and teenager. These days, both of you are confronting new challenges—retirement or career changes, health issues, concerns about the future. It's to be expected these issues will affect your relationship, but as you change, so, too, must your relationship with your parents change.

Part of that evolution requires forging a new relationship, one between mature adults rather than "parent" and "child." You already have the basic underpinnings—love and shared memories. Add mutual respect and common interests and you may find a more fulfilling relationship with your mother and your father than any you've had since childhood.

Of course, some things never change—Mom might still offer her unsolicited opinions on your weight and wardrobe, and Dad might still only start a conversation if it has to do with your car. The key is to love the best parts of them and learn to accept the rest. Here are 14 Stealth Healthy ways to forge an adult relationship with your parents and enhance what might not always have been the strongest of bonds.

 1 Think of them as fellow adults, rather than as your parents. If your parents still treat you like a kid, despite the fact that you have kids of your own, you may have to help them let you "grow up." "Feeling and acting like an adult around your parents is the cornerstone of having an adult relationship with them," says Tina B. Tessina, Ph.D., a licensed psychotherapist in Long Beach, California, and author of *It Ends With You: Grow Up and Out of Dysfunction* and *The 10 Smartest Decisions a Woman Can Make Before 40.* "If you treat them as fellow adults, they're more likely to treat you like one." A simple way to do this is to ask yourself a question before each interaction with them: "How would I act in this situation if Mom or Dad was a friend or an acquaintance?" Then behave accordingly.

2 Talk to your parents as friends. If your parents still treat you like you're 6 or 16, it may feel funny to give up your role as the child. A good start is to model your conversations with Mom and Dad on those you have with friends, says Dr. Tessina. "Don't limit your conversations strictly to family memories, or gossip about family members, or your personal life," she advises. There's a whole wide world out there—why not explore it with

Mom and Dad as you would with a friend? Current events, sports, work, local neighborhood issues, or national politics (if you happen to share the same views) are all fair game.

3 **Keep your sense of humor.** When you're dealing with your parents, laughter can be a lifesaver—both to help you handle the stress of dealing with sometimes crotchety individuals and to help you bond together. Tell a few jokes you know they'll enjoy, share some comics from the paper or e-mail with them, watch the Letterman show together. If you can laugh together, you're doing okay.

4 **Tell your parents what bothers you.** If you love your mom and dad but they drive you batty, your resentment can eat away at your relationship. So don't seethe silently. Communicate, with gentleness and respect. For instance, if your mom keeps calling you at work, tell her that your boss is starting to notice and, while you love talking to her during the day, it's beginning to affect your job performance. Arrange a call you can both count on at a mutually convenient time.

5 **Don't ask your parents' advice or opinion unless you really want it.** Sometimes, asking for a parent's advice is really a way of asking for Mom or Dad's approval. If that's the case, remember that you're an adult now, perfectly capable of choosing a living room carpet or a car on your own. If your parents are bent on offering you advice whether asked or not, smile, nod, and take it in (who knows—it may actually be helpful!). Focus on the fact that they have your best interest at heart. Then make your own choice—without guilt.

Two-Second **Quiz**

Your Spouse's or Your Mother's Chicken Soup?

Answer: *Your spouse's.*
Once you marry, your spouse is the most important person in your world, your life partner, and your number one love. No matter how much you love your parents—or how much better your mom's soup tastes—turn to your spouse for the healing and nourishment you need. (But get your mom's recipe for the next time your spouse gets sick.)

6 **Don't ask your parents to help straighten out your latest personal or financial crisis.** While you may depend on their emotional support, relying too much upon their resources, rather than your own, can lead to mutual resentment, says Dr. Tessina. So get used to solving your problems, big or small, on your own. You'll be amazed how good doing it all by yourself can make you feel—and what a positive effect it can have on your relationship with your parents.

7 **Create opportunities for exploring and uncovering memories.** If your parents are older, look through old scrapbooks with them, asking them for stories about the people in the photos. "We help our parents discover the meaning in their lives by encouraging them to talk about their accomplishments, the high points in their lives, and the joys and sorrows they have experienced," says Tom Swanson, Ph.D., director of support services education at VistaCare, a hospice care provider in Scottsdale, Arizona.

8 Help your parents preserve their memories on video, audiocassette, or in a scrapbook. The finished product will not only be a testament to a renewed closeness between you, but also provides a wonderful legacy.

9 Express your appreciation for all your parents have done for you. Yes, Mom may be a buttinsky, but she always makes your favorite Christmas cookies. Dad is a bit of a stuffed shirt, but just the other day, he came to your rescue when your car died at the mall. The point is, your parents still do things for you that deserve your notice—and gratitude.

10 Rediscover and share mutual interests. When you were a kid, did you and your dad share a passion for a particular football team? Did you and your mother spend time each summer canning tomatoes? Make these happy memories the foundation for new, shared activities.

11 Be honest about who you are and what you want. Maybe there are things about your growing up that your parents regret. But as long as *you* don't regret it, they have to adjust. Be clear about who you want to be and help your parents accept you on your terms.

12 Look for common activities. Baking, shopping, hiking, skiing, carpentry, etc. At any age, sharing a common task or activity, and the stories it engenders, is a great way to build closeness.

13 Do not allow them to channel guilt at you. If your parents are the type to complain about you never calling, never visiting, forgetting an uncle's birthday, not sending enough pictures, or whatever irks them that day, don't take the bait and feel guilty—unless you honestly regret the oversight. In which case, apologize immediately and seek a way to make amends. Otherwise, let it roll off your back. You have no obligation to play parent-child guilt games. You are a mature, independent adult, and act on your own volition. For more on this, see "Dealing With Guilt," page 312.

14 Grant them their independence too. Sometimes it's the grown-up kid who doesn't want to cut the nurturing relationship off. If you are past 25 and still find it necessary to talk to Mom every night, or immediately turn to your dad for a house repair rather than your spouse, or automatically assume your parents will baby-sit the children whenever you need to be out, then you may be the problem, not your folks. They deserve freedom too.

Eight Great Ways to Get Closer

1. Teach your parents to use e-mail or surf the Web.

2. Introduce your parents to your friends, and include them in social gatherings when appropriate.

3. Eat out together. Try a cuisine you have never tried before.

4. Join a book or investment club together.

5. Read the same books and talk about them in your own book club.

6. Start a new family tradition with the grandchildren.

7. Challenge your parents to a round of golf or a hand of gin rummy.

8. Go bike riding or for a walk together.

Neighbors and Friends

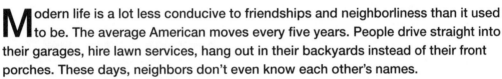

11 WAYS TO MAINTAIN A HEALTHY CIRCLE AROUND YOU

Modern life is a lot less conducive to friendships and neighborliness than it used to be. The average American moves every five years. People drive straight into their garages, hire lawn services, hang out in their backyards instead of their front porches. These days, neighbors don't even know each other's names.

Good neighbors and good friends are a lot like electricity or running water: We don't know how much we depend on them until we don't have them. They make our lives more pleasant and give us a sense of who we are, both as an individual and as a member of the community. In fact, the authors of a recent book, *Refrigerator Rights*, claim that refrigerators are gauges of intimate relationships—after all, you wouldn't snatch a drumstick from the refrigerator of a stranger.

The surprising thing is that all it takes to enhance your relationship with friends and neighbors is respect for their feelings, concern for their property, and a helping hand when it's needed. Here's how to nurture your relationships with two types of vitally important people in your life.

To Be a Popular Neighbor

1 Strike up a conversation over the fence or on the sidewalk. It's okay to be the one to break the ice, even if you've lived next door for years. Most neighbors enjoy making small talk with the folks on the other side of the fence. So as you see them at work in their yards or at play in their pool, smile, wave, and say hello. Ask how their kids are (whether they're toddlers or in college), whether they could use an extra zucchini from your garden, or what they think of the prices at the local supermarket.

2 Extend yourself to the new family down the block. These days, the old Welcome Wagon is a thing of the past. But your new neighbors may be feeling lonely and unsure, especially if they're far from home, and might appreciate a friendly face bearing fresh-baked brownies. If they have kids, tell them where the children in the neighborhood live. Clue them in to the best places to eat and shop. Invite them over for coffee when they get settled, give them your number, and point to your house as you say good-bye.

3 **Be considerate, especially of elderly neighbors.** Return anything that you borrow from a neighbor, such as tools, in good repair and as soon as you're finished with them. Replace anything that belongs to your neighbor that you, your children, or your pets break or soil. If your neighbor hasn't brought in his garbage cans yet, roll them back into his yard. Random acts of consideration will have your neighbors talking—and the talk will be good.

4 **Invite your neighbors to your next bash—or throw one in their honor.** What better way to meet your neighbors than to invite them to an informal barbecue, pool party, or holiday open house? Better yet, you might even consider throwing a get-together just for them. Deliver the invitations in person to everyone who lives on your street and chat with each for five minutes before moving on to the next house. This way, you will get an idea of what your neighbors are like so that you can plan for appropriate food and music.

To Be a Better Friend

5 **On your computer at home or at work, make "call friends" a standing appointment.** Don't have a computer? Keep a Post-it note on the phone, the bathroom mirror, the car dashboard, anywhere you're likely to see it. Also make sure your friends' phone numbers are programmed into your cell phone. Then call that friend when you're stuck in traffic or waiting in line and chat for 10 minutes. Alternatively, schedule a standing once-a-month lunch—same time, same place.

6 **Make time for friendships.** Nothing makes closeness fade away than never talking with or seeing each other. While some bonds of friendships may be strong enough to span long silences, most aren't. If you cherish a person's friendship, make time for him or her, whether it's just the occasional phone call or a weekly get-together.

DoThreeThings

If you do only three things to be a good neighbor, make it these three, our experts tell us:

1. **Be house-proud.** Part of what makes a "good neighborhood" is that the neighbors have a common interest—and a personal and financial investment—in keeping their neighborhood looking neat and clean. So do your part to maintain your lawn and the outside of your home. If yard work or home repairs aren't your thing, hire someone to do it. You might even ask a neighbor for a recommendation for painting or landscaping.

2. **Don't park in your neighbor's parking space.** On-street parking can be a sensitive issue for neighbors who don't have a garage, so don't thoughtlessly take "their space." And don't let any of your visiting friends do it either.

3. **Understand that not all your neighbors love kids or animals.** Don't assume it's acceptable for your children to run wild on the streets with their skateboards, or your dog to roam free. Teach your children the neighborhood boundaries they must live by, be it noise, geography, or time of day. Likewise, promptly clean up any messes your pet may make, either on your property, theirs, or on the sidewalk. Check in with your neighbors occasionally to make sure your clan isn't infringing on them inappropriately, and you'll make a lasting impression.

7 **Remember: A true friend doesn't flee when changes occur.** Nothing is sadder for new parents than to find that their single friends have abandoned them because of the baby. The sign of a good friend is one who stays true through it all—marriage, parenthood, new jobs, new homes, the losses. Just because situations change doesn't mean the person has.

8 **Make sure you aren't being a burden to a friend.** Friendships fade away if there isn't an equilibrium between the give and the take. Be sensitive to how much your friend can and can't offer you—be it time, energy, or help—and don't step over the line. And vice versa: Friendships that drain you will not last. If a friendship is out of balance in this way, you'll need to talk the situation through.

9 **Sweat the small stuff.** Yes, there are times when it doesn't pay to sweat the details, but in a friendship, it's the little things that count. Notice her new haircut. Remember to ask about her mother's surgery or her daughter's new baby. And if you're truly a good friend, you'll know when she needs some cheering up—a simple arrangement of flowers if you can afford it, a simple card or e-mail if you can't. It really is the thought that counts.

 10 **Be a good listener.** It can be the hardest thing in the world to do—to simply listen as he or she pours it all out or is seeking your advice or opinion. To be a better listener, follow this advice:

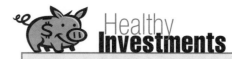

Healthy Investments

A Power Washer

You only use a power washer two or three times a year, but being able to lend your tools to neighbors and friends comes back a hundred times in terms of benefits. Everyone needs a power washer: for cars, the outside of the house, decks, patios, and sidewalks.

▶ Maintain eye contact. Offer nods and murmurs that indicate you understand her point of view.

▶ Don't finish your friend's sentences. If you catch yourself planning your response while your friend is still talking, gently remind yourself to focus on him.

▶ Minimize distractions—don't type, open mail, or watch television while you're on the phone with your friend. Your friend will undoubtedly hear your disinterest in your responses.

▶ Be careful with advice. Assume your friend wants to vent, not necessarily ask for a plan of action.

11 **Be in her corner if she's not there to defend herself.** If you're at a gathering at which someone mentions your friend disparagingly, defend her against gossip or criticism. Say, "Mary is my friend, and it makes me feel bad to hear you talk this way." Sooner or later, news of your loyalty will travel back to her, and it will deepen your friendship.

REMINDER

 Fast Results
These are bits of advice that deliver benefits particularly quickly—in some cases, immediately!

Easy Gains
These are tips that give the biggest value for the least amount of effort.

 Super Effective
These are tips proven to be particularly effective through scientific research or widespread usage by experts.

Coworkers

16 WAYS TO MAINTAIN PEACE AND FUN AT WORK

You can pick your friends, but you can't pick your coworkers. Yet you need these guys in more ways than one. First, you need their goodwill and cooperation in order to perform your own job well. Second, studies find that disagreements with coworkers and bad interoffice relationships deflate morale and impair performance even more than rumors of layoffs.

And third, if you're like most people, you spend more waking hours at work than anywhere else. Reaching out to your colleagues—or extending an olive branch, if need be—can make your work environment a much nicer place in which to spend eight (or 10 or 12 or 14) hours a day even as it increases your job security. (In the event of a layoff, chances are the office loner or grouch is among the first to go.)

You don't have to be *friends* with your coworkers, but you do need to be *friendly*. Read on for fresh ways to make work a kinder, gentler place.

1 Give a happy "Hello!" in the morning. Do you plod into the office, eyes down, shoulders slumped, and immediately start work? If so, you're likely to find that coworkers ignore you (at best) or avoid you (at worst). Get into the habit of smiling and greeting your colleagues as you arrive in the morning or begin your shift. It's really amazing how fast this little courtesy can thaw chilly workplace relations.

2 Learn the art of small talk. Ask your coworkers about their interests—their favorite music, movies, and books, as well as their hobbies, suggests Larina Kase, Ph.D., a psychologist at the Center for Treatment and Study of Anxiety at the University of Pennsylvania in Philadelphia. "Showing a genuine interest in them will make them feel comfortable around you," she says.

Once you know what floats their boat, clip items from newspapers or magazines to help start conversations. "John, I saw this article about that singer you like," or, "Mary, you like to knit, don't you? I found this great new knitting store not too far from here, and thought of you right away."

3 Join the office bowling or softball team. Many offices have them, and they're a great way to get some exercise while you get to know your coworkers in an informal setting.

4 Accept good-natured teasing. Other workers sometimes play jokes and tease to test what kind of person you are. So if they poke fun at your new shoes or mischievously put a racy screensaver on your computer, don't get angry. Let them know that you love a good joke—even if it's sometimes on you. Of course, if the teasing is personal (about your weight or ethnicity, for example), makes it difficult for you to do your job, or makes you feel uncomfortable because of its sexual implications, you may need to take up the matter with your supervisor.

5 **Ask what they think.** People love to be asked their opinion, so go out of your way to ask, "What do you think belongs in this report?" or, "How do you think I should handle this situation with client X?" Then give the advice giver a sincere thank-you, even if the ideas are less than helpful.

6 **Sidestep the gossip mill.** You don't want anyone talking about you behind your back, right? So return the favor. When a coworker sidles up to you bearing a juicy tidbit of gossip about Betty's office romance or Bill's impending firing, respond with, "Really?" and then change the subject or get back to work. If

you don't respond, the gossiper will move on—and you'll retain the trust and respect of your colleagues.

7 **When dealing with a difficult coworker, pretend your kids are watching.** This neat little visualization will help you keep a cool head. After all, you've taught your children to be mannerly. With them "watching" you, it will be difficult to stoop to the level of your infuriating colleague.

8 **Ladle out the compliments.** Did Tom fix the office copier—again? Has the quiet secretary in the cubicle behind you lost 25 pounds? By all means, compliment your coworkers on their achievements— personal or professional. Too often, we focus on what people are doing wrong.

9 **Spread your good cheer.** You don't have to be a Pollyanna, but try to perform one act of kindness a week, choosing a different coworker each time. For example,

In**Perspective**

Office Friendships Benefit Your Work

Do you have a best pal at work? Chances are, if you do, you're a better, more productive worker than the office loner or grouch. That's according to the Gallup Organization, which conducts an annual poll on how employee attitudes relate to workplace performance.

Gallup's poll finds that employees who strongly agree with statements such as "My supervisor cares about me as a person," and,

"I have a best friend at work" are more fully engaged in their jobs, meaning they feel more content and are more productive than those who are less engaged. These are type 1 workers, says Curt Coffman of Gallup. Type 2 are disengaged employees, those who do just enough to get by; and type 3 are actively disengaged, both unhappy and unproductive.

According to Gallup, 63 percent of employees

without a good office pal are disengaged, and 29 percent are actively disengaged. Only 8 percent of those without a good work friend are content and productive at work.

While folks who have a best friend at work don't necessarily experience less stress, says Coffman, it appears they have a better way of coping with that stress in a healthy, productive manner.

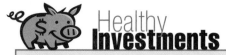

Healthy Investments

A Nerf Gun

Keep it in your office or cubicle and use it to break the tension when a big project is due or people are feeling overwhelmed.

one week you might bring in doughnuts for no reason. Another week, it might be a card for a colleague—maybe a thank-you note for helping you out last week, or a light, humorous card for a colleague who seems down. It can be fun—and rewarding—to see a colleague's face light up for no other reason than you picked them out of the crowd for a special kindness.

10 Return calls and e-mails promptly. To win friends at work, start with good office etiquette. There's nothing more frustrating to busy coworkers than to have their emails and phone messages ignored. Your silence doesn't just make their jobs harder; it also conveys an unpleasant message: You're unimportant to me.

11 Give credit where credit is due. Don't withhold credit from deserving coworkers. You'll alienate them, and they won't be there for you when you need them (or when they all go out for lunch). Embrace the attitude that we all win together, and let others know when a colleague has done something above and beyond on a project. Also, if someone incorrectly gives you credit and praise, acknowledge the coworker who deserves the accolades.

12 Here's one for the boss: Always work at least as hard as anyone working with or for you. Make it clear that you would never ask anyone to do a

level of work you wouldn't be willing to take on yourself.

13 Always be on time to show you respect other people's time.

14 Express your good ideas in a way that makes it clear they are not the only good ideas, but that others may have equally good insights to add.

15 Talk about your life outside the office when it's appropriate. This will remind the people you work with that you're a person first, not just an employee or employer.

16 Assume the positive about what you don't know. Funny how a team of workers always think they're working harder than those yahoos down the hall, and that the bosses are clueless. Don't subscribe to that kind of toxic thinking, even if it's rampant. It's a negative attitude that makes work become miserable. Instead, assume that everyone else is working hard and doing their best, even if you don't know what their work is. You should believe both in the work you're doing and the organization you're doing it for. If you can't, perhaps it's time to move on.

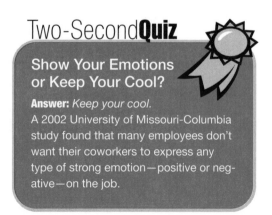

Two-Second Quiz

Show Your Emotions or Keep Your Cool?

Answer: *Keep your cool.*
A 2002 University of Missouri-Columbia study found that many employees don't want their coworkers to express any type of strong emotion—positive or negative—on the job.

On an Airplane

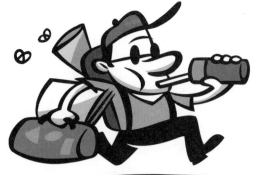

18 STEALTHY STRATEGIES FOR A HEALTHY FLIGHT

There's only one way to really enjoy flying: Buy your own plane. The rest of us are stuck with missed and canceled flights, sardine-can cabins, and humiliating security procedures, all of which are enough to send our stress levels soaring. Add to that the physical tolls extracted by cabin air literally drier than the air in the Sahara, changing cabin pressure, and hours of sitting in a chair seemingly no wider than your hips, with someone's seat back in your lap, and you'll understand why the following Stealth Health tips are so critical when you take to the skies.

1 **Three days before your trip, start boosting your immune system with doses of echinacea and vitamin C.** There are more germs circulating in the air on planes than you can shake a stick at. Don't ruin your trip by getting sick.

2 **Take an aspirin the day before a long flight, the day of the flight, and for three days afterward.** Have you heard of deep-vein thrombosis, also known as economy-class syndrome? When you sit without moving around for long hours, the blood pools in the legs. That could lead to a blood clot, and if that blood clot travels to your lungs or another important organ, it could be deadly. Aspirin thins the blood, making clots less likely.

3 **Pack three chamomile tea bags in your carry-on bag.** When the airline attendant comes around with drinks, ask for a cup of hot water and dunk the tea bag. The herbal tea will soothe your travel jitters and relax you enough so you can get some sleep on the plane, arriving refreshed.

4 **Use a backpack for your carry-on so you can take the stairs** in airports instead of the elevator or escalator. You'll probably have the stairs all to yourself, and it's a great way to stretch your legs and burn a few calories before you get onboard. As you wait for your flight, power walk through your terminal. "I can rack up a couple of miles just by ambling to and from the gates and circling the baggage carousel," says Ian Adamson, an exercise physiologist and adventure athlete who spends roughly seven months of the year traveling to races.

5 **Get up and walk between meals, and use that time to stretch.** Do the following stretching exercises at least once every hour during the flight, courtesy of Adamson:

- Standing in the aisle, stretch your calves by taking a large step back with one leg and reaching into the floor with your back heel.
- Also while standing, stretch your torso and back by twisting gently from side to side.
- Then, when seated, stretch your arms, shoulders, and upper back by extending one arm overhead, bending it, and placing your palm against your shoulder blade. You can use the other arm to increase the stretch.

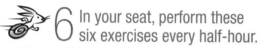 **6** In your seat, perform these six exercises every half-hour. They will keep the blood flowing and help prevent stiffness.

- Raise your shoulders and rotate front to back, then back to front.
- Drop your chin to your chest. Nod yes, then nod no, pointing your chin to one shoulder, then the other.

- Clasp your fingers together, palms facing each other, then stretch your arms out straight in front of you, palms facing out.
- With your heels on the floor, pull your toes up as far as possible. Hold for a few seconds, then release.
- Lift one foot slightly off the floor and make small circular motions in each direction with your foot. Repeat with the other foot.
- Lift one heel as high as possible while keeping your toes on the floor. Hold for a few seconds, then release. Repeat with the other foot.

7 Avoid sitting with your legs crossed. Instead, prop your feet on some carry-on luggage to make yourself more comfortable.

8 Get to the airport two hours early so you can request a seat change to the exit row. You will have oodles more room to stretch your legs, reducing your risk

 In**Perspective**

Jet Lag

Nothing's worse than arriving in Europe for a vacation only to spend the first three days feeling like you've been hit by a truck as you try to recover from jet lag. To reset your internal clock more quickly, follow this advice:

- Allow a day for every time zone you've passed through to fully recover from your jet lag.

- If you're flying east, book an early flight. If you're flying west, however, book a later flight.

- Begin preparing for time changes a few days before your departure by getting up a half hour to an hour earlier or by going to bed later (depending on where you're heading).

- When you get on the plane, immediately adjust your watch to the time of your destination. If it's nighttime, try to sleep.

- Use sunlight to reset your clock. After flying west, spend a few hours out-doors in the afternoon; after heading east, take a half-hour walk outside in the morning.

- Consider taking melatonin when you get on the plane to help you sleep, and then again after arrival when it's time for bed to help reset your body clock.

of blood clots and improving your mood throughout the entire flight. Unfortunately, you can only book the exit row seat at the airport. Use those extra two hours to get in some power walking through the airport. In case you don't get there early enough, book an aisle seat. At least you'll be able to get up and walk around without climbing over your neighbor.

9 **If you can afford it or arrange it, travel business class.** The fabric seats in economy class are perfect havens for dust mites and other allergens and germs. Often, seats in business class are leather, which are more hygienic.

10 **Bring a fully charged cell phone preprogrammed with airline reservation telephone numbers.** If your flight is delayed or canceled, you can immediately call reservations to rebook. Much quicker (and thus less stressful) than standing in the customer service line.

11 **Bring a bottle of water and a bag of healthy snacks** in your carry-on bag even for what should be a short flight. Not only do fewer airlines serve food these days, but unexpected delays (like sitting on the tarmac for 90 minutes while the wings are de-iced) can send your blood sugar plummeting.

12 **Carry a large, empty plastic coffee mug (the kind with a top you can sip through).** Ask any restaurant in the airport to fill it with ice and water. Bingo! Free water to maintain hydration. On the plane, have the attendant refill it. Much better than the tiny cups of water they usually provide.

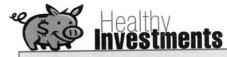

13 **When booking flights, book the first flight of the day.** It's most likely to be on time, so you're less likely to get stressed. It's also most likely to be freshly cleaned.

14 **Keep your nasal passages and ears clear** by taking a decongestant as directed for 24 hours before your flight. This will shrink the membranes in your sinuses and ears.

15 **Chew gum, swallow vigorously, or yawn widely** when the plane is taking off or landing. This will equalize the pressure in your middle ear.

16 **Skip the alcohol during the flight.** The air in the plane is dry enough; alcohol just dehydrates you even more. Same with caffeinated drinks.

17 **Resist the temptation to remove your shoes during the flight.** You'll end up with swollen feet due to the low air pressure in the cabin, and your shoes will be uncomfortable when you put them back on.

18 **Dress in layers.** Planes are often too hot or too cold. Stay in control of your own temperature by having layers to add or subtract.

In a Hotel

20 WAYS TO STAY HEALTHIER AND SAFER

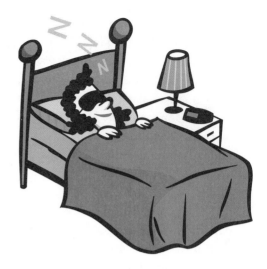

Let's say you're lucky enough to get to take two weeks of vacation away from home each year. Maybe your job sends you to a training session or trade conference for a few days. Then there's your niece's wedding, Thanksgiving with the family, a weekend getaway or two with your spouse to the hills—or Las Vegas. For many adults, a typical year may have us sleeping in a hotel room 10-20 nights per year. That's nothing to sneeze at.

Or more accurately, that's *a lot* to sneeze at. Although we'd all love to stay at five-star hotels that offer plush bathrobes, superb security, and immaculate cleanliness, the reality is most of us can only afford chain hotels with minimal charm, so-so construction, and plenty of hidden mildew and germs.

However, there are ways to make your home away from home not only more pleasant, but healthier and safer too. Here are 20.

1 **Pack your own sheets.** If you have any concerns about your hotel's cleaning practices, pack a queen-size sheet to throw over the bedspread so you're not exposed to dust mites, germs, or allergens lurking in the cover.

2 **Pack a long-sleeved sleep shirt and long sleep pants.** Again, if you are concerned about the hygiene of the bedding, reduce contact by wearing body-covering pajamas and light socks to bed.

3 **Use your bed for sleeping only.** Don't do work on it, eat on it, and don't watch movies or TV on it. Not only is that more hygienic, but you'll likely find it easier to fall asleep that way.

4 **Ask for an allergy-free room.** Some hotels are now offering rooms that are built and furnished to minimize the amounts of dust mites and other allergens. Even if you don't have allergies, this might be a good choice for people prone to colds and flus. Other hotels provide allergy packs, including face masks, special pillows, and mattress covers. But you have to ask for them.

5 **Choose modern over old.** Yes, Victorian bed-and-breakfasts are far superior in terms of charm and personal touches. But they also lead in the amount of allergens and dust you are likely to encounter in the rooms and public sitting areas. So if health is a real concern

while traveling, go for good-quality modern hotels.

6 Ask for a room on the third floor or higher. Most thefts occur on the first two floors. Stay below the seventh floor, however; few fire engine ladders can reach above it.

7 Choose a hotel over a motel. This is mostly for safety reasons: Burglaries are easier when your room's door is quickly accessible from the parking lot. You also get more dirt and allergens coming through the doorway when it opens directly to the outside. You wouldn't want to sleep eight feet from the front door at home, would you?

8 If you're going to be staying for several days, book a hotel with a pool or exercise room—and use them. Exercising will exorcise the traveler's stiffness from your body and burn off some of the calories from that breakfast buffet, business lunch, or wedding cake.

9 Split your breakfast and lunch schedules in two. Use half for eating and the other half for walking outside. Just like you should be doing at work.

10 Check the bed for bedbugs before you unpack. Have you ever woken up in a hotel room, felt itchy, and assumed you'd been bitten by mosquitoes in your sleep? It might have been bedbugs. Growing pesticide resistance has resulted in outbreaks of bedbugs in even some of the best hotels. These brown bugs, which are the size of an apple seed, can leave itchy welts on the skin. One veteran traveler suggests pulling back the comforter quickly and watching closely to see if any

Two-Second Quiz

Hotel or Relative's Home?

Answer: *Hotel.*
Relationship issues aside, a modern, well-run hotel likely will have less dust, mildew, and germs than the rarely used guest bedroom or den futon at your relative's house.

bugs scamper. Also look for bloodstains on pillows or mattress liners and carefully check the seams of mattresses. If you see anything suspicious, ask for another room—then repeat the process. Even if you don't find any bugs, move the bed away from the wall, tuck in the sheets, and keep the blanket from touching the floor. Just in case!

11 Check your luggage for bedbugs when you get home—and do it in the laundry room. If you find any, dump the clothes right into the washing machine, then dry them on high heat for at least 15 minutes. Anything that isn't washable should be put into the freezer for a couple of days.

12 Light a scented candle in your room. The scent will help to hide the antiseptic stale smell of the hotel room as well as provide some stress-relieving aromatherapy. (But use common sense: Never leave a burning candle unattended, or light one if you think there's a chance you might fall asleep.)

13 Moisten the dry air with the help of a teakettle. If your room has a kitchen area, fill the teakettle with plenty of water, heat it until it steams, and let the steam escape into the room until the water's almost gone. Your sinuses will thank you.

14 **Pack a photograph of someone you love (even your dog).** When you come back to your room after a stressful day, begin to feel lonely, or get that "What city am I in?" confusion that often comes with long trips, you can anchor yourself by looking at the picture and reminding yourself of home.

15 **Bring along your own battery-operated travel alarm.** You'll fall asleep better and sleep better all night if you don't have to worry that you set the hotel alarm wrong and will miss that important appointment.

16 **Pack a pair of rubber thongs, a.k.a. flip-flops.** Use them in the bathroom, on the carpet (who can guess the last time the carpet was cleaned?) and in the pool area to prevent any fungal (or worse) infections.

17 **Stay out of the hotel's hot tub.** Okay, now you think we've gone totally nuts. There's no doubt that hot tubs are luxuriously soothing, and if you're willing to take a slight chance, go ahead and plunge in. Just be aware that hot tubs can foster bacteria such as the one that causes folliculitis (itchy red bumps). And some people have developed bronchitis and even serious forms of pneumonia from breathing in air contaminated by bacteria growing in the water.

18 **Play it safe.** One of the easiest ways to stay healthy is to make sure that you're not physically attacked in a strange place. And hotels are strange places.

Two-Second**Quiz**

Sagging Mattress or Sleeping on the Floor?

Answer: *The floor.*
If you have back problems of any kind and the hotel bed has seen better days, pull the mattress onto the floor. You'll get better support and be less likely to wake up with a crick in your back that could cramp your style for days.

Here are some important tips on how to protect yourself:

- When registering, make sure the front-desk person doesn't say your room number aloud, but instead writes it down and hands it to you. If he does say it aloud, ask for another room and ask that he write down the number.
- Ask who is at your door and verify before opening. If you didn't order room service, or don't know why the "employee" is there, call the front desk and verify that they sent someone.
- Use the main entrance of the hotel when returning in the evening.
- Use all locking devices for your door, and lock all windows and sliding glass doors.

19 **Don't leave the Please Make Up Room sign outside your door unless you want to tell the whole world you're not there.** Instead, put the Do Not Disturb sign on the door. If you want your room made up while you're out, call housekeeping and let them know.

20 **Make sure hotel operators don't give out room numbers.** Try it by calling the front desk from your cell phone, giving your name, and asking for your room number.

In the Garden

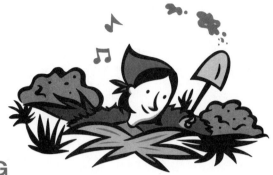

15 SECRETS FOR HEALTHIER DIGGING

Quick: what is one of the best ways to reduce your risk of hypertension, osteoporosis, and depression? How about digging in the dirt? Studies find that gardening is one of the best physical activities going when it comes to preventing or improving chronic health conditions. Plus, the stress-relieving benefits of watching something grow, of breathing in the scent of flowers, of picking a sun-kissed tomato from your own backyard, are legion.

The key is not to overdo it or do it wrong. These 15 Stealth Health tips will enable you to remain healthy while gardening for health.

1 Stretch for five minutes before heading out to the garden. Focus on your hamstrings, back, and arms. For specific moves, see "Stretching," page 148.

2 Dress for gardening. That means wearing sunscreen of SPF 30 or higher and reapplying it every couple of hours. Also put on bug spray, a hat, sunglasses, and a light, long-sleeved shirt that covers most of your neck, says Kathleen W. Wilson, M.D., an internist at the Ochsner Health Center in New Orleans and author of *When You Think You Are Falling Apart*.

3 Call 800-222-1222 to request free magnets or stickers bearing the local Poison Control hotline number. Keep them by the telephone and with your gardening supplies in case you or someone near you is bitten by a snake or contaminated with pesticides or other garden chemicals.

4 Bend with your knees and take frequent breaks from bending over. Back strain is a common gardening injury, says fitness expert Mare Petras. Other good options to avoid strain are to carry a small stool with you to sit or lean on while weeding, and to use knee pads to protect your kneecaps from rocks and hard ground.

5 Check the pollen index before heading outdoors. This is particularly important if you suffer from allergies or asthma. Also, forgo gardening on days of high heat and humidity, when many areas issue ozone alerts. The heavy air could cause problems if you have any respiratory issues.

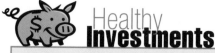

Healthy Investments

Raised Gardening Beds

They require less stooping, are easier to maintain, and generally produce higher yields.

6 Choose gardening tools with padded handles to protect the joints in your hands and fingers from excess pressure. Tools like shears or clippers with a spring-action, self-opening feature are particularly helpful if you have a weak grasp, notes the American Occupational Therapy Association.

7 Divide large bags of mulch, dirt, or fertilizer into smaller, more manageable loads and use a cart or wagon to move materials. When lifting, use the muscles in your legs, not your back.

8 Vary your tasks so that you avoid overstressing any one part of your body. For instance, don't spend the entire day stooping and weeding. Instead, pick one section of the garden to weed, then lay mulch and rake. Tackle another section the following day.

9 Take time after gardening to sit in a shady spot and rest your eyes on your accomplishments. Sip a cool drink and just enjoy the beauty around you.

10 Plant at least one vegetable in your garden. You'll be more likely to eat it. Also plant some herbs to use in place of salt for flavoring food.

11 Always order/buy twice as much mulch as you think you'll need. The more mulch you put down in the garden, the more weed control you'll

have (and the less tempted you'll be to use poisonous weed killers).

12 Keep all your gardening tools, gloves, and so on, in a backpack that you can carry with you as you move from bed to bed.

13 Keep your garden manageable. That might even mean container gardening. If you take on too much too soon, not only will you find yourself sore the next morning (and risk a more serious injury) but you'll quickly become overwhelmed and quit altogether.

14 Carry a water bottle slung around your body and be sure to sip on it every 30 minutes or so. It's easy to become dehydrated when you're working in the yard.

15 Emphasize flowers, not bushes, in your landscape. The pollen in flowers rarely causes allergies, due to its large size. It's the microscopic pollens from many bushes and trees that are culprits for people with allergies.

Two-Second Quiz

Power Mower or Manual?

Answer: *For most yards, manual.* You'll get a much better workout every time you cut the grass, and the intensity isn't that great if your yard is small- to medium-sized. If you have a larger yard, you can go with electric or gas powered, but make it a walking, not riding, mower.

In a Crowd

12 WAYS TO STAY SAFE AND HEALTHY

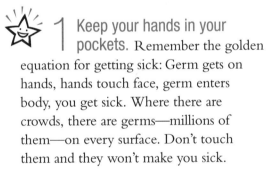

You're seated in a venue with a thousand other people. Which do you feel more threatened by: a fire, or a stranger sneezing on you?

Chances are, most of us aren't very concerned about either. Which is an acceptable attitude to have—both pose relatively minor health risks. But they pose risks nonetheless. And with a little more mindfulness, Stealth Health style, you can better protect your health and safety in the rare case that something goes wrong at the concert hall or football game. We're not suggesting you avoid crowds. Just be sure to follow these tips to keep yourself and your loved ones safe and healthy while you're out living life to the fullest.

1 Keep your hands in your pockets. Remember the golden equation for getting sick: Germ gets on hands, hands touch face, germ enters body, you get sick. Where there are crowds, there are germs—millions of them—on every surface. Don't touch them and they won't make you sick.

2 Carry a bottle of hand sanitizer. Use it after porta-potty visits, before eating, and anytime you feel contaminated by the microbes of the masses.

3 Stick a pair of earplugs in your purse or pocket. If the event gets too loud, or you get stuck standing next to the speakers, stick 'em in your ears.

4 Look for the emergency exit signs as you enter a large venue. It takes only seconds—and those seconds could turn out to be the best you ever spent.

One study found that more than half of fatalities at concerts occurred when people were trying to get out of the building or concert setting.

5 Note how many people the building can safely hold (the figure should be on a sign near the front door). If you feel that number is exceeded, reduce it by one—yourself.

6 Arrange a place to meet your family or friends in case you get separated. Actually, you should choose two places: one inside and one outside.

7 In the rare event of a stampede, try to move sideways to the crowd until you get to a wall. Then press yourself against it until the crowd dissipates, or you find a better exit. It doesn't happen often, but people do get trampled to death. If you've memorized the emergency exits, you'll have better luck getting to one that the rest of the crowd may not have noticed.

8 Pack your own lunch. Peanut butter and jelly sandwiches and apples will keep for the whole day and will help forestall your kids' pleas for junk food from the vendors at the event site. If you can't avoid buying from food carts, check out the vendor. Does his cart look clean? Are his hands clean? Is he handling the food with gloves? Does he handle money and then touch the food? It's hard to tell just by looking at it if food will make you sick, but you should definitely avoid undercooked (pink) meats and meat that is not hot when served. The last thing you need when you're in a place that only has porta-potties is food poisoning.

9 Remember to put a wad of tissues in your purse or pocket. Now you have emergency toilet paper if you have to hit those porta-potties.

10 Put water bottles in the freezer the night before the event. You'll save money on overpriced bottled water at the event, and as the ice melts, you'll have nice cold water on hand to stay hydrated.

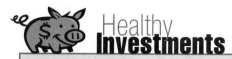

Healthy Investments

A Flu Vaccination

If you're planning to join the crowd during flu season, get the shot (or opt for the nasal spray). You'll be thankful later.

11 Dress in layers. The crowd is pressing in around you, you feel overly warm ... and suddenly the ground comes up to meet you. Don't let it happen. If you've dressed in layers, you can shed one of them if you get too hot. If you only have one layer to start with, you might just get arrested! Of course, layers work the other way too. If the temperature drops as the game goes into overtime, you'll be prepared.

12 Leave before the curtain call. You'll beat the crowd, get out of the parking garage more quickly, and avoid ruining your lovely time out with an evening-ending bout of blood-pressure-raising stress.

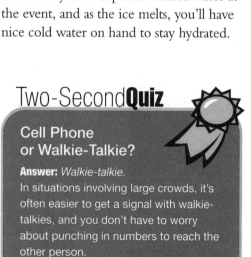

Two-Second Quiz

Cell Phone or Walkie-Talkie?

Answer: *Walkie-talkie.*
In situations involving large crowds, it's often easier to get a signal with walkie-talkies, and you don't have to worry about punching in numbers to reach the other person.

Out in the Snow

12 WAYS TO KEEP SAFE AND WARM

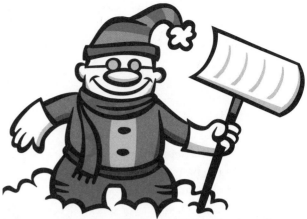

What is it about a snowstorm that brings out the child in all of us? Suddenly we're ready to bundle up and head outside to play. Plus, snow is great for a mid-winter workout, what with all the sledding, skiing, snowboarding, and snowshoeing you can do. Whether you're out in the weather shoveling your walk, driving, or just making snow angels, follow our tips below to keep safe and warm.

1 **Apply a Vaseline shield.** If it's cold *and* windy, your face may suffer a case of windburn. A thin coating of Vaseline on exposed skin—particularly your cheeks, nose, chin, ears, and neck—will help prevent it.

2 **Don't walk with your hands in your pockets.** It's pretty basic advice, but this way, you can use your arms to regain your balance if you slip.

3 **Buy a pair of Yaktrax.** These amazing rubber and wire devices slip over the bottom of your boots and help prevent you from slipping on the ice. (Even see a yak slip and fall? We didn't think so.) They are available at sporting goods stores and on the Internet.

4 **Remember snow's first cousin: ice.** So wear rubber-soled boots with good traction, go slowly, don't carry too many packages, and give yourself extra travel time to get wherever you're going, whether that's on foot or by car.

5 **Look for patches of white or pale gray, waxy-textured skin.** These are signs of frostbite. Get indoors and get immediate medical attention. (Read more about frostbite in the sidebar on page 401.)

6 **It might look silly, but pull large rubber dishwashing gloves over woolen gloves.** This will keep your gloves dry whether you're shoveling snow or making snowballs.

7 **Make sure your boots aren't too tight,** either because they're too small or because you've stuffed them with too many pairs of bulky socks. You won't have enough blood circulating to your feet and they'll get even colder. Wool or polypropylene socks are a good choice for your feet.

8 **Smear on some sunscreen and lip balm if you're out in the snow on sunny days.** And slip on a pair of sunglasses or goggles to protect your eyes from the snow's glare. A sunny

day in winter is often brighter and more dangerous to your eyes than the same sun in summer, thanks to the reflection off ice and snow.

9 **Dress in layers, and make your first layer a shirt or long underwear made of synthetic microfibers,** such as polypropylene. These wick sweat away from the body so you don't get too chilled. Avoid cotton, which gets wet and stays wet. Top your first layer with a fleece top and then a windproof jacket.

10 **Equip your car for driving in snowy conditions.** That means cleaning snow off the car before you start driving, making sure your windshield wipers work well, cleaning off your headlights, and using snow tires or chains if you need them. And stock your trunk with a

---

When Cold Sets In

One of the best ways to guard against hypothermia (lowered body temperature) is to recognize the early warning signs. If someone you're with exhibits any of these, get him to a warm place right away. Severe cases require medical attention.

- Shivering. An early sign of hypothermia, shivering starts mildly, but can become more severe and finally convulsive before ceasing.
- Slurred speech.
- Loss of coordination. This might begin as difficulty tying your shoelaces or zipping your jacket, and eventually include stumbling or falling.
- Confusion.
- Apathy (for example, not caring about your own needs).
- Irrational behavior.

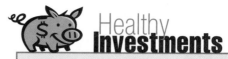

Healthy Investments

A Snowblower

Just two minutes of shoveling wet snow can make your heart rate soar above the zone recommended for aerobic exercise. One study found 10 minutes of shoveling brought heart rates to within 97 percent of their maximum capacity, and resulted in a higher blood pressure than when participants ran to the point of exhaustion. If, however, you're in great shape, then by all means—shovel. It's a wonderful workout!

---

shovel, tow rope, ground sheet (for fitting chains), rubber gloves, plastic ice scraper, blanket, and flashlight.

11 **If you're not in shape to shovel, hire a neighborhood kid to do it for you.** Shoveling snow is very strenuous work. People who should think twice before doing it are those with a history of heart disease, heart attack, or high blood pressure.

12 **Stretch for five minutes and walk outside for 5-10 minutes** before you start shoveling. Here are some other shoveling tips:

- **Drink plenty of water so that you're well hydrated.** Don't drink caffeine or alcohol, or use nicotine products immediately before shoveling.
- **Shovel early and often.** Newly fallen snow is lighter than heavily packed or partially melted snow. And starting out early allows you extra time to take frequent breaks.
- **Take your time.** Never remove deep snow all at once. Shovel a layer that's an inch or two thick and then take off another inch or two.

- **Pick the right shovel.** A smaller blade will require you to lift less snow, putting less strain on your body.
- **Protect your back with good shoveling technique.** Stand with your feet about hip-width apart for balance, and keep the shovel close to your body. Bend from the knees, not the back, and tighten your stomach muscles as you lift the snow. Avoid twisting movements. If you need to move the snow to one side, reposition your body so your feet face the direction the snow will be going. Always throw the snow in front of you, not over your shoulder.
- **Listen to your body.** If you experience any shortness of breath, dizziness, or chest discomfort, stop immediately and seek medical care.

In Perspective

Frostbite

The idea that your fingers and toes fall off if you get frostbite is a myth; quite often, the worst that happens might be permanent numbness. But you can also wind up with gangrene—and lose a toe or finger or ear or nose—if you're not careful. First, recognize the symptoms of frostbite:

- A pins-and-needles sensation, then numbness.

- Hard, pale, cold, numb skin. When frostbitten skin has thawed, it becomes red and painful (early frostbite). More severe frostbite results in white and numb skin because the tissue has started to freeze.

If you or someone you're with has frostbite:

- Get the person to a warmer place. Remove any constricting jewelry and wet clothing.

- If possible, wrap the affected areas in sterile dressings (remember to separate affected fingers and toes) and get the person to the nearest emergency room.

- If immediate care is not available, immerse the affected areas in warm—never hot—water or repeatedly apply warm cloths to affected ears, nose, or cheeks for 20-30 minutes. Keep circulating the water to aid the warming process. Warming is complete when the skin is soft and sensation returns.

- Move thawed areas as little as possible.

- If the frostbite is extensive, give warm drinks to the victim in order to replace lost fluids.

- Don't thaw out a frostbitten area if it cannot be kept thawed. Refreezing may make tissue damage even worse. Also, don't use direct dry heat (such as a radiator, campfire, heating pad, or hair dryer). Direct heat can burn already damaged tissues.

- Don't rub or massage the affected area, or disturb blisters on frostbitten skin.

- Don't smoke or drink alcohol during recovery, as both can interfere with blood circulation.

Index

About the Authors

DAVID L. KATZ, M.D., is associate clinical professor of public health and medicine, and director of medical studies in public health, at the Yale University School of Medicine. He cofounded and directs Yale's Prevention Research Center, a clinical research facility devoted to chronic disease prevention. In addition, Dr. Katz founded, and now directs, the Integrative Medicine Center in Derby, Connecticut, where conventionally trained and naturopathic physicians work collaboratively to provide patients with holistic health care. Dr. Katz has published over 60 scientific articles and seven books to date. Elected to the governing boards of both the American College of Preventive Medicine and the Association of Teachers of Preventive Medicine, Katz was recognized in 2003 as one of America's top physicians in preventive medicine by the Consumer Research Council of America. He is the nutrition columnist for *O, the Oprah Magazine*, and a frequent contributor to newspapers and magazines. He has also appeared on *Good Morning America, 20/20, 48 Hours,* and *World News Tonight With Peter Jennings.*

DEBRA GORDON is an award-winning journalist who has been writing about health and health care for more than 15 years. She cut her teeth on the medical beat while a reporter at the *Virginian-Pilot* newspaper in Norfolk, Virginia, then carried her expertise across the country as the medical reporter at the *Orange County Register,* in Southern California. She currently lives in northeastern Pennsylvania, where she is a full-time freelance writer specializing in health and medicine. She is also the author or coauthor of the consumer health books *Allergy and Asthma Relief, Cut Your Cholesterol, Eat to Beat High Blood Pressure, 7 Nights to a Perfect Night's Sleep,* and *Maximum Food Power for Women.* Her work has also appeared in *Family Circle, Better Homes and Gardens, Good Housekeeping, Reader's Digest,* and *Diabetes Today* magazines.

Acknowledgments

Working on *Stealth Health* was my second opportunity to collaborate with my coauthor, Deb Gordon. I felt privileged the first time, and doubly so now. Deb is creative and constant, efficient and energetic, professional and productive. Deb sent me material before I could ever ask, answered my questions practically as they occurred to me, and just plain dazzled me with her humor, insight, and dedication. I cannot imagine a better partner.

I am very grateful to Neil Wertheimer, editor-in-chief and publishing director of Home & Health Books at Reader's Digest. *Stealth Health* is Neil's brainchild. I thank him for recognizing the need to fit prevention into people's lives, rather than vice versa, and I thank Reader's Digest for selecting me to convey this perceptiveness.

I thank my colleagues in preventive medicine, and in particular fellow members of the American College of Preventive Medicine, for constantly striving at the very mission to which *Stealth Health* is devoted: the improvement of health, and the prevention of disease.

Finally, and foremost, I thank my family. My wife, Catherine. My daughters, Rebecca, Corinda, Valerie, and Natalia. And my son, Gabriel. I recall the adage: If you love something, set it free. If it comes back to you, it belongs to you. If it doesn't, it never did. I know they love me. They set me free again and again to put the hours that should by all rights be theirs into projects such as this. In profound gratitude and permanent debt to them, I can only say: I do, always have, and always will belong to you. I am so very eager, now and always, to come back.

—DAVID L. KATZ, M.D.

This is the second book I've worked on with Dr. David Katz, and, as with the first, he was a joy to work with. Despite the length of *Stealth Health,* and the feeling that we'd never be finished, he never lost his patience or, even more important, his sense of humor.

But David brought much more than his expertise to this project; he also brought his wife, Catherine, herself a Ph.D. and published author. Catherine was a fountain of advice and recipes for the food chapters, helped review the marriage and libido chapters (she and David have five children, so she knows what she's doing), and provided good cheer and support when both David and I were flagging. Thanks so much, Catherine.

Speaking of a sense of humor—I must thank our editor, Neil Wertheimer. He never failed to come up with a clever tip or sidebar, never let the tried-and-true get past his "freshness" radar, and always asked for revisions with unfailing good humor topped with a compliment.

Then there are the hidden Reader's Digest people on the book—Jeanette Gingold, who copyedited and proofed it, Rich Kershner and Elizabeth Tunnicliffe, who designed it. They deserve a great big thanks for making what are, in the end, just words look and sound so great (and accurate).

Finally, my thanks to the dozens of experts who graciously contributed their own suggestions, tips, and ideas to make *Stealth Health* what it is today.

—DEBRA L. GORDON

More Health Advice from Reader's Digest

Reader's Digest is among the world's top providers of health information, advice, programs, recipes, and resources, with more than 100 million book and magazine readers each month, spread across more than 60 countries. Here are other Reader's Digest health books available by visiting our Web site (www.rd.com), by calling 800-846-2100, or at most bookstores.

Allergy and Asthma Relief

ChangeOne: Lose Weight Simply, Safely, and Forever

Curing Everyday Ailments the Natural Way

Cut Your Cholesterol (featuring the exclusive Live It Down Plan)

Doctors' Guide to Chronic Pain

Eat to Beat Diabetes

Eat to Beat High Blood Pressure

Eat Well, Stay Well

Foods That Harm, Foods That Heal

Improve Your Brainpower

Know Your Options: The Definitive Guide to Choosing the Best Medical Treatments

Medical Breakthroughs 2005

1,801 Home Remedies

Reader's Digest Guide to Drugs and Supplements

Stopping Diabetes in Its Tracks

The Natural Solution to Diabetes

The Everyday Arthritis Solution

Also, visit our recipe center on the number one health Web site in the United States, www.webmd.com.